P9-DVF-719

THE INFLAMMATORY PROCESS

Second Edition

VOLUME II

CONTRIBUTORS

J. R. Casley-Smith
Hubert R. Catchpole
Christian Crone
Lester Grant
John H. Luft
R. G. Macfarlane
Nathaniel F. Rodman
Roe Wells
D. L. Wilhelm
D. A. Willoughby
Benjamin W. Zweifach

THE INFLAMMATORY PROCESS

SECOND EDITION

EDITED BY

Benjamin W. Zweifach, M. D.

Department of Applied and
Mechanical Engineering Sciences
University of California, San Diego
La Jolla, California

Lester Grant, M. D.

Department of Medicine
School of Medicine
New York University
New York, New York

Robert T. McCluskey, M. D.

Department of Pathology
Harvard Medical School and
The Children's Hospital Medical Center
Boston, Massachusetts

VOLUME II

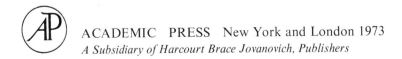
ACADEMIC PRESS   New York and London 1973
A Subsidiary of Harcourt Brace Jovanovich, Publishers

ACADEMIC PRESS, INC.
111 Fifth Avenue, New York, New York 10003

United Kingdom Edition published by
ACADEMIC PRESS, INC. (LONDON) LTD.
24/28 Oval Road, London NW1

LIBRARY OF CONGRESS CATALOG CARD NUMBER: 73-8250

PRINTED IN THE UNITED STATES OF AMERICA

CONTENTS

PART I. VASCULAR EVENTS IN THE INFLAMMATORY PROCESS

Chapter 1. Microvascular Aspects of Tissue Injury

Benjamin W. Zweifach

Chapter 2. Capillary Permeability

I. Structural Consideration

John H. Luft

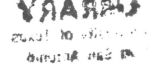

v

LIST OF CONTRIBUTORS

J. R. CASLEY-SMITH (161), The Electron Microscope Unit, The University of Adelaide, Adelaide, South Australia

HUBERT R. CATCHPOLE (121), Department of Pathology, University of Illinois at the Medical Center, Chicago, Illinois

CHRISTIAN CRONE (95), Institute of Medical Physiology, Department A, University of Copenhagen, Copenhagen, Denmark

LESTER GRANT (205), Department of Medicine, School of Medicine, New York University, New York, New York

JOHN H. LUFT (47), Department of Biological Structure, School of Medicine, University of Washington Seattle, Washington

R. G. MACFARLANE (335), Sir William Dunn School of Pathology, University of Oxford, Oxford, England

NATHANIEL F. RODMAN (363), Department of Pathology, College of Medicine, University of Iowa, Iowa City, Iowa

ROE WELLS (149),* Department of Medicine, Harvard Medical School, Peter Bent Brigham Hospital, Massachusetts General Hospital, and Massachusetts Rehabilitation Hospital, Boston, Massachusetts

D. L. WILHELM (251), School of Pathology, University of New South Wales, Kensington, Australia

D. A. WILLOUGHBY (303), Department of Experimental Pathology, St. Bartholomew's Hospital Medical College, West Smithfield, London, England

*Present address: Massachusetts Rehabilitation Hospital, Boston, Massachusetts 02114

BENJAMIN W. ZWEIFACH (3), Department of Applied and Mechanical Engineering Sciences, University of California, San Diego, La Jolla, California

PREFACE

Since publication of the first edition of "The Inflammatory Process," investigators have unearthed an enormous amount of basic information about inflammation, much of it relevant to clinical states. In addition, the biologic probe has moved closer and closer to the cell, its wall and contents, which has brought some insight into molecular mechanisms and their derangements in inflammatory states. In a sense, in the last decade the direction of research in the inflammatory reaction seems to have changed, with a shift toward molecular biology, but this is more apparent than real. Research has been moving in this direction not only in this field but in others as well for many years.

These would be reasons enough for a second edition of this treatise which deals with the commonest pathologic reaction in the animal kingdom. The first edition received favorable critical comment, characterizing it as a scholarly work that made a reasonably successful attempt to synthesize a sprawling literature and to invest the subject with some directional guidelines.

Fortified by this encouraging response we had no difficulty in reaching a decision that a second edition of this work was necessary. In planning this edition it became clear that new material on a subject as broad as inflammation could not possibly be compressed into a single volume without running the risk of superficiality. Space had to be reserved for an analysis of cell surface phenomena; for a fuller treatment of connective tissue; for an extensive discussion on the role of the formed elements of the blood in inflammatory states, particularly in the light of the rapidly burgeoning literature on platelet physiology; for an extended discussion of the life history and functional capacities of the leukocytes; for a synthesis of the vast inchoate bits and pieces of literature dealing with chemotaxis; for a summation of phagocytosis, which biochemists have been exploring vigorously for a decade and which is now yielding new insights at a molecular level, many of them carrying strong clinical implications; and for an analysis of the mechanisms responsible for tissue damage in inflammation, especially in immunologically induced reactions. These are among the aspects of the subject that demanded special treatment over and above briefer references to them in the first edition. Thus, the second edition is comprised of three volumes.

It is fitting to conclude such an edition with a chapter by Dr. Lewis Thomas, who offers the laconic suggestion that there is some question about whether there does exist in Nature an inflammatory process as commonly understood. There are inflammatory reactions to be sure, and this could mean only that there are inflammatory processes. In our zeal to put trees together in well-tended and nicely pruned forests, we may have succumbed to the occupational hazard, a pitfall for scientists and theologians alike, of rearranging Nature as we imagine was intended in the first place but conceivably setting on a construction quite wide of the mark.

Benjamin W. Zweifach
Lester Grant
Robert T. McCluskey

PREFACE TO FIRST EDITION

At a time when journals and textbooks are proliferating so rapidly that the scientific community is hard pressed to keep up with them, it is fair to ask why another book is needed now in an area where the literature is voluminous. Since the early nineteenth century, the inflammatory process has been one of the most intensively investigated fields of experimental medicine. At the turn of the century textbooks of pathology devoted fully one third of their contents to the subject of inflammation, and today it still bulks large in most texts. Yet it is a curious commentary that, aside from relatively short review articles, few attempts have been made to sort out the extensive literature in this important field to bring it up to date in a critical and coherent way. The last such effort, indeed, was that of Adami, of McGill, who in 1909 brought out a monograph, "Inflammation—An Introduction to the Study of Pathology" in an effort to deal with, and unify, the many interrelated and often contradictory aspects of this subject. It is of some interest that the monograph was 249 pages long, carried 226 references and, most remarkable of all, was written without collaboration. In the intervening half-century a substantial number of symposia and treatises emerged but these were directed largely to special viewpoints and circumscribed aspects of the problem. Perhaps the closest approach to a current, objective review can be found in Florey's "General Pathology," in which the subject is covered in many of its significant aspects.

The editors and publishers of "The Inflammatory Process" believe that with the enormous multiplication of research in this field the need exists for a more comprehensive volume which would include analyses of the major immunologic mechanisms which give rise to inflammatory reactions. Investigations of the immune process tend, in a sense, to move toward a common meeting ground with studies of inflammatory mechanisms, one supporting the other. One of the major objectives of the present volume is to explore areas where these two approaches converge.

Aside from the convenience of an encyclopedic background for research in this field, the value of this volume depends in part on its success in correlating new and old facts. The contributors were asked, therefore, to organize the material in such a way that pressing questions could be raised against a background of the apparent acceptable, hard core of experimental facts. Such an assignment is a difficult one. The very nature of the research process requires a constant challenging and modifying of hypotheses; new facts are accepted as significant or are discarded, depending on whether they provide a further insight into biologic mechanisms. Inevitably, in dealing with a sprawling literature, a selection of data has to be made. The editors know that the choices of each essayist were thoughtful ones and appropriate in the design of this volume.

The realization that much current material may not stand the test of time seemed no deterrent for a work that runs to more than 800 pages. It is intended that the treatment be comprehensive enough to serve as a reference work, with the main lines of research in the field placed in an historical perspective. This militated against a treatise of monograph size. In its present form, the volume can serve equally well as an authoritative reference for graduate students and medical students, for experimental biologists, and for others who wish to examine the experimental background of current theories of inflammation. Inevitably there is an overlap in some of the chapters, but where this serves to maintain continuity in the development of the author's theses, it has been considered important to preserve it. The book covers comprehensively both the morphologic and the dynamic aspects of the problem. It starts with a discussion of the experimental approach to the study of inflammation in which the emphasis is on the importance of a changing technology in providing new viewpoints on old problems. An attempt is made then to establish the morphologic basis of the problem as a prelude to a discussion of dynamic events and an analysis of the participation of white blood cells in the inflammatory process. The roles of mast cells, chemical mediators, lysosomes, and hemostatic mechanisms lead to two general chapters on fever and wound healing, as expressions of inflammation, followed by a discussion of anti-inflammatory agents and their contributions to an understanding of inflammatory reactions. The later chapters deal with the complexities of complement and the mechanisms of inflammation resulting from immunologic processes. It is hoped that the emphasis on pathophysiology and mechanisms of the inflammatory process will cast the discussion in a meaningful context for serious students and at the same time provide others who are interested in this area of experimental pathology with an authoritative introduction to the subject.

The editors would like to thank the publishers and the contributors for an extraordinary sense of responsibility in meeting a tight deadline for this volume, the revisions and editing of which, including new bibliography, continued almost to the point of publication.

Benjamin W. Zweifach
Lester Grant
Robert T. McCluskey

CONTENTS OF OTHER VOLUMES

Part I

VASCULAR EVENTS IN THE INFLAMMATORY PROCESS

Chapter 1

MICROVASCULAR ASPECTS OF TISSUE INJURY

BENJAMIN W. ZWEIFACH

I. General Aspects of Reaction

The method that best reflects the dynamic nature of the inflammatory process is microscopic examination which reveals the sequence of events in living tissues. The somatic representations of the injury reaction form the framework into which must be incorporated all other information, on whatever level—ultrastructural, biochemical, or biophysical. The essential details of the phenomenon were documented with singular insight as far back as the nineteenth century by Lister (1858), Cohnheim (1867), and Metchnikoff (1905). Early workers were quick to recognize that irrespective of the initiating stimulus diverse forms of local injury progressed through a similar sequence of vascular changes involving vasoconstriction, arteriolar dilation, edema, blood cell aggregation, sticking and emigration, and stasis. Lister (1858) clearly perceived that some form of tissue impairment over and above blood stagnation was an important contributor to the reaction to injury. One cannot but be impressed by the fact that Cohnheim in 1867 had concluded that the injury reaction involved a change in the "physico-chemical makeup of the vessel wall."

Despite the fact that the injury reaction is one of the most intensively studied aspects of pathology, it has not been possible to put into proper perspective the cellular and vascular events which are responsible for the separate facets of the inflammatory process. Some of the difficulties stem from the fact that the visual sequelae are, in substance, only outward manifestations of a whole family of homeostatic readjustments. Emphasis has been placed on the overall similarity of the vascular events, without proper regard for the fact that vascular and cellular components are, per force, limited in the number of ways in which they can react to any stimulus.

For the most part, attempts to unravel the evolution of the visible process have centered about the identification of chemical principles which are believed to be released during the cellular reaction and to be responsible for its seemingly unremitting course. During the past 15 years, ultra-structural information, through the application of the electron microscope, has put to test many previously accepted tenets and has challenged their validity. The current resurgence of microcirculatory research using sophisticated quantitative techniques promises to put our concepts of the dynamic aspects of inflammatory reaction to an even more severe test.

A keystone of the inflammatory reaction is the degradation of the blood–capillary barrier to the extent that the tissues become infiltrated with blood proteins and cells. Equally important in the genesis of tissue injury, but far less adequately documented, are the factors which uncouple the balance of vasomotor adjustments acting to keep local blood flow and fluid exchange in accord with tissue needs. Lewis, in his 1927 monograph, pointed out that the development of the inflammatory reaction is influenced to a considerable extent by biological agents, which under normal circumstances act as regulators of physiological processes.

A. Local Regulatory Influences

Our discussion of microcirculatory events will deal first with vasomotor aspects, since these must be recognized and separated from other intrinsic derangements affecting the blood–tissue barrier and the blood cellular elements. In effect, the terminal vascular bed represents the only access that the general population of cells has to the circulation. Capillary blood flow under physiological conditions is believed to be modulated by locally elaborated by-products which counteract the vasomotor tone imposed at the tissue level by intrinsic myogenic activity of vascular smooth muscle and at the systemic level via the blood stream and nervous system (Folkow, 1955). The final muscular subdivisions of the arterial tree, the terminal arterioles, are 20- to 25-μm endothelial tubes covered by a single discontinuous layer of muscle cells. Thus, the minute vessels—the terminal arterioles and their branches, the true capillaries, and the venules—are an integral part of the tissue proper, and, as such, are directly exposed to the continous shifting in the milieu of the parenchymal cell environment. At this level of organization, in contrast to the larger blood vessels, a new regulatory mechanism is brought into play by chemical materials which are either liberated from cellular stores or formed in the tissue compartment (Zweifach, 1957).

The principal aspects of local homeostasis are shown in Table I. Nervous regulation of the circulation is substantially less in the terminal vascular bed than in the feeding arteries or veins. Conventional staining techniques do not reveal any consistent distribution of terminal nerve fibers to the smallest arterioles, precapillaries, or capillaries (Nelemans, 1948; Berman et al., 1972). The current consensus (see Fulton and Zweifach, 1958; Mellander and Johansson, 1968; Zweifach, 1969) is that the microvasculature is regulated primarily by the interaction of humoral factors introduced via the blood stream and the tissue. It is obvious that chemical products released during local injury will be disseminated primarily by diffusion, and will have a direct effect only on directly contiguous microscopic vessels (Zweifach, 1964). In contrast, vasomotor changes in the large blood vessels (arteries or veins) which occur after injury are probably activated secondarily by the nervous system (Fulton et al., 1961) or by ascending propagation in a retrograde direction (Folkow and Neil, 1971).

TABLE I

Local Control of Terminal Vascular Bed

Function	Mechanism
Volume of blood	Tone of arterioles (neurogenic)
Intracapillary pressure	Resistance in collecting venules (neurogenic and humoral)
Nutritional surface area ⎫ Intercapillary distance ⎭	Activity of precapillary sphincters (humoral)
Reactivity of smooth muscle	Local chemical environment
Venous outflow from tissues	Rheologic properties of blood and vasomotion

B. Sequence in Injury

The sequence of events in tissue injury depends more upon the severity of the initiating stimulus than upon the nature of the irritant. Studies on blue dye–protein accumulation in the skin [see Chapter 8 by Wilhelm, Chapter 9 by Willoughby, and reviews by Sevitt (1958) and Spector (1969)] suggest that the response to injury develops in two distinct stages—an immediate vasodilator reaction accompanied by an increased permeability to plasma protein which reaches its maximum within 8–10 minutes and a delayed phase which unfolds over a period of hours and culminates in the infiltration of the tissue with leukocytes, vascular stasis, and local hemorrhage.

The evidence is reasonably convincing that the successive phases are mediated by different factors (see Chapters 8 and 9): the first phase is mediated by a histaminelike agent and the second by a derivative which can arise either by enzymic degradation of the plasma globulins or of tissue components. As indicated in their chapters, Wilhelm and Willoughby believe that the phasic nature of the reaction in the skin is due to redistribution of blood and the involvement of different vessels. Wells and Miles (1963) have gone as far as to state that the initial phase is relatively unimportant in determining the eventual course of the injury reaction. This point of view should be tempered by noting, for example, that we do not as yet understand the preparative action of an amine such as epinephrine which has no demonstrable long-range effects, but which leads to hemorrhagic necrosis in the skin when bacterial endotoxin is introduced up to about 4 hours later. It should also be pointed out that even on the basis of protein exudation per se not all inflammatory processes are outwardly biphasic. Wilhelm (1962) believes this may be a matter of degree since, with relatively severe stimuli, the two phases overlap and fuse. With a continuing stimulus, such as xylene, the reaction is outwardly monophasic (Aschheim and Zweifach, 1961). It remains to be demonstrated the extent to which aspects of the injury reaction, other than protein exudation, are discontinuous.

Visually, the earliest event in most forms of acute tissue injury is a short-lived contraction (from 10–20 seconds up to several minutes) of the feeding arterioles in the immediate vicinity of the phlogen (Spector and Willoughby, 1963). When a large area is damaged, the arterioles along the periphery of this circumscribed zone remain partially narrowed. Frequently, the resulting ischemia is complete, as in the case of the response to localized thermal injury in the rabbit ear chamber (Allison *et al.*, 1955).

Lewis and Grant (1925) have described arterial constriction in human skin after mechanical stroking. The arterioles and small arteries in the mesentery narrow when they are stroked with a glass microneedle (Zweifach, 1955). Recently, a focused laser beam has been used to induce highly circumscribed (3–4 μm) thermal injuries adjacent to the microvessels in the rabbit ear (Grant and Becker, 1966) and mesentery (Kochen and Baez, 1965). Vasodilation was the predominant feature. Injuries which are more gradual in their onset, as with ultraviolet light (Grant et al., 1962) or xylene (Aschheim and Zweifach, 1961), are not associated with a significant constrictor episode. Most investigators place little importance on this particular manifestation, although Spector and Willoughby (1960) believe an adrenalinelike substance may serve a protective function by reducing local blood flow.

Blood flow through the affected tissue may be increased by as much as tenfold (Aschheim and Zweifach, 1962). At first, blood courses more rapidly through the most direct avenues leading to the venous vessels. A stage is then reached where increased amounts of blood are diverted into previously inactive capillary side channels as the precapillary sphincters are opened maximally (Zweifach, 1961a). Up to this point, the response is essentially that of an ordinary reactive hyperemia (Zweifash, 1966). It is this phase which can be suppressed by blocking agents such as antihistamines (see Wilhelm, 1962).

Recently developed microtechniques (Intaglietta et al., 1970) have made it possible to obtain continuous recordings of arteriolar, capillary, or venular pressures during the progression of the local inflammatory process. Representative readings made in the mesentery of the cat after the application of a microdrop of zylene are shown in Table II. The values shown during the injury are peak values. It should be noted that the pressures in the capillaries and venules are greater than the colloid osmotic pressure of the plasma (26 cm H_2O). Therefore, fluid filtration predominates and contributes

TABLE II

PRESSURE DISTRIBUTION IN CAT MESENTERY[a]

Vessel	Ischemia (cm H_2O)	Normal (cm H_2O)	Local hyperemia (cm H_2O)
Artery (100)	50	50	85
Arteriole (30)	30	40	65
Capillary (10)	24	30	37
Venule (25)	15	20	29

[a]Values represent average of twenty direct micropressure readings: ischemia after local application of cold irrigating fluid (18°C); local hyperemia, 20–30 minutes after application of xylene. Diameter of vessel (in μm) indicated in parentheses in first column.

significantly to the resulting edema. As leukocyte palisading becomes more prominent in the collecting venules, pressures in the capillaries and post-capillaries climb to near-arteriolar levels because of the increased venular resistance. It is interesting to note that capillary and venular pressures remain high even when the increase permeability to protein is not as prominent. Presumably, fluid filtration is reduced because tissue pressure increases as edema develops.

Shortly thereafter, a number of events herald another phase. The precapillary sphincters become refractory to vasoconstrictor stimuli (Zweifach, 1971). Recent investigations with the various prostaglandins (Horton, 1969) show that the E_1 and E_2 forms suppress adrenergic neurotransmission, and a similar effect on precapillary vessels is not unlikely. Despite the continued arterial dilation, the outflow of blood via the collecting venules slows progressively. Conheim (1889) and Metchnikoff (1893) focused attention on the vasodilation during tissue injury, believing the distention of the venous vessels to be secondary to the widening of the small arteries and arterioles. It is unfortunate that no accurate quantitative data are available to compare the relative increases in blood flow under different experimental circumstances. The total increase in flow is the result of two distinct mechanisms: a direct, local increase in blood flow limited to the affected site and a secondary spread or arterial flare, especially striking in the skin (Lewis, 1924).

Coincident with the local accumulation of vasocative materials and the attendant acidosis, hyperkalemia, etc., the terminal vascular bed develops signs of a disorganized pattern of reactivity. This is manifested not only by bizarre venular responses to constrictor stimuli, such as serotonin and bradykinin, but by heightened reactions of the arterioles to doses of catecholamines which normally affect only the precapillary vessels (Zweifach and Nagler, 1961).

The term vasodilation is used freely in descriptions of the inflammatory response, but, in fact, it refers primarily to the feeding arterioles and precapillaries and to the corresponding effluent veins. Although the number of capillaries with an active circulation is progressively increased, the true capillaries do not become significantly dilated. The collecting venules, which for the most part are nonmuscular, are also only moderately dilated. The vulnerability of the venules during the inflammatory reaction may, to a considerable degree, be a reflection of their inability to undergo distention beyond a limited point.

The increased blood flow is accompanied by visual evidence of an increase in the permeability of the microvascular barrier. Within 30–60 seconds, blue dye–protein complexes leak out of the circulation, particularly in the region of the postcapillaries and small venules (Menkin, 1936; Rigdon,

1941). A similar gradient of permeability to plasma proteins was found by Hauck and Schröer (1969) in the rabbit mesentery using fluorescent-tagged albumin. Measurements based on the extravascular shift of isotopically labeled albumin (Aschheim and Zweifach, 1962) indicate that the protein lost from the circulation at this time has essentially the same relative concentration as normal blood proteins, suggesting bulk leakage of plasma into the tissue compartment.

Krogh (1920) and Ricker (1924) were convinced that the increased blood flow, acting indirectly to distend the capillaries and venules, was the primary factor responsible for the excessive loss of fluid and plasma proteins. When capillary pressures were measured directly with micropipettes (Landis, 1927), it became apparent that an increased driving force provided by the hydraulic pressure of the blood was not sufficient in itself to explain the fluid loss in injury. Changes in the vessel wall proper occur, the precise nature of which have only recently become apparent through the added dimension afforded by electron microscopy.

In situations in which the injury is limited and reversible, increased permeability to protein can develop without a sticking of platelets or leukocytes to the inner vessel wall (Zweifach, 1962). Outwardly, the integrity of the capillary or venular wall does not appear to be compromised. Ultrastructural evidence, however, indicates that contiguous borders of endothelial cells separate sufficiently from one another to allow free movement of plasma and colloidal markers into the subendothelial space (Majno and Palade, 1961; Marchesi, 1961; Movat and Fernando, 1963c; Karnovsky, 1968).

Stasis of red cells can likewise develop in some forms of injury (Fig. 1) with essentially no sticking of leukocytes and platelets to the affected vessels (Florey, 1926). Extravasation of red blood cells between interendothelial cell junctions has been found in electron micrographs of venules subjected to an elevated pressure (Majno, 1965; Skalak et al., 1970). However, in most experiments in which destruction of parenchymal cells or injury of the endothelial cells is involved, leukocyte and platelet sticking are prominent features (for details, see Chapter 7 on leukocyte sticking).

As shown by Clark and Clark (1935), Allison and Lancaster (1959), Cliff (1966), and Grant and Becker (1966) in the rabbit ear chamber, local heat or the local application of a chemical irritant causes the inner surface of the capillary endothelium to become adhesive to leukocytes and platelets within about 10–15 minutes (Fig. 2) and to sequester circulating colloidal particles such as carbon (Fig. 3). The capillary vessels in the affected areas become fragile and are easily disrupted by slight external pressure or mechanical handling. If one applies a calcium chelator (EDTA) to the surface of the exteriorized mesentery, the venules and their feeding capillaries develop

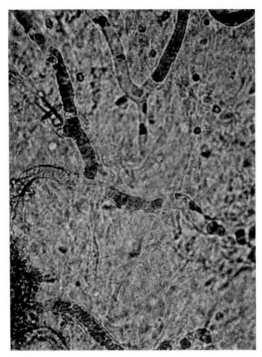

Fig. 1. Stasis in blood capillaries in area of mesentery where local heat has been applied (40°C for 3 minutes). Red cells form a solid mass obstructing flow. There is no evidence of increased adhesiveness of vessel lining. Vessel diameter remains unchanged. (× 300.)

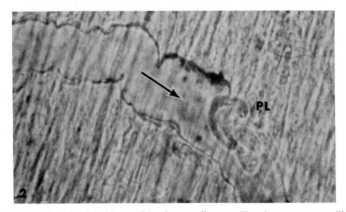

Fig. 2. Effect of mechanical injury with microneedle to capillary in rat mesentery illustrating accumulation of platelets and leukocytes (PL) at damaged wall. Single red blood cell is impaled on endothelial spike which projects upward from below. Arrow indicates direction of blood flow. (× 400.)

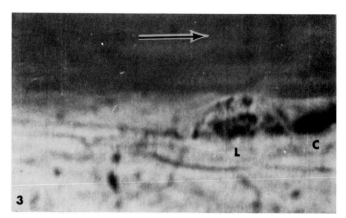

Fig. 3. Wall of venule in rat mesentery several minutes after irritation of wall with micro-needle at point C where carbon has accumulated after injection into blood stream. At L, a leukocyte which has become attached to venular wall also shows carbon adhering to its surface. Arrow indicates direction of blood flow. (× 750.)

petechial hemorrhages and stasis much more readily in injured sites than in normal areas (Zweifach, 1969). Evidence derived from both electron and conventional light microscopy (Sanders *et al.*, 1940; Lecomte and Hugues, 1956) shows that the endothelial cells in the capillaries and venules frequently thicken and swell. The attached leukocytes, after a variable delay, then begin to emigrate rapidly. Here again, the endothelial membrane appears to be the portion of the vessel wall that is affected.

Lewis and Grant (1924) made the interesting observation that the initial period of increased permeability in the skin after histamine administration is followed, in turn, by a period of complete refractoriness to further stimulation by histamine. Burke and Miles (1958) and others (see Spector, 1958) reaffirmed this and showed that, eventually, the vessels again become increasingly permeable to plasma proteins. The palisading of leukocytes and platelets in the venules serves to increase outflow resistance. As a result, the capillary circulation is slowed and areas of stasis appear in many of the branching channels. Petechial hemorrhages develop, for the most part, in the venules (Fig. 4) and in those capillaries in which flow has resumed after a period of stasis (Weber, 1955). Branemark and Ekholm (1968) were able to compare the visually recorded sequelae of capillary stasis with the ultrastructural changes in the same vessels and found the only abnormality to be penetration of red cells between contiguous endothelial borders. In the local Arthus reaction or the dermal Schwartzman phenomenon (Gerber, 1936; Moore and Movat, 1959), red cell lysis frequently appears in conjuction with the development of petechiae and the

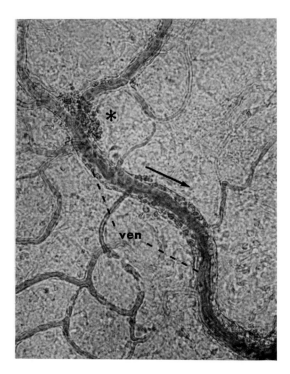

Fig. 4. Petechial hemorrhages form most readily in venules. They are frequently associated with leukocyte adhesion and emigration. As shown here, the venule wall (in mesentery) is most susceptible to rupture close to points of branching (*) where red cells have penetrated into the interstitium proper. Arrow indicates direction of blood flow. (× 200.)

presence of minute thrombi plugging effluent channels. Eventually, nutritive blood flow through the capillary bed is reduced to the point where tissue necrosis sets in.

Microscopic inspection of the acute inflammatory process thus shows essentially the following vascular sequence: arterial vasodilation, increased capillary flow, increased leakage of protein-rich fluid into extravascular compartment (separation of endothelial cells in venules, but no other signs of vessel damage), obstruction of venous outflow, slowed capillary flow, alteration of capillary wall proper, capillary and venular stasis, emigration of white cells in venules, petechial hemorrhages, and eventually vasorrhexis (Fig. 5A–D).

Obviously, this sequence of events does not develop either uniformly or to the same extent under all conditions. Electron microscope studies (Majno *et al.*, 1961; Movat *et al.*, 1963; Peterson and Good, 1962; Cotran, 1967) show that the initial response to injury involves pathology primarily

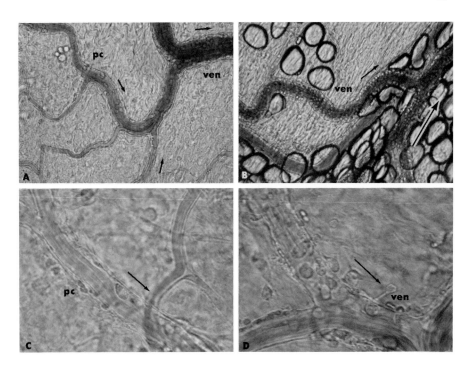

Fig. 5. Increasing severity of leukocyte sticking and emigration in the mesentery. In A, note that under control conditions leukocytes marginate and roll in the direction of flow in the postcapillaries (pc) and collecting venules (ven)(× 130). In B, so-called palisading of leukocytes occurs as local injury develops. These leukocytes adhere tightly and frequently layer on one another (× 130). C, under higher magnification (× 260), shows the earliest manifestation of leukocytic sticking to postcapillary (pc) The polymorphonuclear leukocyte is deformed by the shear of the blood flow and is attached mainly at its posterior contact with the endothelial wall. D shows a more advanced stage of a reversible thermal injury (at 15–20 minutes). Numerous leukocytes are seen adhering to the vessel wall. Three cells (in area where arrow has been placed) have emigrated into tissue proper. Other cells are in the process of diapedesis. (× 260.) Arrows indicate direction of blood flow.

in the venular vessels, whereas damage to the capillaries develops only later during the delayed phase of the process (Wells and Miles, 1963; Cotran and Majno, 1964; Cotran, 1970). Wilhelm, (1970) presented evidence indicating that these varied responses may be ascribed to the involvement of different vessels at different stages. It will become apparent in the subsequent discussion that reactions which have been cited as characteristic of a given process (increased permeability to dye–protein complexes) may involve, under different circumstances, basically different structural changes.

II. Specific Components

A. Behavior of Terminal Vascular Bed as an Organic Unit

It is reasonable to assume that substances which are suspected of being mediators of the vascular events in tissue injury should reproduce, on a microcirculatory level, the basic elements of the reaction. Particular substances have been classified as mediators primarily because of their ability to induce either leukocyte sticking or an increase in permeability to plasma proteins. The mechanism by which such substances produce their effects is difficult to establish since the injection of even a simple saline solution can elicit a mild injury reaction.

Over the years, a seemingly endless number of agents have been proposed as the mediators responsible for the local change in permeability during tissue injury. Lewis (1927) concluded that "there exists a single and organized mechanism of defense against injuries of all kinds and that agent . . . is a chemical derived from tissues." Of the agents that, to date, have been purified or identified chemically not one is able by itself to mimic the serial events characteristic of tissue injury (see Chapters 8 and 9). Substances which have received most attention, vasoactive amines and polypeptides of the kinin class, reproduce the early phase involving vasodilation and local edema (Bhoola *et al.*, 1960). More recently, the C_{20} fatty acids known as prostaglandins have been found to be related to tissue injury and have been proposed as mediators of the delayed phase of the reaction (Melmon and Cline, 1967). Hayashi *et al.* (1967) have been able to extract from burned tissues at least two specific substances which reproduce separately the immediate and delayed phases of the vascular reaction. Inasmuch as any one of a half dozen substances present in tissues can be used to produce the same effects, it is difficult, by this criterion alone, to identify with any degree of certainty the particular mediators involved in the injury reaction.

In experiments in which synthetic mediators such as histamine, serotonin, or bradykinin are injected, inflammation, as such, is not reproduced since both permeability changes and leukocyte emigration appear only when unusually high concentrations of these agents are used. On the other hand, several agents in combination, in addition to their usual vasomotor effects, have been found to lead frequently to capillary and venular stasis and even to tissue hemorrhage (Zweifach and Nagler, 1961; Lewis and Matthews, 1970). Epinephrine, but not other vasoconstrictors, has been shown (Gatling, 1958) to convert local inflammatory reactions into hemorrhagic prototypes [for example, epinephrine and bacterial endotoxin

(Thomas, 1956)]. The common denominator here may be the adenyl cyclase–cyclic AMP mechanism (the so-called second messenger system), which is affected by epinephrine and by mediators such as the prostaglandins, E_2 and $F_{2\alpha}$ (Horton, 1969; Brockelhurst, 1971).

1. PROPENSITY OF VENULES TO INJURY

In practically all tissues examined, the collecting venules and postcapillaries represent the weak points at which the injury reaction is most prominent. This propensity is evidenced by a tendency for contiguous endothelial cells to separate and for plasma proteins to escape into the tissue (Majno et al., 1961; Movat and Fernando, 1963a). The presence of numerous fenestrae in venular endothelium provides another possible mechanism for the exaggerated response to injury in these vessels. Electron microscopy provides no clue to the susceptibility of venular endothelial cells to develop gaps or leaks.

Ancillary evidence indicates that the basement membrane may be structurally defective on the venous side. In nutritional scurvy (Lee et al., 1955), hemorrhages first occur and are most pronounced in the collecting venules of the mesentery. Tests of capillary fragility with negative pressure devices show the venules to be unusually susceptible to this form of deformation (Hare and Miller, 1951). Animals exposed to whole body X irradiation develop petechial hemorrhages in their venules (Zarem and Zweifach, 1965). Keep in mind that the mechanical strength of the vessel depends upon features other than the basement membrane per se, such as the perivascular tissue which contains collagen and reticular fibers. The weakened state of the venules in chronic conditions may be due, in part, to a generalized collagen defect.

Possibly, some of the functional peculiarities of the venulues are the results of their perfusion with venous blood which has the highest concentration of tissue by-products (Zweifach, 1955; see Luft, Chapter 2). Diapedesis of leukocytes, extravasation of red blood cells, and extravascular loss of macromolecules occur most readily in venous vessels. Unlike the true capillaries in which the basement membrane tightly abuts the surrounding tissue, the endothelium of the venules is separated from the perivascular sheath by a space of 1–2 μm, which would allow for approximately a 10% increase in circumference under pressure. The substantial increase in blood flow and pressure during tissue injury leads to disproportionate changes in transmural pressure in the capillaries and venules (Zweifach, 1971). The transmural pressure which develops in blood vessels is a function of their size as indicated by the La Place law in which

$$P(\text{transmural pressure}) = T(\text{wall tension}) \times R(\text{vessel radius})$$

Smaller vessels thus develop less wall tension than do larger ones under the same pressure head. Since venules are from two to three times as wide as the capillaries, they will be subjected to a much greater distending force as the flow and pressure increase during local inflammation.

2. SHUNTING

Under normal circumstances, as I have shown (Zweifach, 1957), the blood flow through the mesentery microvasculature is characterized by the intermittent opening and closing of precapillary sphincters, thereby bringing into the active circulation greater or lesser numbers of "open" capillaries and in this way varying the surface area available for exchange. With the seemingly indiscriminate arteriolar dilation in the immediate area of injury and with the ascending arterial dilation, the bed is perfused with such large amounts of blood that the optimal distributing capacity of the small vessels is exceeded. Initially the blood tends to flow rapidly in some segments of the vascular network, while bypassing others. This effect is most evident in channels which are the most proximal branches of the arteries and arterioles and which, by virture to their location, can serve as functional shunts.

In some tissues, such as the skin and intestinal wall, anatomical shunts between small arteries and veins can divert a considerable fraction of the total flow directly into the venous side of the circulation (Grant *et al.*, 1932; Clark, 1938; Barlow, 1950). Under conditions of local vasodilation, the circulation may not only be below levels needed to nourish the tissues, but shunting leads to a substantial increase in the pressure in the effluent venules, which, in turn, will interfere with proper drainage from capillary vessels entering the veins more distally. Much of the backflow seen in injured tissues (Clark and Clark, 1935) may be attributed to similar shunts between the microscopic vessels.

3. AXON REFLEX

An important difference between ordinary reactive hyperemia and the edema or wheal process following local injury in the skin is the involvement of widespread arteriolar dilation through activation of the so-called antidromic reflex along terminal sensory fibers. Bruce, in 1910, documented in detail the reddening and flushing beyond the area of immediate injury; he found the spread of the reaction to be due to a locally mediated neurogenic reflex. It was possible with local anesthetics to blunt the flare in conjunctival vessels of the eye injured with mustard oil, although local hyperemia and capillary stasis developed as usual. Sensory denervation also suppressed extension of the vasodilation.

In the more recent literature, a complete description and analysis of the flare reaction following local injury is found in the writings of Lewis (1927) and Lewis and Harmer (1927).

Grant and Duckett-Jones (1929) concluded that the dermal wheal which develops under abnormal conditions is essentially an exaggeration of a normal reaction, thus emphasizing the hemodynamic aspect of fluid exchange. It should be noted, however, that in other situations in which an elevated pressure within the terminal vascular bed leads to excess outward filtration the phenomenon is not associated with marked protein loss (Smirk, 1936; Landis and Hortenstine, 1950). The seemingly disproportionate loss of protein resulting from vasodilation per se in the skin may be due to the extensive network of venules in the subdermis.

The local wheal phenomenon consisted of three separate phases according to Lewis and Grant (1925) and Lewis and Harmer (1927): (1) a local vasodilation, independent of nerves; (2) widespread vasodilation of feeding arterioles via a nervous reflex; and (3) a change in permeability of the terminal blood vessels due to the elaboration of a histaminelike substance from the damaged tissue. Little progress has been made in identifying the chemical factors that could initiate the reflex vasodilation (Fleisch, 1935; Hilton and Lewis, 1957; Illig, 1961).

Lewis and Grant (1925) found, as had others before them (Ebbecke, 1917; Hirschfelder, 1924), that the increase in blood flow and edema induced by local irritants in the skin could be minimized by pretreating with a local anesthetic such as cocaine. Although the flush or flare reaction was abolished, local damage to the capillary wall developed as usual, indicating the direct nature of this aspect of the lesion.

The importance of the nervous system in local inflammatory changes is reinforced by reports that sympathetic denervation blunts the dermal hemorrhage and necrosis induced by bacterial endotoxin (Thomas, 1954). Catecholamines may be implicated in the response to injury because of the adrenergic nature of vascular smooth muscle innervation and the demonstrated exacerbation interaction of local tissue damage by epinephrine or norepinephrine (Spector, 1969; Horton, 1969). Serotonin and bacterial endotoxin also have been shown to affect adrenergic-mediated vasomotor responses (Boquet and Izard, 1950).

4. TISSUE EDEMA

A prominent feature of the inflammatory reaction is the swelling of the affected site. Damaged tissue has been shown to take up water readily under both *in vivo* and *in vitro* conditions (Robinson, 1960; Opie, 1956; Hedbys *et al.*, 1963). In the intact animal, the tense swollen appearance of the damaged tissue is, in part, the result of extensive vasodilation and an increased amount of blood in the venous compartment. A substantial leakage of plasma proteins into the extravascular tissue (Aschheim and Zweifach, 1962; Mellander, 1968) represents the major translocation in the inflamed tissue.

The work of Ludwig (1865), Cohnheim (1867), and Starling (1896) led them to conclude that edema develops primarily as a result of excessive filtration through the injured capillary walls. On the other hand, Fischer (1910) believed that, in the main, edema is the result of an increased imbibition of water by the colloidal constituents of injured tissues, presumably because of local acidity (Schade, 1935). Fischer favored the mechanism of hydration of colloids, as opposed to the osmotic forces postulated by Loeb (1923). Changes in the properties of the connective tissue proper under both physiological and pathological conditions have been recently proposed. Hyaluronic acid complexes and the mucopolysaccharides represent important sources of tissue osmotic pressure (Wiederhielm, 1972; Laurent, 1970), and changes in their physicochemical distribution could contribute to the edema process.

It has been known for many years (Menkin, 1956) that dye-labeled plasma albumin complexes tend to accumulate in injured skin. The phenomenon has been visualized by Witte (1957b) in the mesentery with the aid of fluorescent dye–protein complexes. By using isotope-labeled serum albumin, Aschheim and Zweifach (1962) were able to quantitate this aspect of the reaction. They found that extravasated proteins leave the injured area much more slowly than does water or small molecular solutes. This discrepancy is probably due to the relatively rapid flux by diffusion of small molecules, as opposed to the much slower movement of large proteins by convective forces. A complicating feature is the fact that the plasma proteins may become attached to charged groups on connective tissue elements.

From a functional point of view, the end result of tissue damage is a breakdown of compartmental barriers; not only is the blood–tissue barrier compromised, but the cell plasma membrane, which physically delimits intracellular and extracellular compartments, is functionally impaired (Robinson, 1960). Inflammatory reactions have been shown to be attended by cell dysfunction involving serious translocations of sodium, potassium, electrolytes, water, enzymes, and substrates (Cameron, 1952; also see Trump, Volume I, Chapter 3).

The use of protein accumulation per se as a measure of increased permeability requires some comment. With the separation of endothelial cells, plasma moves into the tissue compartment. Inasmuch as the magnitude of such movement depends upon the prevailing hydraulic pressure in the capillaries and venules, protein loss is flow dependent. Witte (1957a) studied the movement of protein-labeled fluorescent material across the capillary wall, and found that protein loss was most prominent in vessels with an active flow through the mesentery. Thus, in the mesentery, there was no appreciable loss of dye–protein complexes from capillaries or venules in which the flow had been mechanically obstructed.

The hydrostatic pressure and tissue osmotic pressure tend to rise in the injured area so that bulk movement of plasma will be retarded and may even stop. A phenomenon of this kind could by itself account for the intermediate phase of "reduced permeability" reported by many investigators (see Miles, 1956). Thereafter, with the gradual movement of protein, water, etc. into lymphatics and with the continued deterioration of the blood capillary and venular walls, plasma protein again will move into the injured site. It is generally agreed that only a small fraction of the extravasated protein returns directly into the blood stream (Wasserman and Mayerson, 1951; Courtice et al., 1964; Casley-Smith, 1970). This can be readily explained by the fact that protein loss from the blood depends upon the convective flow initiated by the prevailing hydrostatic pressure in the microvessels. No comparable inward force from the tissue exists, tissue pressure being comparatively low. Diffusion of proteins in the extravascular compartment is both slower and much more restricted than for smaller molecules.

B. Vascular Permeability

1. NORMAL PERMEABILITY

Most concepts of capillary permeability attempt to account for the exchange of materials across the vessel wall on the basis of a simplified general mechanism. Such an approach cannot be justified, however, in view of the wide range of materials of differing molecular size, solubility, charge, shape, etc., which are believed to be involved. Furthermore, the capillary barrier is not a homogeneous, monostructured unit, but a mosaic of inter-locking elements woven into a tubular shape. It would be more appropriate in discussions on abnormal capillary permeability to refer not only to the permeating substance involved, e.g., water, ions, oxygen, albumin, but also to the specific structural components of the wall.

On a broad conceptual level, the original proposal for fluid exchange by Starling (1896) is probably correct: viz., the mass transfer of fluid across the capillary barrier, in final analysis, will depend upon the balance between the hydraulic force of the blood and the osmotic pressure of the plasma proteins. Such an exchange involves both diffusion and a bulk movement of water (frequently called hydrodynamic flow), which is presumed to occur through aqueous channels or pores (Pappenheimer, 1953). Two physical pathways for such bulk movement of water have been suggested: (1) the porous, hydrophilic, intercellular material and its connecting basement membrance (Chambers and Zweifach, 1947) and (2) the attenuated, outermost extensions of the endothelial cells (Palade, 1953). As indicated by studies with deuterium (Hevesy and Jacobsen, 1940; Edelman, 1952), water apparently moves very rapidly across the surface of cells by diffusion. Indicator dilution studies show that tritiated water, when leaving the blood stream, is distributed as a single exponential function (Neufeld and Marshall, 1970).

Evidence based on the kinetics of exchange of ions and small molecular solutes clearly shows that diffusion is the principal mechanism for transcapillary permeability (Cowie *et al.*, 1949; Chinard *et al.*, 1955; Renkin, 1959; see Crone, Chapter 3). The fact that ions (sodium and potassium) and small molecules (glucose, mannitol), some of which do not penetrate into cells, do traverse the blood capillary wall with equal facility and exchange freely with the extravascular compartment makes it necessary to invoke some special endothelial mechanism to account for this discrepancy—particularly if one assumes that transcapillary diffusion occurs across the entire endothelial surface. An especially favorable site for such exchange would be the attenuated portions of the endothelial cell where the opposing cell membranes appear to have fused into a series of fenestrae or windows (see Luft, Chapter 2). Diffusion across the short distances involved in extremely rapid (as much as 200 times greater than hydrodynamic flow). Water-soluble materials presumably move through a continuous water phase by way of aqueous channels smaller than those involved in the bulk exchange of water between blood and tissue compartments (Zweifach, 1968). Free diffusion is hindered to a variable degree depending on the molecular size, shape, and charge of the material involved (Renkin and Pappenheimer, 1957). The Darcy coefficient for the movement of molecules through the capillary wall and ground substance materials remains to be determined (Zweifach *et al.*, 1968).

Exchange studies of radioactive solutes indicate that substances up to the molecular size of inulin diffuse comparatively freely, whereas large molecules encounter increasing resistance to passage across the capillary barrier (Renkin, 1959). As is well known, plasma proteins are, for the most part, retained within the blood stream under normal circumstances. An increase in the "effective pore size" of the barrier after tissue damage or local hypozia is probably due to a combination of circumstances which includes a tendency for the tightly joined endothelial cells to move apart, an increase in the number of open fenestrae, and a change in the configuration of the filamentous gel making up the basement membrane. The behavior of gases such as oxygen and carbon dioxide suggests that they permeate the capillary wall by virtue of their lipid solubility, so that the entire cell surface is available (Landis, 1934; Duling and Berne, 1970).

There is much speculation concerning the relationship of the endothelial cell vesicles (caveolae intracellularis) to both normal and abnormal exchange processes (Bennett, 1956; see also Chapter 2 by Luft). Marchesi and Barrnett (1963) have described by a combined electron microscope histochemical approach the localization of a nucleosidase in the membranes of these vesicles. They interpret this evidence as demonstrating a specialized secretary function for this type of vesicular transport. When colloidal particles are injected into the blood stream (Farquhar et al., 1961), they frequently become entrapped in these vesicles. Karnovsky (1968) has found that soluble proteins (enzymes of different molecular weight) can also be taken up by the endothelial vesicle system. Another possibility is that the vesicular type of uptake may include certain lipoprotein complexes, which have an affinity for cell surfaces (Courtice, 1959). In this context, the phenomenon of vesiculation at the electron microscope level has certain similarities to the phenomenon of phagocytosis as seen with the conventional light microscope (Cohn and Morse, 1960), an important difference being that phagocytized particles are incorporated into digestive vacuoles, "phagosomes," whereas materials in the pinocytotic vesicles are believed to be simply transported through the cell cytoplasm.

2. ABNORMAL PERMEABILITY

It is obvious that transcapillary movement of materials during injury must occur either through some part of the endothelial cell or between the cells. Both routes have been implicated by both direct visual and electron micrographic evidence. Early workers such as Arnold (1871) described the existence of stigmata or openings between contiguous endothelial cells. Krogh (1920) believed that physical distension of the capillaries as a result of increased intravascular pressure produced temporary defects in the capillary barrier through which plasma proteins and blood cellular elements could pass. The phenomenon of granulopexy or uptake of colloidal particles by endothelial cells has been interpreted by Biozzi et al. (1948), Ovary (1958), Gozsy and Kato (1960), and Jansco (1941), among others (see Jansco, 1955), to represent active endothelial participation in the exchange between blood and tissue compartments. There is some question as to whether it is possible to distinguish with conventional light microscopy endothelial phagocytosis per se from the type of reaction in which the colloidal particles become lodged in the subendothelial space after a separation of endothelial cell junctions (Strock and Majno, 1969).

Chambers and Zweifach (1947) found it difficult to see how the endothelial cells themselves could be sufficiently permeable to ions, electrolytes, and colloidal particles to account for transcapillary exchange and yet still be able to maintain their integrity. The evidence to date leaves no doubt that except for specialized organs—liver, spleen, and kidney—the endothelium in most capillary beds forms a continuous lining even in the most attenuated parts of the vessels, where the wall may be as thin as several hundred angstroms (Fawcett, 1959; Rhodin, 1962). Moore and Ruska (1957) speculated that these vesicles were the transport apparatuses for moving materials from the lumen to the exterior of the vessel. More recently, on the basis of work by Majno and Palade (1961), Marchesi and Florey (1960), Cotran (1970), Marchesi (1961), Florey and Grant (1961), and Movat and Fernando (1963b), the emphasis again shifted to the separation of endothelial cells and the movement of plasma and cells through such defects into the subendothelial space limited on the outside by only the basement membrane.

The demonstration that the increased permeability mediated by histamine, bradykinin, or serotonin is accompanied by the formation of clefts between the endothelial cells (see Chapter 2) suggests that the normal imperviousness of the venular capillary wall to protein can be attributed to the endothelial cell proper. On the one hand, we must take into account the observation that colloidal particles such as ferritin do penetrate into the endothelial cell under certain circumstances by the phenomenon of vesiculation. On the other hand, such colloids can also traverse the blood capillary wall through intercellular pathways. Unfortunately there is no firm basis for estimating the relative magnitude of the exchange through each of these mechanisms. Renkin (1964) has calculated that vesicular transport might account for the transcapillary movement of macromolecules above a molecular weight of 20,000. Most workers envisage the process as a comparatively slow phenomenon. Other workers (Shea *et al.*, 1969; Tomlin, 1969), on the basis of theoretical analyses, believe vesicular transport can occur much faster than hitherto thought possible.

Whether pinocytotic vesicles can move with equal facility in both directions across the endothelial cell remains largely speculative, although Wissig (1958b) claimed that ferritin and even carbon particles that reach the pericapillary compartment of the diaphragm from the peritoneal cavity appear inside the vessel lumen. One cannot be certain that the movements of denatured proteins such as ferritin via the endothelial vesicle system reflect the mechanisms normally used for the transcapillary movement soluble plasma proteins.

Perhaps the strongest argument in favor of the bulk movement of plasma proteins via the intercellular route is the demonstration that the concentration of protein in edema fluids during inflammation is essentially that of the plasma (Aschheim and Zweifach, 1962) and that a reduction in blood flow diminishes or stops such exchange. Under normal conditions, a limited protein loss could occur through a continuously changing population of temporary openings between contiguous endothelial cells (Zweifach,

1961b). It was assumed prior to the advent of electron microscopy, that a continuous endothelial membrane was made possible by a cement material (Chambers and Zweifach, 1947). Some insight into the nature of the factors responsible for intercellular adhesion comes from several sources—the staining of cell outlines with silver (McGovern, 1955; Florey et al., 1959), the presence of a metachromatic staining material between cells (Curran, 1957; Mende and Chambers, 1958), and the separation of adherent cells in calcium-free media (Chambers and Zweifach, 1940).

Classic descriptions of the endothelial vessels in fixed tissues stained with silver indicated a network of silver-stained lines corresponding to the borders of the endothelial cells (Eberth and Schimmelbusch, 1889; Hoyer, 1865; Arnold, 1871). More recent work (Stehbens and Florey, 1960) has laid open to question the precise nature of the silver-stained lines, especially their significance with respect to the intercellular material (Gottlobb and Hoff, 1967). It appears that the thickness of the lines cannot be used as an estimate of the interendothelial cell space. On the other hand, the capacity of the intercellular material to reduce silver probably has some meaning, but the significance still escapes us.

Electron micrographs show the endothelial cells to be closely interdigitated and separated, on the average, by from 100 to 200 Å, a space too small to be resolved with the light microscope. At many points, the adjacent surface membranes of endothelial cells seem to be actually fused, so-called tight junctions, a feature also observed in other epithelial membranes that demonstrate selective permeability to ions and small molecules (Farquhar and Palade, 1963; Bruns and Palade, 1968). These investigators believe that the fusion of cell surfaces along the inner endothelial aspect of the small vessels is sufficiently complete under normal conditions to prevent the movement of colloidal materials and to restrict the movement of smaller molecules from the blood to the tissues by way of potential intercellular pathways.

Fromter and Diamond (1972) propose that the permeability of all cellular membranes depends upon the state of intercellular adhesion and that this feature can be altered selectively to change the permeability properties of the membrane, even to particles as small as ions.

The basement membrane materials and the attenuated interendothelial cellular material are probably a continuum of the same structural elements (Majno, 1965). Thus, when contiguous endothelial cells become separated during injury, they may not only move apart from one another, but from the basement membrane as well. There is no reason to assume that chemical reactions which affect the basement membrane will not have a comparable action on the intercellular components as well.

It is difficult to explain how calcium deficiency or local acidosis leads to a weakening of interendothelial cell binding without implicating some chemical grouping which, in final analysis, acts as a bridging agent. A simple surface charge attraction does not provide an adequate explanation for cell to cell adhesion (Carter, 1965). Work on the aggregation of platelets (Clayton *et al.*, 1963; Born and Cross, 1964; Gaarder and Laland, 1964) indicates that surface sugar groupings involving adenosine triphosphate (ATP) combine with each other to act as a bridging factor for the adhesion of these structures. Calcium may serve a similar function in binding endothelial cells into sheets or cellular membranes (see Chapter 7 for discussion of Bangham's surface charge hypothesis).

C. Adhesiveness

One of the earliest recognized manifestations of the inflammatory response on the microscopic level was the phenomenon of stickiness. Not only did platelets and leukocytes adhere to the vessel lining after local injury (Virchow, 1897), but colloidal dyes and particles such as carbon were sequestered on the walls of the affected vessels (Herzog, 1924). This aspect of the inflammatory process is discussed in detail in Chapter 7. For the sake of completeness, a number of features relative to the microcirculation are included in this presentation.

The older literature (see Anitschkow, 1924; Biozzi *et al.*, 1948; Jansco, 1955) contains repeated references to the sequestration of colloidal dyes and carbon by vascular endothelium after even simple hyperemia (Herzog, 1925). This localization of material during the injury reaction was thought to be a physical attachment to the endothelial surface followed by subsequent uptake into the cell. This kind of localization during injury may, in some cases, merely reflect the increased outward filtration of fluid through defects in the vessel wall and the retention of the larger particles by the basement membrane barrier as suggested by Majno (1964). In experiments where both dye-complexed protein and colloidal carbon were injected intravenously, the protein escaped into the tissue proper, whereas the colloidal carbon was filtered off by the vessel wall (Gozsy and Kate, 1957). Since they were able to influence the blue dye–protein leakage and carbon-sticking phenomena separately, these workers concluded that the two phenomena were not causally related.

On the basis of light microscope observation, the hypothesis was advanced that the surface of the endothelium and of both the leukocytes and platelets become "sticky" so that they are mutually attracted (Fig. 6). It is not clear what was responsible for this phenomenon—the deposition of a coating material, a change in the properties of the polysaccharide–protein complex encasing the cell, or some change in electrical properties of the affected

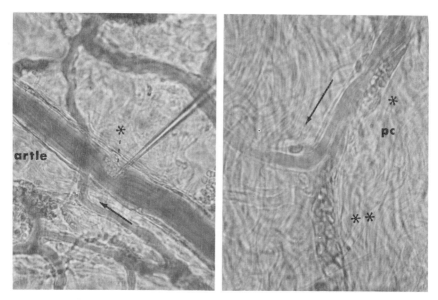

Fig. 6. Left, an arteriole in mesentery into which a fine microneedle has been inserted. Note that a pure platelet thrombus (*) is formed despite rapid flow and high shear rate in vessel. Such platelet aggregates continue to form and break away for about 3–5 minutes after the needle has been withdrawn. Right, the injury reaction to the same mechanical stimulus is much more extensive on the venous side of the circulation. The needle is just in focus (*) in upper part of the postcapillary vessel (pc). The sticking reaction now includes leukocytes and two red blood cells. Downstream in the direction of flow (**) a mass of leukocytes, red cells, and platelets has been washed away from the original site of injury. Arrows indicate direction of blood flow. (× 250.)

surfaces (see Danon, 1971, and discussion in Chapter 7). A number of separate pieces of evidence suggests that the phenomenon of sticking during the injury reaction may be due to a masking of the normally negative surface charge by the release of basic or cationic proteins from damaged cells. For example, Zeya and Spitznagel (1963) were able to separate from granules of polymorphonuclear leukocytes a basic protein which was later shown to be bactericidal in nature. Janoff and Zweifach (1963) found that preparations of such cationic proteins, when injected locally into the mesenteric circulation, produced sticking and emigration of leukocytes despite the fact that these lysosomal extracts possessed none of the known enzymic constituents of these granules. The phenomenon probably reflects some physical property of basic proteins as a class rather than that of a particular cationic protein, since Frimmer and Hegner (1963) were able to produce a typical inflammatory reaction in the rabbit mesentery which involved sticking and emigration of leukocytes by local application of a basic polypeptide derived from thymus nuclei. Katchalsky (1964) reported a similar injury reaction with basic peptides such as polylysines.

Ultrastructural evidence, however, fails to shed light on the mechanism responsible for either the adhesiveness of leukocytcs and platelets to the affected endothelial surface or for the tendency of these blood elements to stick to one another and to attract colloidal particles (Florey, 1961a,b; Marchesi, 1962). Electron micrographs of leukocytes and macrophages during the sequence of phagocytosis show that at first colloidal particles become attached to the cell surface and later appear within the cytoplasm (Farquhar, 1961). Depending on the fixative used, particles of carbon or trypan blue may be seen inside endothelial cells without being enclosed in membranous vesicles (Wissig, 1958a). The material lining the free surface of the endothelial membrane during the injury reaction can be stained *in vivo* with alcian blue (Grant and Becker, 1966).

The evidence to date makes it unlikely that intravascular coagulation per se is a primary factor in the surface stickiness of tissue injury (Allison and Lancaster, 1961; Grant and Becker, 1966), although Jansco (1961) has presented provocative evidence with rare earth anticoagulants to support this thesis.

D. Barrier Function of Basement Membrane

In the majority of microvessels, the outer aspect of the endothelial tube is covered with what is referred to in the literature (Zimmermann, 1923) as the "pericapillary sheath," a condensation of the ground substance containing collagen and reticular fibrils. That investment is clearly visible, and in thin tissues such as the mesentery it is separated from the underlying endothelium by a thin space. Leukocytes which emigrate through the vessel wall at first lie in the perivascular space (Zweifach, 1953; Florey and Grant, 1961; Marchesi, 1961). Farquhar (1961) and others (Ekholm, 1957; Wissig, 1958b) have shown that the vessels in endocrine glands have a split basement membrane which is separated into endothelial and parenchymal components. The extent to which the pericapillary sheath represents a cleavage of the basement membrane or whether it is a completely separate entity has not been established.

The physical appearance of the periendothelial basement membrane, as visualized with the electron microscope (thickness, density, structural configuration), gives no real clue to its functional capacity to serve as a filter. Wide extremes in permeability encountered after injury reactions of all kinds are not associated with obvious structural changes in the basement membrane (Florey, 1961a).

Electron micrographs of the basement membrane surrounding the small blood vessels reveal only an amorphous, poorly defined matrix with occasional fibrils (Bargmann, 1958). Some workers have proposed that the membrane is a mucoprotein secreted by the endothelial cells and epithelial elements (Curran, 1957). Others believe that the acid mucopolysaccharide matrix contains protein-coated fibrils (Bargmann, 1958) which, in effect, represent the aqueous pores through which the plasma constituents are ultrafiltered (Vollrath, 1968). Niessing and Rollhäuser (1954) suggested that the basement membrane contains lipid lamellae as well, but this contention has not been confirmed.

Vessels with a well-defined basement membrane usually have only a limited permeability to protein (Bennett et al., 1959). In contrast, structures such as lymphatic capillaries or sinusoids of the liver and spleen do not have a continuous basement membrane and are collectively much more permeable to plasma proteins than are capillary barriers (see Chapter 6 by Casley-Smith). It is interesting that venules, despite the presence of prominent basement membranes, are more prone to develop an increased permeability during injury reactions than are the capillaries (Majno et al., 1961).

Although electron microscope findings suggest a barrier function for the capillary basement membrane, direct studies of the microcirculation (Fulton et al., 1960; Zweifach, 1962) reveal that under many circumstances red blood cells and carbon are extruded through the basement membrane into the tissue. Such openings are not permanent and are sealed off quickly, e.g., when caused by hypertonic agents (Zweifach, 1962). In other situations, such as depletion of calcium, local heat, irritation with bacterial endotoxins or histamine, the small venules may develop a collar of red blood cells and carbon, presumably a reflection of the fact that these elements have been trapped between the endothelium and the basement membrane. When a microbolus of dye-labeled albumin is injected directly into the connective tissue, the material diffuses uniformly throughout the interstitium. From a functional standpoint, the basement membrane surrounding small vessels can be considered to serve primarily as a structural support and it acts as a filter only for a very large macromolecules [antibody–antigen (Ab–Ag) complexes] and for blood cells.

E. Red Blood Cells

1. VASCULAR STASIS

Stasis in its simplest form occurs when the fluid component of blood is rapidly filtered off while the cellular elements are retained (Fig. 7) until a compacted mass of red blood cells interrupts flow. The phenomenon is

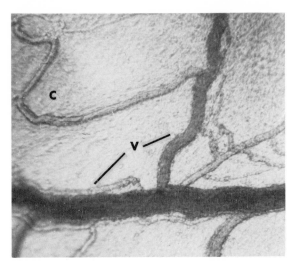

Fig. 7. Mesentery of rat irrigated with hypotonic saline (0.7%). Within 10–15 minutes, a close packing of red blood cells in the capillaries (C) results in complete stasis with no evidence of platelet or leukocyte sticking. The collecting venule (V) running vertically continues to show decreased flow, whereas the large venule (V) running horizontally is not affected. (×90.)

usually reversible with flow resuming within 10 minutes to an hour, depending upon the severity of the insult. At least two mechanisms leading to this type of stasis have been identified (Klemensiewicz, 1916; Tannenberg, 1925; Krogh, 1922; Landis, 1927; Illig, 1955). The first involves some form of endothelial cell damage, as manifested by adhesion of platelets, leukocytes, dye particles, or carbon. A second mechanism may occur either when the intercellular junction is weakened and endothelial cells move apart temporarily to create a leak between the contiguous borders or when an intrinsic disturbance in the cells themselves causes contiguous cells to separate so that bulk fluid movement occurs more readily (Zweifach, 1961b). The basement membrane does not appear to be involved in either of these circumstances since there is no evidence that this barrier significantly retards the outward passage of plasma proteins.

Krogh (1920) and Jacoby (1920) originally expressed the belief that stasis resulted from a dilation of the small blood vessels and a consequent increase in their permeability. The presumption here is that stretching of the vessel wall increases the number of aqueous channels or available pores. In line with this explanation, it should be pointed out that physical distension of venules could lead not only to a separation of endothelial cells, but also to a thinning of the cell proper and to opening of the many fenestrae present in venular endothelium (Rhodin, 1962). Landis (1927) reexamined Krogh's experiments and concluded that capillary stasis is the result of two separate factors—an elevation of the intravascular pressure and a change in the vessel wall. He explained the stasis which develops locally with toxic substances such as urethane on the basis of osmotic effects and concurrent damage to the vascular endothelium. Subsequent studies by Illig (1953), Baron and Chambers (1936), and Zweifach (1963) again emphasized a change in the vascular barrier as the central factor in the genesis of true stasis. The endothelial cell is the primary structure involved (Zweifach, 1963).

Witte (1957c) believed that changes in blood coagulation mechanisms represent a fundamental aspect of the stasis reaction, especially where immunological factors are involved. Intravascular coagulation is known to be associated with profound changes in vascular integrity (see Chapter 10 on hemostasis). It remains to be demonstrated to what extent an activation of coagulation leads to the release of vasoactive agents which affect the capillary wall, or whether some component of the clotting mechanism which is normally attached to the lumen surface of the vessel is removed during the injury reaction (Jensen, 1956; Copley et al., 1960).

2. SLUDGED BLOOD

The development of local areas of stasis, their resolution, and the release of blood cell masses into the blood stream brings into focus another aspect of the problem: the presence in the circulation of what has been referred to by Knisely et al. (1947) as "sludged blood." Actually, the term is purely descriptive, referring to a phenomenon noted after a whole array of seemingly unrelated circumstances. Clumps of red cells are formed which are sufficiently cohesive to circulate as a solid mass, but yet are pliable enough to be squeezed through microscopic blood vessels much smaller than the mass itself. There is some question as to whether it is justifiable to apply a single term, "sludge," to a condition which probably is not a single entity in terms of its causation and morphological characteristics (Laufman, 1951; Lutz, 1951).

Harding and Knisely (1958) presumed that during sludging the red blood cells become coated with a proteinaceous material which causes them to adhere to one another. There is no evidence that under these conditions red blood cells are altered enough to adhere to the vessel wall as in the inflammatory process. Knisely et al. (1947), Bloch (1956), and Harders (1957) believe that the reaction develops independently of the coagulation system and is a reversible process. Hardaway and Johnson (1963) and Robb (1963) believe that the phenomenon can progress to the point where actual microthrombi are formed. The deleterious consequences of sludging are attributed to an altered flow property of the blood, especially at low shear rates, and to impaction of many small vessels to the point where key tissues cannot be perfused effectively with blood (Gelin and Zederfeldt, 1961). Dintenfass (1968) described the "high viscosity syndrome" in which the red cells become less deformable and thereby disrupt the normal flow and distribution of blood cells through the microscopic vessels. The rheologic aspects of tissue injury are discussed in Chapter 5 by Wells.

In many conditions in which sludging has been described (see Bloch, 1956; Branemark, 1969), such as burns or traumatic shock, agglutinated masses of red cells are frequently enmeshed with platelet masses. In other situations, such as acute endotoxemia, aggregates of red blood cells, which are not simple rouleaux, can be seen in the circulation without evidence of actual fibrin or platelets in the clumps (Hugues and Lecomte, 1944). It is interesting to note that under the latter conditions carbon particles in the blood stream were not observed to adhere either to the endothelial wall or to the red blood cells (Zweifach, 1953).

F. Platelets and Vascular Permeability

In addition to their well-established role in intravascular coagulation and thrombosis (see MacFarlane, Chapter 10), blood platelets are believed to contribute to the maintenance of normal capillary permeability. Some investigators believe the permeability of the vascular barrier in injured sites is due, in part, to a loss of some endothelial cell supporting function of the platelets (Cronkite *et al.*, 1952; Johnson *et al.*, 1964; see also Volume I, Chapter 9 by Zucker). Suspensions of washed platelets, when added to the perfusion medium, were found by Danielli and Stock (1950) to counteract the increased permeability leading to edema in hindlimb preparations. They postulated that platelets, by plugging leaky "pores," serve to decrease the permeability of the vascular barrier. No attempt was made to define precisely the nature or location of these pores. Although such a mechanical explanation is probably an oversimplification, the waterproofing action by platelets could be explained as a filling either of gaps between cells or of openings in the basement membrane.

Wilbrandt *et al.* (1956), on the basis of the perfusion of isolated preparations, found that a protein extract of platelets restored the permeability of the small blood vessels which had become edematous after treatment with Versene, a calcium chelator. Such evidence makes less acceptable a simplified explanation such as the mechanical aspects of platelet plugging, but does not completely rule out such a possibility. In other conditions of increased permeability, as in animals exposed to whole body X irradiation

(Cronkite and Brecher, 1964) or in patients with thrombocytopenia purpura (Woods *et al.*, 1953), administration of platelet suspensions has had a striking ameliorative effect. The thrombocytopenia precedes the alteration in the blood–tissue barrier in these conditions. It is clear that the reduced number of platelets does not represent the critical factor, but that it is some qualitative change in these elements. Spaet (1952) emphasized that in addition to the thrombocytopenia the vessel wall itself must be damaged before permeability defects become apparent. One cannot dismiss the possibility that the two mechanisms may be interrelated.

Although it may appear paradoxical, the reaction to injury, in effect, is associated locally with a thrombocytopenia because of the clumping and intravascular coagulation which may occur. Copley (1957) points out that large doses of anticoagulants such as heparin can by themselves cause clumping of blood platelets, a phenomenon which, in turn, predisposes to a bleeding tendency. Local tissue injury in heparinized animals usually leads to an untoward bleeding in the small vessels. Visually, this shows up as failure of a platelet–fibrin plug to form and to seal off the capillary defect (Zweifach, 1963). It is likely that in an immediate emergency situation the platelets may serve as a temporary seal until the structural elements involved—endothelium and basement membrane—are able to repair themselves. Baumgartner *et al.* (1971) believe that the deposition of a layer of platelets over a denuded or damaged portion of vascular endothelium serves a protective function and blocks the chain of events leading to a viscious cycle.

Platelet adhesion and accumulation in the small vessels occur most prominently at the point of direct injury. In turn, leukocyte adhesion develops immediately adjacent to these sites and downstream in the direction of flow. At first, the platelets adhere only fleetingly to the vessel surface, then more firmly, and eventually to one another; this suggests a generalized process since the endothelium and leukocytes are also affected at this time (Clark and Clark, 1935; Arendt *et al.*, 1953; Allison *et al.*, 1963; Stehbins, 1967).

Since carbon particles at this time also ahere to all three elements—endothelium, platelets, and leucocytes (Zweifach, 1961b)—there is a good possibility that some common surface interaction is involved. When platelet adhesion is manifested in living preparations under the microscope, electron microscope photographs show no clear-cut evidence of any sticky layer on the cell surface (Florey, 1961b). This may be due to technical difficulties, since, as suggested by Pease (1966), materials of this kind may be washed out during the fixation and preparation of tissues for electron microscopy (Mende and Chambers, 1958). It should be noted that the electron micrograph data of Luft (see Chapter 2) show an endocapillary layer even under normal conditions; ruthenium chloride was used to stain the material.

Platelets have also been implicated in the local vasoconstriction that occurs when vessels are severed or torn. Several investigators (Zucker, 1947; Born *et al.*, 1958) have extracted from platelets a constrictor principle which they believe is responsible for contraction of damaged blood vessels. Serotonin (5-hydroxytryptamine) has been suggested as the mediator (Zucker and Borrelli, 1955). Inasmuch as the accumulation of platelets during inflammation occurs mostly in the collecting venules and distal capillaries, which are nonmuscular and do not exhibit active contraction, this feature is not an especially critical aspect of the local injury reaction.

A purpura-like syndrome has been described after the injection of anti-platelet serum into animals (Katsura, 1928; Clark and Jacobs, 1950; Shulman, 1958; Shimizu, 1959). Experiments of this kind should be repeated with purified antigens since the anti-platelet antibody is produced with relatively crude tissue extracts. Intravenous injection of such antibodies invariably causes diffuse endothelial damage as shown by adhesion of colloidal carbon and dyes to the lumen surface in the living circulation and by swelling of these cells as seen in fixed preparations (Katsura, 1928).

The acute inflammatory reaction has been found to proceed in thrombocytopenic animals essentially as in controls (Johnstone and Howland, 1958; Page and Good, 1958). Damaged vessels bleed somewhat more readily, presumably because of the inability to seal off defects in the walls. The production of thrombocytopenia and leukopenia in experimental animals is a drastic procedure and so difficult to control that the implication of data of this kind must be carefully weighed (Allison and Lancaster, 1960).

G. Ground Substance

Most discussions of the injury reaction do not emphasize sufficiently the fact that a major component of the hematoparenchymal barrier is the tissue ground substance interposed between the vessel and the parenchymal cells. Histological inspection of injured tissues reveals the intercellular compartment to be distended with fluid and many of the fibrillar elements to be swollen and even fragmented (Movat *et al.*, 1960). Since the ground substance complex is a gel (Hvidberg, 1960; Gersh and Catchpole, 1960; Laurent, 1970), it has been suggested that local sequestration of fluid is, in part, due to an increased avidity of the tissue colloids for water (Slack, 1959; Wegelius and Asboe-Hansen, 1956). Lansing (1959) found that injury is associated with an absorption of cations, such as calcium, onto collagen and reticular fibers. There is good evidence that other large molecular complexes, including plasma proteins, are bound to connective tissue elements in damaged areas (Higginbotham, 1959). Dyestuffs injected in the blood stream stain injured fibers much more heavily than usual (Rigdon, 1939). In fact, it is difficult, even by drastic chemical means, to extract dyes such as Evans' blue or water blue from injured tissues for quantitative measurements (Ridgon, 1939; Judah and Willoughby, 1962). Measurements of the leakage of plasma proteins into tissue and their return from these sites show that with time despite an increased lymph flow the concentration of protein is increased in injured sites over and above that of water (Aschheim and Zweifach, 1962).

As previously pointed out, Fischer, in 1910, proposed that physicochemical changes in the colloidal constituents of tissue are of basic importance in the formation of local edema, a view not too far removed from current concepts of connective tissue properties (Gersh and Catchpole, 1960; see Chapter 4 by Cathchpole). Several authors (see review by Duran-Reynals, 1939) have described enzymes of the hyaluronidase type which break down some of the complex polysaccharides making up the ground substance. A number of investigators (Elster *et al.*, 1949) have speculated that the increased permeability during the injury reaction may be due, in part, to hydrolytic enzymes of this type. Experimental studies in which tissue extracts with hyaluronidase activity were applied with micropipettes did not demonstrate a disruptive effect on transcapillary exchange (Zweifach and Chambers, 1950). Other factors, however, may be related to this type of connective tissue change. These include the release of hydrolytic enzymes of the lysosome type (de Duve, 1959; see Cochrane and Janoff, Volume III, Chapter 3), accumulation of metabolic by-products of the adenosine type (Stoner and Threlfall, 1960), or local acidity (Stetson and Good, 1951).

Microscopy in living tissues shows changes in the physical properties of the connective tissue in the inflammatory process. When colloidal particles are injected with a micropipette into arteolar tissue, a sharply localized bleb is formed without spreading (Zweifach, 1963). In contrast, when colloids are injected into a tissue site about 20–30 minutes after injury, the material becomes rapidly dispersed, clearly indicating that the ground substance has been transformed from a gel to a sol state. It has been often reported (see Allison *et al.*, 1955) that leukocytes which have emigrated at first move about freely and randomly until they reach the directly damaged site, whereupon they round up and become confined to a circumscribed area. It is possible that the watery consistency of the injured tissue represents a physical factor which favors the entrapment of leukocytes in the area. Such a phenomenon may account for apparently conflicting data dealing with chemotaxis of leukocytes under *in vivo* and *in vitro* circumstances (Harris, 1954). However, this observation does not exclude chemotaxis as a factor in such reactions (see Chapter 7 by Grant, and Volume I, Chapter 7 by Hirsch).

H. Rheologic Considerations

The physical properties of the blood itself represent an important factor influencing local flow. The alterations during systemic and local injury range from simple aggregations of red blood cells, to formation of discrete masses large enough to fill the lumen of small vessels, to platelet clumping and fibrin formation (Tannenberg, 1925). Disturbances of this kind change the physical characteristics of blood and, in effect, serve to introduce abnormal shear stresses to the point where flow through the small vessels becomes disorganized (see Chapter 5 by Wells).

Danielli and Stock (1950), Jensen (1956), Copley (1957), and Copley and Tsuluca (1962) have postulated an endocapillary vascular lining which is a component of the coagulation system. According to this concept, the blood–tissue barrier has a thin film lining the lumen surface which is presumed to be fibrin in its monomer or dimer form. The deposition and regulation of the film thickness is maintained by an equilibrium with the plasmin fibrinolytic system. The presence of such a fibrin film has not beeen confirmed by electron microscopy. During injury, activation of the coagulation process could alter the nature of such a lining material so that it becomes adhesive and attracts both cells and colloidal particles (Herzog, 1924; Gozsy and Kato, 1960). Jansco (1961), working with anticoagulants derived from rare earth metals, was able to elicit an anti-inflammatory effect without influencing the accompanying hyperemia, and he concluded that fibrinogen in an as yet unresolved way plays an important role in edema formation. In fact, Jansco questions whether or not so-called vasoactive mediators of the inflammatory reaction act directly on the vessel wall, and he believes that they require the intervention of the coagulation system. This concept is not too far removed from one which envisages activation of complement and the Hageman factor as key factors in the liberation of vasoactive mediators of the kinin type (Kaplan and Austen, 1970). Other workers, such as Allison and Lancaster (1961), on the basis of experiments with other anticoagulants and fibrinolytic factors, do not accept the fibrin layer concept.

I. Lymphatic Drainage

An important aspect of the exchange of materials between the tissue compartment and the vascular system resides in the terminal lymphatics. As shown in Fig. 8, the lymphatic capillaries consist of a network of interconnecting vessels (20–40 μm), pouchlike endothelial outpocketings, usually in close proximity to the venules and frequently abutting directly against them (Kraus, 1957; Clark and Clark, 1937; Baez, 1960). It is generally accepted

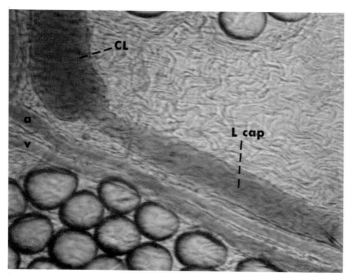

Fig. 8. Terminal lymphatic capillary (L cap) in mesentery is filled with dye by micropipette in lower right corner. The necklike region in the lymphatic contains a valve where capillary enters the larger collecting lymphatic (CL) Small arteriole (a) and venule (v) are below lymphatic. Fat cells are seen at bottom (× 200.)

that plasma proteins, large monomolecular complexes, blood cells, etc., are returned to the circulatory system via the lymphatic capillaries (Wasserman *et al.*, 1955; Mayerson, 1959; Kraus, 1957; Grotte, 1956; Hauck and Schroer, 1971). A continuous slow return of a proteinaceous fluid occurs in the lymph vessels which drain the skin and skeletal musculature. The volume and content of the lymph is considerably altered after injury (Cope and Moore, 1944). The ability of red blood cells, macrophages, and proteins to enter the lymphatic channels freely under these conditions appears to involve a weakening of the endothelium of the lymph capillaries and a separation of these cells similar to that observed in the blood vessels (Casley-Smith and Florey, 1961; Cliff and Nicoll, 1970). Some authors (Guyton *et al.*, 1971) believe that the separation of lymphatic capillary endothelium is facilitated by the attachment of connective tissue fibrils to the outer surface of the cell.

Electron microscope studies have indicated that unlike the blood capillaries the lymphatic vessels consist of a thin endothelial tube with only vestiges of a basement membrane (Fraley and Weiss, 1961; Casley-Smith, 1968). In some areas, the walls of the lymph capillaries have only an attenuated endothelial structure. The endothelial cells lining the lymphatic channels do not differ appreciably from vascular endothelium (Florey, 1961a; see Chapter 6 by Casley-Smith). The extreme perviousness of the lymphatic capillaries is attributed to the absence of a complete basement membrane and the absence of tight intercellular junctions. Contiguous endothelial cells are frequently separated by as much as 1500–2000 Å (Palay and Karlin, 1959). A careful study of the passage of colloidal material and red blood cells from the peritoneal cavity into the lymphatics was made by French et al. (1960). Lymph capillaries were found to come into direct contact with specialized areas of the diaphragm to form lacunae across which the particulate material moves both between the cells and through them. Discrete fenestrations were not seen, each potential space being covered by a thin basement membrane.

De Langen (1952) believed that there is a much greater convective exchange of fluid and dissolved materials between the blood and lymphatic capillaries via the tissue compartment than is generally accepted. He argued for a continuous movement of fluid as a basic mechanism for local tissue homeostasis. Other studies of the response to tissue damage have shown that while blood–lymph exchange at first increases (Hudack and McMaster, 1932) the flux is actually reduced later (Glenn et al., 1943). Some investigators, such as Menkin (1956), described a blockage of the lymphatics during injury and believed the phenomenon to be a protective measure to isolate the affected area. Miles and Miles (1958) were unable to provide evidence of an impaired movement of materials such as dyes and india ink from an injured site into terminal lymphatics. Apparently, the phenomenon of "fixation" in an injured site may be due to physicochemical factors within the tissue proper.

A variety of breakdown products of damaged tissue enters the circulation via the lymphatics (Glenn et al., 1942). More recently, it has been shown that acid hydrolases are released from damaged lysosomes during hemorrhagic shock and appear in high concentration in the thoracic duct lymph (Dumont and Weissmann, 1964). Enzymes such as β-glucuronidase or acid phosphatase, which accumulate in the blood during traumatic shock (Janoff et al., 1962), probably are also disseminated from injured sites by way of the lymphatics (see Volume III, Chapter 3 by Cochrane and Janoff).

III. Summary

The major features of the acute inflammatory process—vasodilation, transudation of plasma proteins, and cellular emigration—appear to develop separately, although, because of structural considerations, the events clearly impinge on one another. Initially, hemodynamic changes predominate: (a) arterial dilation, (b) increased venular resistance, (c) elevated capillary pressure, and (d) increased surface area for exchange through opening up of new capillaries. Simultaneously with the vasodilation, substantial amounts of plasma proteins leak into the tissue to cause manifest edema. Cellular emigration, on the other hand, is usually delayed in appearance and progresses more slowly.

The reaction from its onset thus involves an increased transudation of protein whose magnitude is clearly dependent upon the associated dilation and hyperemia. Landis (1964) and Michel (1970) have found that even under optimal conditions spotty leaks of blue dye–protein complexes are encountered, especially in the minute venules. It is probable that a portion of the escaping plasma protein in the first phase of the injury response is simply an enhanced leakage through defects caused by the increased volume flow and intravascular pressure per se. However, in view of the fact that mediator substances such as histamine, 5-hydroxytryptamine, kinins, and prostaglandins are known to be released at this time, it is equally likely that a separation of endothelial cells occurs, thereby increasing the number of potential leaks through which bulk movement of plasma can occur. Inasmuch as blood flow is increased by a factor of as much as ten, this combination of circumstances can account for the protein loss and edema during the first part of the reaction to injury.

Most observers are convinced that the early permeability response is predominantly venular, whereas the subsequent delayed reaction also involves the extensive network of true capillaries. The thesis advanced by Krogh (1920) and Ricker (1924) that vasodilation per se could account for the appearance of gaps between endothelial cells and the outpouring of plasma may be applicable to the venules. The capillaries, on the other hand, are much more resistant to distention by the intravascular pressure, and do not under normal circumstances develop additional leaks when blood flow alone is increased. They are, in fact, tunnels in a gel, and as such they are supported by the surrounding ground substance—a feature which makes them much less distensible than venules (Fung *et al.*, 1971). The fact that leakage of plasma proteins does occur in the capillaries later in the syndrome suggests that either the capillary wall proper or the surrounding tissue has been weakened in some way.

Protein transudation continues throughout the remainder of the inflammatory process, although the loss of blue dye–protein complexes falls off rapidly after the first 15–30 minutes, and then, after a variable time course, increases again. This waxing and waning is probably due to several factors: a reduction in blood flow, an increased tissue pressure, the bypassing of many capillaries, and a slowing of flow in small vessels because of change in rheologic properties of the blood. The subsequent increase in permeability to protein may be due to alterations in the vascular barrier itself, and it eventually encompasses the basement membrane.

It would be unwise to attempt to distinguish between separate phases of the inflammatory process on the basis of blue dye–protein loss alone. There is no evidence that the separate phases of the syndrome are, in fact, due to comparable changes in the vascular barrier. For example, electron microscope studies show a separation of contiguous endothelial cells of the venules only during the immediate reaction to a phlogen. Increased vesicular transport or cytopempsis does not appear to be a contributing factor at this time. It is not known whether or not gaps or stomata in the capillaries are the primary defects responsible for the subsequent phase of increased permeability during the injury process.

It is doubtful that physical distention of the vessels during the early phase would, by itself, lead to the formation of new openings. We cannot say with any assurance that the leakiness produced by histamine, bradykinin, serotonin, or prostaglandin E_1 is the result of vasodilation and an increased intravascular pressure alone, nor can we say that it requires a concomitant weakening of the surface bonds between adjacent endothelial cells, which is in turn exacerbated by the elevated intravascular pressure. Recent evidence presented by Landis and Pappenheimer (1963) favors the latter explanation. Majno *et al.* (1969) interpret the endothelial cell separation after histamine administration as a reflection of the potential contractility of the cells.

Certain experimental modalities such as heat, hypertonicity, and urethane lead to rapid capillary stasis without the accumulation of platelets and leukocytes characteristic of more conventional inflammatory situations. Under these conditions, the loss of plasma is most likely due to a separation of endothelial cells at numerous points. The altered permeability at this stage does not involve either alterations in the basement membrane or activation of the vesicular transport mechanism.

Most discussions of the inflammatory process consider the increased perviousness of the barrier per se to be a major event. Undoubtedly, this feature is the keystone of the reaction which sets it apart as a pathological phenomenon, but, by itself, it is only one of several contributory aspects. In most situations, one can only guess at the extent to which various factors become involved over and above the markedly increased blood flow. Included are features such as separation of endothelial cell borders, vesicular transport, physicochemical deterioration of the basement membrane, or a change in an endocapillary lining material.

From a teleologic point of view, the initial phase of the reaction may be looked upon as an attempt to counteract the deranged local homeostasis by flushing the tissue with blood and by increasing blood protein exchange between blood and lymph systems via the tissue compartment. Later, cellular elements are introduced into the tissues to remove and to neutralize abnormal materials—both exogenous and endogenous in origin. Cellular extravasation cannot be carried out on any significant scale without compromising the exchange function of the vascular barrier, and blood flow is disrupted for a variety of reasons ranging from excessive filtration to actual plugging of the vessel by blood cell aggregates.

An especially vexing problem is that of blood cell sticking and emigration, which is discussed in detail in Chapter 7. The sticking reaction can be attributed to changes in at least three components—blood plasma, blood cells, and vascular endothelium—so that generalizations based on visual recording of events are especially hazardous. Some authors have placed major emphasis on the physical disruption of blood flow by the phenomenon of sludging or aggregation. This point of view at best represents an oversimplication. Identification of the chemical principles responsible for the sequelae of the inflammatory process is made all the more difficult by the fact that, as yet, we have not been able to pinpoint the contribution of specific tissue constituents to normal regulatory adjustments.

The neurogenic aspect of the inflammatory reaction has been treated only cursorily because of the paucity of meaningful information on this problem. The axon or anti-dromic reflex exists as a well-established descriptive phenomenon, but little is known about its activation except that the reaction is independent of the hyperemia, sticking, etc. Equally important is the extent to which the nervous system is responsible for the bizarre pattern of reactivity of the small blood vessels after injury, especially in infectious conditions or antigen–antibody interactions (Delauney *et al.*, 1948). Reflexes originating in the muscular venules and small veins are believed to affect tissue blood flow. Such a mechanism may contribute to the increased resistance to venous drainage during injury. Certainly, the blunting of local tissue reactions to immunological stimuli after denervation or chemical sympathetic blockade is suggestive of a neurogenic contribution to the inflammatory process.

The tendency to implicate *a mediator* of the inflammatory reaction is not as prevalent today as in the past (Schachter, 1969). Ultrastructural information has shown that several separate mechanisms can account for outwardly similar manifestations. It has become increasingly apparent that major disagreements concerning the structural basis for transcapillary permeability phenomena cannot be resolved by the electron microscope approach alone.

Ultrastructural studies show the basement membrane to be a barrier to the outward passage of blood cells and colloidal particles. There is no evidence that the basement membrane encasing the capillaries or venules is an effective hindrance to the outward movement of dissolved materials, with the possible exception of glomerular capillaries. It presumably is a factor contributing to the physical strength or compliance of the vessel wall, although the basement membrance shares this distinction with the surrounding connective tissue which contains, in addition, collagen and reticular fibers. The basement membrane material is presumed to be produced by the endothelial cells which are responsible for its maintenance and repair. The contribution of pericytes to basement membrane activity remains to be defined.

Many investigators are convinced that an important constituent of the blood vessel barrier is the so-called endocapillary layer. Originally conceived on the basis of purely circumstantial evidence, its presence was at first disputed by electron microscopists. Two types of substances have been proposed in this regard: a monomolecular layer of monomer fibrin or some mucopolysaccharide complex. It may be that the blood platelets are in some way related to such a layer. Although the original suggestions envisaged such a lining only on the innermost surface of the endothelial cell facing the lumen, it is equally possible that such materials could be deposited on the inner surface of the basement membrane as well. There is reasonably good evidence that the basement membrane deteriorates during the delayed phase of the injury reaction, possibly through enzymic degradation by hydrolytic enzymes.

A discussion of microvascular aspects of the inflammatory process can best be concluded by reaffirming the need for continued reexamination of the visual sequence of events in the light of newer information on biophysical and biochemical levels. Such an appraisal would serve not only to establish the relative contribution of specific reactions, but would also permit us to analyze the microscopic changes from an entirely different aspect under more adequately controlled conditions.

References

Allison, F., Jr., and Lancaster, M. G. (1959). *Brit. J. Exp. Pathol.* **40**, 324.
Allison, F., Jr., and Lancaster, M. G. (1960). *J. Exp. Med.* **111**, 45.
Allison, F., Jr., and Lancaster, M. G. (1961). *J. Exp. Med.* **114**, 535.
Allison, F., Jr., Smith, M. R., and Wood, W. B., Jr. (1955). *J. Exp. Med.* **102**, 655.
Allison, F., Jr., Lancaster, M. G., and Crosthwaite, J. L. (1963). *Amer. J. Pathol.* **43**, 775.
Anitschkow, N. (1924). *Klin. Wochenschr.* **3**, 1729.
Arendt, K. A., Shulman, M. H., Fulton, G. P., and Lutz, B. R. (1953). *Anat. Rec.* **117**, 595.
Arnold, J. (1871). *Arch. Pathol. Anat. Physiol. Klin. Med.* **53**, 7.
Aschheim, E. and Zweifach, B. W. (1961). *Circ. Res.* **9**, 349.
Aschheim, E., and Zweifach, B. W. (1962). *Amer. J. Physiol.* **202**, 554.
Baez, S. (1960). *In* "Flow Properties of Blood and Other Biological Systems" (A. L. Copley and G. Stainsby, eds.), p. 398. Pergamon, Oxford.
Bargmann, W. (1958). *Deut. Med. Wochenschr.* **83**, 1704.
Barlow, T. E. (1950). *J. Anat.* **84**, 405.

Baron, H., and Chambers, R. (1936). *Amer. J. Physiol.* **114**, 700.
Baumgartner, H. R., Stemerman, M. B., and Spaet, T. H. (1971). *Experientia* **27**, 283.
Bennett, H. S. (1956). *J. Biophys. Biochem. Cytol.* **2**, Suppl. 9, 99.
Bennett, H. S., Luft, J. H., and Hampton, J. C. (1959). *Amer. J. Physiol.* **196**, 381.
Berman, H. J., McNary, W., Ausprunk, D., Lee, E., Weaver, S., and Sapawi, R. (1972). *Microvasc. Res.* **4**, 51.
Bhoola, K. D., Calle, J. D., and Schachter, M. S. (1960). *J. Physiol. (London)* **152**, 75.
Biozzi, G., Mene, G., and Ovary, Z. (1948). *Rev. Immunol.* **12**, 320.
Bloch, E. H. (1956). *Ergeb. Anat. Entwicklungsgesch.* **35**, 1.
Boquet, P., and Izard, Y. (1950). *Proc. Soc. Exp. Biol. Med.* **75**, 254.
Born, G. V. R., and Cross, M. J. (1964). *J. Physiol. (London)* **170**, 397.
Born, G. V. R., Ingram, G. I. C., and Stacey, R. S. (1958). *Brit. J. Pharmacol.* **13**, 62.
Brånemark, P-I. (1969). "Intravascular Anatomy of Blood Cells in Man." Karger, Basel.
Brånemark, P-I., and Ekholm, R. (1968). *Blut* **16**, 274.
Brocklehurst, W. E. (1971). *Proc. Roy. Soc. Med.* **64**, 4.
Bruce, A. N. (1910). *Naunyn-Schmiedebergs Arch. Exp. Pathol. Pharmakol.* **53**, 424.
Bruns, R. R., and Palade, G. E. (1968). *J. Cell Biol.* **37**, 244.
Burke, J. F., and Miles, A. A. (1958). *J. Pathol. Bacteriol.* **76**, 1.
Cameron, G. R. (1952). "Pathology of the cell." Thomas, Springfield, Illinois.
Carter, S. B. (1965). *Nature (London)* **208**, 1183.
Casley-Smith, J. R. (1968). *Lymphology* **1**, 77.
Casley-Smith, J. R. (1970). *Experientia* **26**, 852.
Casley-Smith, J. R., and Florey, H. W. (1961). *J. Exp. Physiol.* **46**, 101.
Chambers, R., and Zweifach, B. W. (1940). *J. Cell. Comp. Physiol.* **15**, 255.
Chambers, R., and Zweifach, B. W. (1947). *Physiol. Rev.* **27**, 436.
Chinard, J. P., Vosburgh, G. J., and Enno, T. (1955). *Amer. J. Physiol.* **183**, 221.
Clark, E. R. (1938). *Physiol. Rev.* **18**, 242.
Clark, E. R., and Clark, E. L. (1935). *Amer. J. Anat.* **57**, 385.
Clark, E. R., and Clark, E. L. (1937). *Amer. J. Anat.* **60**, 253.
Clark, W. G., and Jacobs, E. (1950). *Blood* **5**, 320.
Clayton, S., Born, G. V. R., and Cross, M. J. (1963). *Nature (London)* **200**, 138.
Cliff, W. J. (1966). *J. Exp. Med.* **124**, 543.
Cliff, W. J., and Nicoll, P. A. (1970). *Quart. J. Exp. Physiol. Cog. Med. Sci.* **55**, 112.
Cohn, Z. A., and Morse, S. I. (1960). *J. Exp. Med.* **111**, 667.
Cohnheim, J. F. (1867). *Arch. Pathol. Anat. Physiol. Klin. Med.* **40**, 1.
Cohnheim, J. F. (1889). *In* "Lectures on General Pathology," Sect. I, Chapter 3, pp. 109–171. New Sydenham Society, London.
Cope, O., and Moore, F. O. (1944). *J. Clin. Invest.* **23**, 241.
Copley, A. L. (1957). *Aerztl. Forsch.* **11**, 114.
Copley, A. L., and Tsuluca, V. (1962). *Proc. Int. Pharmacol. Meet. 1st, 1961* Vol. 10, p. 67.
Copley, A. L., Scott-Blair, G. W., Balca, T., and Staple, P. H. (1960). *In* "Flow Properties of Blood" (A. L. Copley and G. Stainsky, eds.), p. 418. Pergamon, Oxford.
Cotran, R. S. (1967). *Mol. Pathol.* **6**, 143.
Cotran, R. S. (1970). *In* "Physical Bases of Circulatory Transport" (E. B. Reeve and A. C. Guyton, eds.), p. 249. Saunders, Philadelphia, Pennsylvania.
Cortran, R. S., and Majno, G. (1964). *Amer. J. Pathol.* **45**, 261.
Courtice, F. C. (1959). *Aust. J. Biol. Med. Sci.* **37**, 451.
Courtice, F. C., Muñoz-Marcus, M., and Garlick, O. G. (1964). *Quart. J. Exp. Physiol. Cog. Med. Sci.* **49**, 441.
Cowie, D. B., Flexner, L. B., and Wilde, W. S. (1949). *Amer. J. Physiol.* **158**, 231.
Cronkite, E. P., and Brecher, G. (1954). *Acta Radiol., Suppl.* **116**, 376.

Cronkite, E. P., Jacobs, G. J., Brecher, G., and Dillard, G. (1952). *Amer. J. Roentgenol., Radium Ther. Nucl. Med.* **67**, 796.
Curran, R. C. (1957). *J. Pathol. Bacteriol.* **74**, 347.
Danielli, J. F., and Stock, A. (1950). *J. Cell. Comp. Physiol.* **15**, 255.
Danon, D. (1971). *Eur. Conf. Microcirc., 6th, 1970* p. 415.
de Duve, C. (1959). *In* "Subcellular Particles" (T. Hayashi, ed.), p. 128. Ronald Press, New York.
De Langen, C. D. (1952). *Wien. Med. Wochenschr.* **102**, 933.
Delauney, A., Lebrun, J., Kerneis, J. P., and Delauney, M. (1948). *Rev. Immunol.* **12**, 23.
Dintenfass, L. (1968). *Haematologia* **2**, 19.
Duling, B. R., and Berne, R. M. (1970). *Circ. Res.* **27**, 669.
Dumont, A. E., and Weissmann, G. (1964). *Nature (London)* **201**, 1231.
Duran-Reynals, F. (1939). *J. Biol. Med.* **11**, 601.
Ebbecke, U. (1917). *Pfluegers Arch. Gesamte Physiol. Menschon Tiere* **169**, 1.
Eberth, J. C., and Schimmelbusch, C. (1889). *Arch. Pathol. Anat. Physiol. Klin. Med.* **116**, 327.
Edelman, I. S. (1952). *Amer. J. Physiol.* **171**, 279.
Ekholm, R. (1957). *Z. Zellforsch. Mikrosk. Anat.* **46**, 139.
Elster, S. K., Freeman, M. E., and Dorfman, A. (1949). *Amer. J. Physiol.* **156**, 429.
Farquhar, M. G. (1961). *Angiology* **12**, 270.
Farquhar, M. G., and Palade, G. E. (1963). *J. Cell Biol.* **17**, 375.
Farquhar, M. G., Wissig, S. L., and Palade, G. E. (1961). *J. Exp. Med.* **113**, 47.
Fawcett, D. W. (1959). *In* "The Microcirculation" (S. M. R. Reynolds and B. W. Zweifach, eds.), p. 1. Univ. of Illinois Press, Urbana.
Fischer, M. H. (1910). "Oedema." Wiley, New York.
Fleisch, A. (1935). *Arch. Int. Physiol.* **41**, 141.
Florey, H. W. (1926). *Proc. Roy. Soc., Ser. Bup.* **100**, 269.
Florey, H. W. (1961a). *Nature (London)* **192**, 908.
Florey, H. W. (1961b). *Quart. J. Exp. Physiol. Cog. Med. Sci.* **46**, 119.
Florey, H. W., and Grant, L. H. (1961). *J. Pathol. Bacteriol.* **82**, 13.
Florey, H. W., Poole, J. C. F., and Meek, G. A. (1959). *J. Pathol. Bacteriol.* **77**, 625.
Folkow, B. (1955). *Physiol. Rev.* **35**, 629.
Folkow, B., and Neil, E. (1971). "Circulation," p. 285. Oxford Univ. Press, London and New York.
Fraley, E. E., and Weiss, L. (1961). *Amer. J. Anat.* **109**, 85.
French, J. E., Florey, H. W., and Morris, B. (1960). *Quart. J. Exp. Physiol. Cog. Med. Sci.* **45**, 88.
Frimmer, M., and Hegner, D. (1963). *Naunyn-Schmiedebergs Arch. Exp. Pathol. Pharmakol.* **245**, 355.
Fromter, E., and Diamond, J. (1972). *Nature (London) New Biol.* **235**, 9.
Fulton, G. P., and Zweifach, B. W. (1958). "Factors Regulating Blood Flow." Amer. Physiol. Soc., Washington, D. C.
Fulton, G. P., Lutz, B. R., and Kagan, R. (1960). *Circ. Res.* **4**, 133.
Fulton, G. P., Lutz, B. R., and Callahan, A. B. (1961). *Physiol. Rev.* **40**, 57.
Fung, Y. C., and Zweifach, B. W. (1971). *Annu. Rev. Fluid Mech.* **3**, 189.
Gaarder, A., and Laland, S. (1964). *Nature (London)* **202**, 909.
Gatling, R. R. (1958). *J. Exp. Med.* **108**, 441.
Gelin, L. E., and Zederfeldt, B. (1961). *Acta Chir. Scand.* **122**, 343.
Gerber, I. (1936). *Arch. Pathol.* **21**, 331.
Gersh, I., and Catchpole, H. R. (1960). *Perspect. Biol. Med.* **3**, 282.
Glenn, W. W. L., Peterson, D. K., and Drinker, C. K. (1942). *Surgery* **12**, 685.
Glenn, W. W. L., Muus, J., and Drinker, C. K. (1943). *J. Clin. Invest.* **22**, 451.

Gottlob, R., and Hoff, H. F. (1967). *Vasc. Surg.* **1**, 92.

Gozsy, B., and Kato, L. (1957). *J. Physiol. (London)* **139**, 1.

Gozsy, B., and Kato, L. (1960). *Ann. N. Y. Acad. Sci.* **88**, 43.

Grant, L. H. Palmer, P., and Sanders, A. G. (1962). *J. Pathol. Bacteriol.* **83**, 127.

Grant, L. H., and Becker, F. F. (1966). *Arch. Pathol.* **81**, 36.

Grant, R. T., and Duckett-Jones, T. (1929). *Heart* **14**, 337.

Grant, R. T., Bland, E. F., and Camp, P. D. (1932). *Heart* **16**, 137.

Grotte, G. (1956). *Acta Chir. Scand., Suppl.* **211**, 1.

Guyton, A. C., Granger, H. J., and Taylor, A. E. (1971). *Physiol. Rev.* **51**, 527.

Hardaway, R. M., and Johnson, D. G. (1963). *Mil. Med.* **128**, 198.

Harders, H. (1957). *Thromb. Diath. Haemorrh.* **1**, 482.

Harding, F., and Knisely, M. H. (1958). *Angiology* **9**, 317.

Hare, F. W., Jr., and Miller, A. J. (1951). *AMA Arch. Dermatol. Syphilol.* **64**, 449.

Harris, H. (1954). *Physiol. Rev.* **34**, 529.

Hauck, G., and Schröer, H. (1969). *Pfluegers Arch.* **312**, 32.

Hauck, G., and Schröer, H. (1971). *Eur. Conf. Microcirc., 6th, 1970* p. 203.

Hayashi, H., Tasaki, I., and Yoshinaga, M. (1967). *Nature (London)* **215**, 759.

Hedbys, B. O., Mashima, S., and Maurice, D. M. (1963). *Exp. Eye Res.* **2**, 99.

Herzog, F. (1924). *Z. Exp. Med.* **43**, 79.

Herzog, F. (1925). *Virchows Arch. Pathol. Anat. Physiol.* **256**, 1.

Hevesy, G., and Jacobsen, C. F. (1940). *Acta Physiol. Scand.* **1**, 11.

Higginbotham, R. D. (1959). *Int. Arch. Allergy Appl. Immunol.* **15**, 195.

Hilton, S. M., and Lewis, G. P. (1957). *Brit. Med. Bull.* **13**, 189.

Hirschfelder, A. D. (1924). *Amer. J. Physiol.* **70**, 507.

Horton, E. W. (1969). *Physiol. Rev.* **49**, 122.

Hoyer, H. (1865). *Arch. Anat. Physiol.* p. 244.

Hudack, L., and McMaster, P. D. (1932). *J. Exp. Med.* **56**, 223.

Hugues, J., and Lecomte, J. (1944). *Acta Haematol.* **12**, 177.

Hvidberg, E. (1960). *Acta Pharmacol. Toxicol.* **17**, 267.

Illig, L. (1953). *Klin. Wochenschr.* **31**, 366.

Illig, L. (1955). *Virchows Arch. Pathol. Anat. Physiol.* **326**, 501.

Illig, L. (1961). "Die terminale Strombahn." Springer-Verlag, Berlin and New York.

Intaglietta, M., Pawula, R. F., and Tompkins, W. R. (1970). *Microvasc. Res.* **2**, 212.

Jacoby, W. (1920). *Naunyn-Schmiedebergs Arch. Exp. Pathol. Pharmakol.* **68**, 49.

Janoff, A., and Zweifach, B. W. (1963). *Science* **144**, 698.

Janoff, A., Weissmann, G., Zweifach, B. W., and Thomas, L. (1962). *J. Exp. Med.* **115**, 451.

Jansco, N. (1941). *Ber. Physiol. Lab. Versuchsanst. Landuirt. Inst. Univ. Halle* **126**, 475.

Jansco, N. (1955). "Speicherung." Akademiai Kiado, Budapest.

Jansco, N. (1961). *J. Pharm. Pharmacol.* **13**, 597.

Jensen, H. (1956). *Exp. Med. Surg.* **14**, 189.

Johnson, S. A., Balboa, R. S., and Dessel, B. H. (1964). *Exp. Mol. Pathol.* **3**, 115.

Johnstone, D. E., and Howland, J. W. (1958). *J. Exp. Med.* **108**, 431.

Judah, J. D., and Willoughby, D. A. (1962). *J. Pathol. Bacteriol.* **83**, 567.

Kaplan, H. P., and Austen, K. F. (1970). *J. Immunol.* **802**, 91.

Karnovsky, M. J. (1968). *J. Cell Biol.* **52**, 64.

Katchalsky, A. (1964). *Biophys. J.* **4**, Suppl. 9, 41.

Katsura, H. (1928). *Trans. Jap. Pathol. Soc.* **14**, 152.

Klemensiewicz, R. (1916). *Beitr. Pathol. Anat. Allg. Pathol.* **63**, 321.

Knisely, M. H., Bloch, E. H., Eliot, T. S., and Warner, L. (1947). *Science* **106**, 431.

Kochen, J. A., and Baez, S. (1965). *Bibl. Anat.* **7**, 46.

Kraus, H. (1957). *Z. Zellforsch. Mikrosk. Anat.* **46**, 446.

Krogh, A. (1920). *J. Physiol. (London)* **53**, 399.

Krogh, A. (1922). "The Anatomy and Physiology of Capillaries." Yale Univ. Press, New Haven, Connecticut.

Landis, E. M. (1927). *Amer. J. Physiol.* **81**, 124.

Landis, E. M. (1934). *Physiol. Rev.* **14**, 404.

Landis, E. M. (1964). *Ann. N. Y. Acad. Sci.* **116**, 765.

Landis, E. M. and Hortenstine, J. C. (1950). *Physiol. Rev.* **30**, 1.

Landis, E. M., and Pappenheimer, J. R. (1963). *In* "Handbook of Physiology" (Amer. Physiol. Soc., J. Field, ed.), Sect. 2, Vol. II, Chapter 29, p. 961. Williams & Wilkins, Baltimore, Maryland.

Lansing, A. I. (1959). *In* "The Arterial Wall" (A. I. Lansing, ed.), p. 136. Williams & Wilkins, Baltimore, Maryland.

Laufman, H. (1951). *AMA Arch. Surg.* **62**, 486.

Laurent, T. C. (1970). *In* "Capillary Permeability" (C. Crone, ed.), p. 261. Munksgaard, Copenhagen.

Lecomte, J., and Hugues, J. (1956). *Int. Arch. Allergy Appl. Immunol.* **8**, 72.

Lee, R. E., Goebl, D., and Fulton, L. A. (1955). *Ann. N.Y. Acad. Sci.* **61**, 665.

Lewis, G. P., and Matthews, J. (1970). *J. Physiol. (London)* **207**, 15.

Lewis, T. (1924). *Heart* **11**, 119.

Lewis, T. (1927). "The Blood Vessels of the Human Skin and Their Responses." Shaw, London.

Lewis, T., and Grant, R. T. (1924). *Heart* **11**, 209.

Lewis, T., and Grant, R. T. (1925). *Heart* **12**, 73.

Lewis, T., and Harmer, I. M. (1927). *Heart* **14**, 19.

Lister, J. (1858). *Phil. Trans. Roy. Soc. London* **148**, 645.

Loeb, L. (1923). *Medicine (Baltimore)* **2**, 171.

Ludwig, C. (1865). "Die physiologischen Leistungen des Blutdruckes." Hirzel, Leipzig.

Lutz, B. R. (1951). *Physiol. Rev.* **31**, 107.

McGovern, V. J. (1955). *J. Pathol. Bacteriol.* **69**, 283.

Majno, G. (1964). *In* "Injury, Inflammation and Immunity" (L. Thomas, J. W. Uhr, and L. Grant, eds.), p. 58–93. Williams & Wilkins, Baltimore, Maryland.

Majno, G. (1965). *In* "Handbook of Physiology" (Amer. Physiol. Soc., J. Field, ed.), Sect. 2, Vol. III, p. 2293. Williams & Wilkins, Baltimore, Maryland.

Majno, G., and Palade, G. E. (1961). *J. Biophys. Biochem. Bytol.* **11**, 571.

Majno, G., Palade, G. E., and Schoefl, G. I. (1961). *J. Biophys. Biochem. Cytol.* **11**, 607.

Majno, G., Shea, S. M., and Leventhal, M. (1969). *J. Cell Biol.* **42**, 647.

Marchesi, V. T. (1961). *Quart. J. Exp. Physiol. Cog. Mêd. Sci.* **46**, 115.

Marchesi, V. T. (1962). *Proc. Roy. Soc., Sar. B* **156**, 550.

Marchesi, V. T., and Barrnett, R. J. (1963). *J. Cell Biol.* **17**, 547.

Marchesi, V. T., and Florey, H. W. (1960). *Quart. J. Exp. Physiol. Cog. Med. Sci.* **45**, 343.

Mayerson, H. S. (1959). *In* "The Microcirculation" (S. M. R. Reynolds and B. W. Zweifach, eds.), p. 129. Univ. of Illinois Press, Urbana.

Mellander, S. (1968). *Proc. Roy. Soc. Med.* **61**, 55.

Mellander, S., and Johansson, B. (1968). *Pharmacol. Rev.* **20**, 117.

Melmon, K. L., and Cline, M. J. (1967). *Nature (London)* **213**, 90.

Mende, I. J., and Chambers, E. L. (1958). *J. Biophys. Biochem. Cyol.* **4**, 319.

Menkin, V. (1936). *J. Exp. Med.* **64**, 485.

Menkin, V. (1956). *Science* **123**, 527.

Metchnikoff, E. (1905). "Immunity in Infective Diseases" (transl. by F. G. Binnie). Cambridge Univ. Press, London and New York.

Michel, C. C. (1970). *In* "Capillary Permeability" (N. A. Lassen and C. Crone, eds.), Chap. 10, p. 628. Academic Press, New York.

Miles, A. A. (1956). *Ann. N. Y. Acad. Med.* **66**, 356.

Miles, A. A., and Miles, E. M. (1958). *J. Pathol. Bacteriol.* **76**, 21.

Moore, D. H., and Ruska, H. (1957). *J. Biophys. Biochem. Cytol.* **3**, 457.

Moore, R. H., and Movat, H. Z. (1959). *AMA Arch. Pathol.* **67**, 679.

Movat, H. Z., and Fernando, M. P. (1963a). *Exp. Mol. Pathol.* **2**, 549.

Movat, H. Z., and Fernando, N. V. P. (1963b). *Amer. J. Pathol.* **42**, 41.

Movat, H. Z., and Fernando, N. V. P. (1963c). *Lab. Invest.* **12**, 895.

Movat, H. Z., Moore, R. H., and Wolochow, D. (1960). *Brit. J. Exp. Pathol.* **41**, 97.

Movat, H. Z., Fernando, N. V. P., Uriuhara, T., and Weiser, W. J. (1963). *J. Exp. Med.* **118**, 557.

Nelemans, F. (1948). *Amer. J. Anat.* **83**, 43.

Neufeld, G. R., and Marshall, B. E. (1970). *Proc. Eng. Med. Biol.* **121**, 36.

Niessing, K., and Rollhäuser, H. (1954). *Z. Zellforsch. Mikrosk. Anat.* **39**, 431.

Opie, E. L. (1956). *J. Exp. Med.* **104**, 897.

Ovary, Z. (1958). *Progr. Allergy* **5**, 459.

Page, A. R., and Good, R. A. (1958). *Amer. J. Pathol.* **34**, 645.

Palade, G. E. (1953). *J. Appl. Phys.* **24**, 1424.

Palay, S. L., and Karlin, L. J. (1959). *J. Biophys. Biochem. Cytol.* **5**, 363.

Pappenheimer, J. R. (1953). *Physiol. Rev.* **33**, 387.

Pease, D. C. (1966). *J. Ultrastruct. Res.* **15**, 555.

Peterson, R. D. A., and Good, R. A. (1962). *Lab. Invest.* **2**, 507.

Renkin, E. M. (1959). *In* "The Microcirculation" (S. R. M. Reynolds and B. W. Zweifach, eds.), p. 28. Univ. of Illinois Press, Urbana.

Renkin, E. M. (1964). *Physiologist* **7**, 13.

Renkin, E. M. and Pappenheimer, J. R. (1957). *Ergeb. Physiol., Biol. Chem. Exp. Pharmakol.* **49**, 59.

Rhodin, J. A. G. (1962). *J. Ultrastruct. Res.* **6**, 171.

Ricker, G. (1924). "Pathologie als Naturwissenschaft." Springer-Verlag, Berlin and New York.

Rigdon, R. H. (1939). *Proc. Soc. Exp. Biol. Med.* **42**, 43.

Rigdon, R. H. (1941). *J. Lab. Clin. Med.* **27**, 1554.

Robb, H. J. (1963). *Ann. Surg.* **158**, 685.

Robinson, J. R. (1960). *Physiol. Rev.* **40**, 112.

Sanders, A. G., Ebert, R. H., and Florey, H. W. (1940). *Quart. J. Exp. Physiol. Cog. Med. Sci.* **30**, 281.

Schachter, M. (1969). *Physiol. Rev.* **49**, 509.

Schade, H. (1935). "Die Molekularpathologie der Entzundung." Steinkopff, Darmstadt.

Sevitt, S. (1958). *J. Pathol. Bacteriol.* **75**, 27.

Shea, S. M., Karnovsky, M. J., and Bossert, W. H. (1969). *J. Theor. Biol.* **24**, 30.

Shimizu, H. (1959). *J. Nagoya City Univ. Med. Ass.* **80**, 807.

Shulman, N. R. (1958). *J. Exp. Med.* **107**, 711.

Skalak, R., Brånemark, P-I., and Ekholm, R. (1970). *Angiology* **21**, 224.

Slack, H. G. B. (1959). *Amer. J. Med.* **26**, 113.

Smirk, F. H. (1936). *Clin. Sci.* **2**, 317.

Spaet, T. H. (1952). *Blood* **7**, 641.

Spector, W. G. (1958). *Pharmacol. Rev.* **10**, 475.

Spector, W. G. (1969). *Int. Rev. Exp. Pathol.* **8**, 1.

Spector, W. G., and Willoughby, D. A. (1960). *J. Pathol. Bacteriol.* **80**, 271.

Spector, W. G., and Willoughby, D. A. (1963). *Bacteriol. Rev.* **27**, 117.

Starling, E. H. (1896). *J. Physiol. (London)* **29**, 312.

Stehbens, W. E. (1967). *Quart. J. Exp. Physiol. Cog. Med. Sci.* **52**, 150.

Stehbens, W. E., and Florey, H. W. (1960). *Quart. J. Exp. Physiol.* **45**, 252.

Stetson, C. A., Jr., and Good, R. A. (1951). *J. Exp. Med.* **93**, 49.

Stoner, H. B., and Threlfall, C. J. (1960). *In* "The Biochemical Response to Injury" (H. B. Stoner and C. J. Threlfall, eds.), p. 105. Thomas, Springfield, Illinois.

Strock, P. E., and Majno, G. (1969). *Surg., Gynecol. Obstet.* **129**, 1213.

Tannenberg, J. (1925). *Frankfurt. Z. Pathol.* **31**, 173.

Thomas, L. (1954). *Annu. Rev. Physiol.* **16**, 467.

Thomas, L. (1956). *J. Exp. Med.* **104**, 865.

Tomlin, S. G. (1969). *Biochim. Biophys. Acta* **183**, 559.

Virchow, R. (1897). *Arch. Pathol. Anat. Physiol. Klin. Med.* **149**, 381.

Vollrath, L. (1968). *Deut. Med. Wochenschr.* **93**, 360.

Wasserman, K., and Mayerson, H. S. (1951). *Amer. J. Physiol.* **165**, 15.

Wasserman, K., Loeb, L., and Mayerson, H. S. (1955). *Circ. Res.* **3**, 594.

Weber, H. W. (1955). *Klin. Wochenschr.* **33**, 387.

Wagelius, O., and Asboe-Hansen, G. (1956). *Exp. Cell Res.* **11**, 437.

Wells, F. R., and Miles, A. A. (1963). *Nature (London)* **200**, 1015.

Wiederhielm, C. A. (1972). *In* "Biomechanics: Its Foundations and Objectives" (Y. C. Fung, N. Perrone, and M. Anliker, eds.), p. 273. Prentice-Hall, Englewood Cliffs, New Jersey.

Wilbrandt, W., Lüscher, E., and Aspier, H. (1956). *Helv. Physiol. Pharmacol. Acta* **14**, C81.

Wilhelm, D. L. (1962). *Pharmacol. Rev.* **14**, 257.

Wilhelm, D. L. (1970). *Rev. Can. Biol.* **30**, 153.

Wissig, S. L. (1958a). *Anat. Rec.* **130**, 467.

Wissig, S. L. (1958b). *J. Biophys. Biochem. Cytol.* **7**, 419.

Witte, S. (1957a). *Z. Gesamte Exp. Med.* **129**, 181.

Witte, S. (1957b). *Z. Gesamte Exp. Med.* **129**, 358.

Witte, S. (1957c). *Folia Haematol. (Frankfurt am Main)* [N.S.] **1**, 320.

Woods, M. C., Gamble, F. N., Furth, J., and Bigelow, R. R. (1953). *Blood* **8**, 545.

Zarem, H., and Zweifach, B. W. (1965). *Proc. Soc. Exp. Biol. Med.* **119**, 248.

Zeya, H. I., and Spitznagel, J. K. (1963). *Science* **142**, 1085.

Zimmermann, K. (1923). *Z. Anat, Entwicklungsgesch.* **68**, 29.

Zucker, M. B. (1947). *Amer. J. Physiol.* **148**, 275.

Zucker, M. B., and Borrelli, J. (1955). *J. Appl. Physiol.* **7**, 432.

Zweifach, B. W. (1953). *Rev. Can. Biol.* **12**, 179.

Zweifach, B. W. (1955). *Conf. Connect. Tissues, Trans. 1954* Vol. 5, p. 37.

Zweifach, B. W. (1957). *Amer. J. Med.* **23**, 684.

Zweifach, B. W. (1961a). "Functional Behavior of the Microcirculation." Thomas, Springfield, Illinois.

Zweifach, B. W. (1961b). *Angiology* **12**, 507.

Zweifach, B. W. (1962). *Angiology* **13**, 345.

Zweifach, B. W. (1963). *Fed. Proc., Fed. Amer. Soc. Exp. Biol.* **22**, 1351.

Zweifach, B. W. (1964). *Ann. N.Y. Acad. Sci.* **116**, 831.

Zweifach, B. W. (1966). *Fed. Proc., Fed. Amer. Soc. Exp. Biol.* **25**, 1784.

Zweifach, B. W. (1968). *Fed. Proc., Fed. Amer. Soc. Exp. Biol.* **27**, 1399.

Zweifach, B. W. (1969). *In* "Dynamics of Thrombus Formation and Dissolution" (S. A. Johnson and M. M. Guest, eds.), p. 45. Lippincott, Philadelphia, Pennsylvania.

Zweifach, B. W. (1971). *Circ. Res.* **28**, Suppl. II, 129.

Zweifach, B. W., and Chambers, R. (1950). *Ann. N.Y. Acad. Sci.* **52**, 1047.

Zweifach, B. W., and Intaglietta, M. (1968). *Microvasc. Res.* **1**, 83.

Zweifach, B. W., and Nagler, A. N. (1961). *In* "Hahnemann Symposium on Inflammation and Diseases of Connective Tissues" (L. C. Mills and J. H. Moyer, eds.), p. 84. Saunders, Philadelphia, Pennsylvania.

Chapter 2

CAPILLARY PERMEABILITY

I. Structural Considerations

JOHN H. LUFT

I. Introduction

Capillaries exist to assist the exchange of certain material required by, or detrimental to, the cells of the organism. There is active convection of a central reservoir of fluid, namely blood, throughout the vertebrate tissues by way of the vascular system, but it is mainly in the smallest divisions of this system of conduits that the exchange of these materials takes place. These finest tubes measure about 20 μm or less in diameter, and include capillaries as well as venules (Majno and Palade, 1961). The exchange of substances across the walls of these vessels is conveniently treated in terms of the physiological concept of permeability.

The thinness of the capillary wall has hindered morphologists who tried to provide a substantial structural foundation on which to base physiological

47

experiments. The wall thickness is close to the limit of resolution of the light microscope, so that fixed, embedded, and stained sections convey disappointingly little information about capillary structure. On the other hand, the light microscope is a nondestructive analytical tool and can be used with living preparations. Unfortunately, most tissues, including capillaries, are quite transparent, but optical tricks such as oblique or dark-field illumination or phase contrast in the hands of a skilled biologist can demonstrate a remarkable sensitivity to tenuous detail. By a stroke of good fortune, it is possible to demonstrate junctions between endothelial cells of capillaries as dark lines by simply treating the vessel with silver nitrate solution. By 1950, various optical and staining procedures, the use of micromanipulation to disturb capillaries in a controlled manner, and the use of colloidal pigments as tracers to detect cellular boundaries, leak pathways, and sticky surfaces had provided a wealth of morphological knowledge about capillaries (Zimmermann, 1923; Krogh, 1930; Danielli and Stock, 1944; Chambers and Zweifach, 1947). Residual problems seemed to be related to capillary contractility, the nature of the endothelial cement between cells, and the location and structure of the pores predicted by physiological experiments. It was natural, therefore, that when the electron microscope became available attention should have been directed toward capillaries, but the past 15 years have shown this instrument to be more a key to Pandora's Box than a magic sword to slay dragons still lurking in dim vascular recesses. Despite numerous papers devoted to the ultrastructure of capillaries, the increasing complexity of the subject seems to have engendered a spirit of submission to the idea that one must take into account each of the several layers of the capillary wall, and "specify the type of capillary present in each organ before its physiology can be discussed with profit" (Farquhar, 1961; Fawcett, 1963). In the introduction to the recent conference on capillary permeability in Copenhagen, Crone listed as one of the points of general agreement, "... that there is a vast spectrum of ways in which capillary walls are constructed with the liver and intestinal capillaries at one end and the brain capillaries at the other ..." (Crone, 1970). The extensive review of capillary ultrastructure by Majno (1965) amply documents the great variety of capillaries. The complementary approach, using Occam's Razor, is to derive a capillary model which can rationalize the most variation with the fewest assumptions, and this is the intent of this chapter.

II. Permeability of Capillaries

A. Definition from Physiology

Before going further, it would be well to define the term "permeability" as used in the title, for it will recur throughout the chapter. Used in the biological sense, the concept of permeability is a physiological phenomenon and is a measure of the rate of penetration of a substance through some sort of barrier. As derived from Fick's law, which describes the movement of material in response to forces imposed upon it, the amount of substance is represented by ds, and it passes through a barrier in time dt. The amount of material passing in any given time is directly proportional to the area, A, of the barrier and to the pressure difference (hydrostatic or osmotic) between the two sides of the barrier, but inversely proportional to the thickness of the barrier and the viscosity of the fluid. This relationship is expressed by Eq. (1) (Davson and Danielli, 1952),

$$ds/dt = KA(P_i - P_o) \tag{1}$$

where P_i and P_o are the pressures inside and outside the barrier, and K is a constant of proportionality which contains the thickness of the barrier and the viscosity when these remain constant during the experiment. K is thus the permeability constant or the permeability. The model required for the concept of permeability requires at least two well-stirred compartments each separated by barriers. Equation (1) is a differential equation in time, so that K is a rate-of-change quantity in terms of so many grams or so many milliliters per second (per unit area and unit pressure). It is a proper concept for dynamic biology, namely physiology, but is excluded by definition from the complementary facet of biology, namely morphology. The title of this chapter then, in the strict sense, is a contradiction in terms. However, in the broad sense, there is a fundamental relationship wherein the same phenomenon can be described in more than one way, such as the wave–particle "duality" of light, and it is in this sense that the chapter will proceed. We will examine the structure of the compartments and particularly the barriers with the electron microscope in light of the permeability known from physiological measurements with full realization that the structural data alone cannot provide the quantitation required to verify or challenge the physiological measurements. It can, however, substantiate, contradict, or fail to find the structures assumed in the various quantitative theories proposed to explain the experimental measurements.

B. Summary of the Permeability Data in the Normal Vertebrate

At the turn of the century, Starling (1896, 1909) proposed that material passed across capillary walls according to recognized principles of diffusion and that all the components of plasma could pass unrestricted except for the plasma proteins. The simplification which resulted from ignoring any active function of the endothelial cells, as had been suggested by Heidenhain

(1891), permitted Starling to make his classic statement about conditions in the capillaries which regulate the movement of water. Thus, the force of internal capillary (hydrostatic) pressure, which tends to drive fluid outward, was pictured as opposing the osmotic pressure of the plasma proteins, which draws water inward from the extracellular fluid outside the capillary. When the two forces are equal, there would be no net transfer of fluid, and any imbalance would relieve itself by fluid movement toward new concentrations and a new equilibrium. The physiological measurements, however, were averages over extensive capillary beds, and conditions in a single capillary were uncertain.

Landis (1927) attacked the problem of capillary permeability directly by measuring the internal hydrostatic pressure inside individual capillaries as well as measuring fluid movement. In his review of capillary pressure and permeability (Landis, 1934), he concluded that the evidence permits a summary of the general nature of endothelium as follows:

1. Capillaries possess an enormous total area for interchange between blood and tissue spaces.

2. The endothelium reveals a permeability to fluid many times greater than that of certain cell membranes (which had been studied quantitatively up to that time).

3. The endothelium demonstrates the physical characteristics of an inert (in the sense of nonsecreting) membrane permeable to water and crystalloids, but relatively impermeable to plasma proteins.

Pappenheimer and his co-workers (1951) have reexamined the literature relating to fluid movement through capillaries. Their paper opens with the sentence, "The penetration of capillary walls by water and dissolved substances appears to take place solely by processes which require no energy transformation on the part of the capillary endothelial cells." They mention the Starling hypothesis and continue to the effect that the

> striking similarities between the permeability characteristics of living capillaries, on one hand, and artificial porous membranes on the other, have given rise to the 'Pore Theory' of capillary exchange. In its simplest form, the pore theory supposes that the capillary walls are pierced with numerous ultramicroscopic openings which are, in general, too small to allow the passage of plasma protein molecules, but are of sufficient size and number to account for the observed rate of passage of water and non-protein constituents of plasma.

In this classic paper they assembled an abundance of excellent physiological data on the conditions, molecular selectivity, and magnitude of capillary fluid exchange in the perfused hindlimb of cats—predominantly, therefore, in the capillaries of skeletal muscle. Their calculations from experiments on the permeability of these capillaries to small, lipid-insoluble molecules and from physical principles of fluid flow indicated that their measurements were those to be expected of a membrane perforated with either (1) uniform circular pores of radius 30 Å and length 0.3 μm (3000 Å) at a frequency of 2×10^9 pores/cm^2; or (2) uniform rectangular slits of half-width (corresponding to radius) 18.5 Å, 0.3 μm thickness, and slit length about ten times that of the length of the capillary itself. They felt that their data slightly favored pores over slits, but that is was not decisive for either.

Pappenheimer *et al.* (1951) also compared the filtration ratio in mammalian muscle with that in glomerular capillaries, and then compared both with a collodion membrane of thickness and pore diameter nearly equivalent in dimensions and molecular selectivity to these capillaries. For equal areas, the glomerular capillaries pass fluid 100 times more rapidly than the muscle capillaries, but the collodion membrane, with its large percentage of open pore area, allows fluid to pass 35 times faster than even the glomerular capillaries. Thus, they reached the following important conclusions:

> The discovery that only a minute fraction of the capillary wall is involved in the capillary exchange of water and lipoid-insoluble molecules provides a simple explanation for the fact that glomerular capillaries may be many times more permeable to water than peripheral capillaries without losing their impermeability to plasma protein.

The interpretation of Pappenheimer and his co-workers required some revision with respect to the penetration of the capillary bed in muscle by large molecules. Pappenheimer used an osmotic method that had a limiting sensitivity of about 5% of the effective pore area available for smaller molecules, and the results indicated that the capillaries were impermeable to hemoglobin or larger molecules within this uncertainty. Subsequently, more sensitive procedures, such as measuring the leakage of tracer molecules from the blood into the lymphatic fluid draining from the capillary bed under test, have shown that small amounts of large molecules also get through the capillary walls. Grotte (1956), using dextrans of various molecular weights as well as polymethylmethacrylate spheres about 800 Å in diameter, confirmed the Pappenheimer figures for molecules below 30,000 mw. For larger molecules, the data were felt to be consistent with the presence of infrequent but large leaks (radius greater than 120 Å, but less than 350 Å). Mayerson *et al.* (1960), using carefully calibrated dextran molecules up to 400,000 mw, also obtained evidence for the small pores as well as for the penetration of the largest dextran molecules which they suggested could be accounted for by either large pores (greater than 140-Å radius) or by vesicular transport.

This work was expanded in an extensive review by Landis and Pappenheimer (1963). By then, improvements in the treatment of the osmotic properties of nonideal (leaky) membranes required consideration of an "osmotic reflection coefficient," and, as a consequence, they revised upward their equivalent pore radius to 40–45 Å (Landis and Pappenheimer, 1963, pp. 1010–1011). Although values were not given for slits, the revised values for them would have been about 50–55 Å (Luft, 1966; Karnovsky, 1967). There is still some variability in the pore or slit sizes as calculated from physiological data, which formed an important theme in a recent conference on capillary permeability (Crone and Lassen, 1970). A current paper (Perl, 1971) develops these concepts further, and concludes that additional factors cancel out to predict equivalent pore or slit widths back to the dimensions originally calculated by Pappenheimer *et al.* (1951).

C. Altered Permeability in Pathological and Inflammatory States

This topic is covered thoroughly in the other chapters of these volumes. It is sufficient to remark that it has long been known that inflammation or tissue damage produces an increase in capillary permeability to both water and the plasma proteins. Starling (1909) stated that the lymphatic flow in an inactive limb of a normal animal is slight, is of low protein content, and is little effected by moderate changes in blood pressure. Massage or muscular activity increases the flow. However, if the limb of an anesthetized animal is scalded by several minutes exposure to water at 50°–60°C, the following occurs: (1) its lymph flow is increased; (2) its lymph is more concentrated in protein, showing that the permeability of the capillary wall has been increased; and (3) its response to any changes in capillary blood pressure is immediate, whether caused by arterial dilatation or venous obstruction. Similar effects occur upon readmitting blood to a limb deprived of blood for 1 hour. Renkin and Garlick (1970) recently employed controlled heating (45°C) in an attempt to localize the mechanism and to perhaps identify both the pores and the leaks in capillary permeability.

III. Capillary Structure

A. Summary of Capillary Structure by Light Microscopy

In 1852, Kölliker described capillaries in the following manner:

> Their structureless membrane is perfectly clear and transparent, sometimes delicate, and presenting a simple contour, sometimes thicker and bordered by a double line. In its microscopical reactions, it corresponds entirely with older cell membranes and the sarcolemma of the transversely striped muscles, and as regards its other properties, it is perfectly smooth on both aspects, and notwithstanding its tenuity, tolerably resistant

and elastic, although very probably not contractile. It invariably presents a certain
number of elongated cell nuclei which are disposed with wide interspaces, usually at
opposite sides of the vessel . . . .

Most of the details which had been recognized through light microscopy were
collected by Zimmermann (1923) and by Benninghoff (1930). From these
papers, it is apparent that cytologists were handicapped by a harsh reality.
Good as their microscopes were, they were not adequate for the task of
revealing the fine details of endothelial structure. Secondly, many of the
papers were concerned with the form and distribution of the pericytes, which
were thought to be capable of movement. This preoccupation with capillary
contractility persisted as late as Krogh and Vimtrup's article (1932) in
Cowdry's "Special Cytology."

The review by Chambers and Zweifach (1947) added new information
obtained by intravascular injection of aqueous suspensions of carbon black,
by alterations in the capillary ionic environment and pH, and by micro-
trauma (Chambers and Zweifach, 1940), particularly as it related to the
endothelial cement which they identified at endothelial cell junctions. In
their 1947 paper they suggested that

> There is good evidence for the existence of 3 structural components of the capillary
> wall, variations of each of which may alter conditions affecting the passage of materials
> through the wall. These are: the endothelium *per se*; consisting of pavement-like cells,
> and an intercellular cement; an endocapillary lining which is non-cellular and is pos-
> sibly derived from the circulating blood proteins; and third, a pericapillary sheath which
> serves as an outer supporting layer with characteristics common to the surrounding con-
> nective tissue matrix.

They regarded the movement of water and crystalloids as occurring *between*
endothelial cells at the intercellular junctions and as being filtered by the
intercellular cement and possibly by components of the endocapillary layer
together with the pericapillary sheath. The endothelial cells themselves were
considered necessary for secretion, repair, and regeneration of the various
filtration layers.

Along with the capillaries, it has long been realized that venules are
particularly sensitive to insults and that these respond first by an increased
permeability to fluid, protein, and even pigment. Since the positive identification of venules as distinct from capillaries is not always possible, they have
frequently been included in the operational definition of capillaries, either
implicitly or explicitly (Bennett *et al.*, 1959). Recently, however, Majno *et al.*
(1961), in a superb light microscope study, have emphasized the selectivity
which venules of 20- to 30-μm diameter display toward histamine or serotonin. The excellent review by Majno (1965) should be consulted for further
details and references.

To conclude this section, four figures are introduced to show the advance made possible by the electron microscope. Figure 1* illustrates a capillary from mouse diaphragm, fixed for electron microscopy, but cut $\frac{1}{2}$ μm thick and stained for light microscopy. The details are blurred and vague, and they illustrate the optical limitation which existed before 1950. Phase contrast microscopy adds little; Fig. 2 is the same section examined before staining under phase illumination. Even a poor electron microscope provides more detail than the best light microscope; Fig. 3 is an electron micrograph of a section serial to that illustrated in Figs. 1 and 2, but defocused to provide similar resolution. There are differences, but the density distribution roughly corresponds to that obtained by light microscopy. Figure 4 is the same section as Fig. 3, but printed in focus; there is considerable improvement.

B. The Compartments and Their Limits

As mentioned previously, the notion of permeability requires at least two compartments separated by one barrier. It is obvious that the barrier itself forms one boundary for the compartments, so that awkwardness develops in discussing one without the other. Worse still, as will become apparent later, there is some uncertainty as to which lamina of the several concentric layers constituting the capillary wall is *the* membrane in the sense of defining its permeability properties. Electron micrographs of capillaries show that there is a succession of compartments and barriers. For simplicity, only the capillary lumen and the tissue extracellular space will be considered here.

Figs. 1–4. Capillary from mouse diaphragm. ($\times$ 5000.)

Fig. 1. Epon section ($\frac{1}{2}$ μm) with resin removed (Mayor *et al.*, 1961) and stained with toluidine blue, 1.32 NA apochromat.

Fig. 2. Same section, plastic removed but unstained, in water, 1.15 NA phase contrast apochromat. Phase contrast accentuates fine detail showing collagen bundles (C), the endothelial wall, and the muscle mitochondria better than the stained section, although the "halo" from the adjacent muscle tissue interferes.

Fig. 3. This figure has been defocused in printing to match the resolution in the light micrographs; thus, the resolution is aberration-limited, rather than diffraction-limited as in Figs. 1 and 2, but the resemblance is close.

Fig. 4. An electron micrograph, in focus, of an 800-Å thick section lightly stained with lead. The capillary is closely confined by the cross-sectioned muscle cells. The large space (Ex) is edematous extracellular space.

*The tissue shown in all figures (except Fig. 15) was taken from frog or mouse, fixed in buffered glutaraldehyde and/or OsO_4, and embedded in Epon epoxy resin (Luft, 1961). Light microscopy employed Leitz equipment and the electron microscopy was done with a Siemens Elmiskop I at 40 or 60 kV.

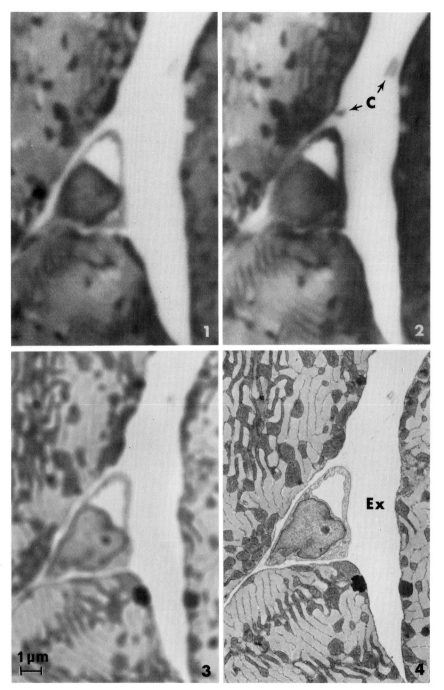

Figs. 1–4

55

1. The Capillary Lumen

The capillary lumen is a simple compartment normally filled with plasma in which are suspended various cells and cell fragments. It is limited by the cell membrane (and derivatives) of the endothelial cells, and, to a reasonable degree and under certain conditions (Pappenheimer, 1953), it represents a sample of the circulating blood. In electron micrographs, the appearance of the capillary lumen depends on the method of tissue fixation. Before 1963, when Sabatini *et al.* introduced glutaraldehyde, osmium tetroxide was the fixative of choice. However, it preserved blood plasma in the capillary lumen weakly and erratically. Glutaraldehyde fixation retains plasma more uniformly (Bruns and Palade, 1968a). Of course, not even glutaraldehyde will preserve luminal contents when the tissue has been fixed by vascular perfusion. In Fig. 5, the lumen (L) contains no precipitate whatever. In Figs. 6–8, the capillary lumens show variable amounts of flocculent material—probably precipitated plasma protein. All of these capillaries were fixed with OsO_4 only, without perfusion. Although fixation has transformed the plasma into a gel where it has been retained, the plasma proteins in life were in solution. Erythrocytes are frequently encountered and, less often, leukocytes and platelets. These cellular elements are completely discontinuous with respect to the capillary lumen, and can have no direct relationship to permeability, although their presence may have secondary or indirect effects. For example, it is necessary that the compartments be well stirred, particularly near the barriers. Prothero and Burton (1961) have discussed the contribution of erythrocytes in promoting mixing in capillaries. Lassen (1970) contributed a vigorous discussion of the necessity for stirring in glomerular capillaries.

2. The Extracellular Space

Unlike the capillary lumen, the extracellular tissue spaces have some structure, i.e., they normally are not fluid, but rather are viscoelastic. There is biochemical or histochemical evidence that this space contains various

Fig. 5. Same as Fig. 4 (mouse diaphragm). The nucleus of the single endothelial cell bulges into the partly collapsed but empty lumen (L), and a process of a pericyte (P) is incorporated into the basement membrane (BM) completely surrounding the capillary. The vesicles (V) in the endothelial cytoplasm range from 300 to 1000 Å in diameter. There are several small mitochondria (arrows). A bundle of collagen fibers (C) and a few fine filaments (F) are seen in the edematous extracellular space (Ex). In several places, the thick-and-thin array of filaments is visible in the muscle. Eight-hundred Å thick section, lightly stained with lead; this procedure gives good representation of cell structure, but fine details are obscured by section thickness. (Compare with Fig. 8.) ($\times 20,000$.)

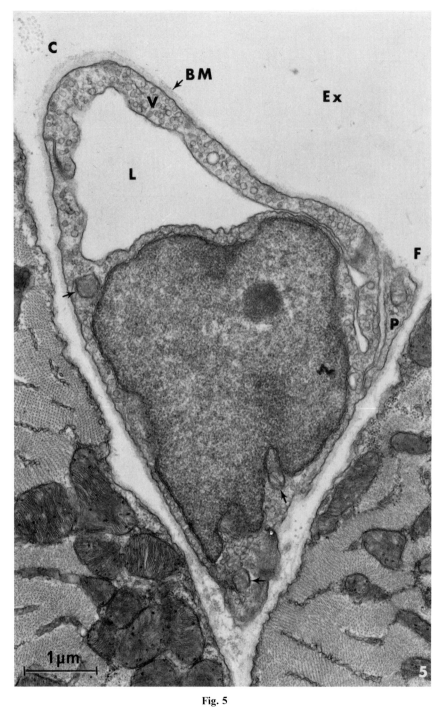

Fig. 5

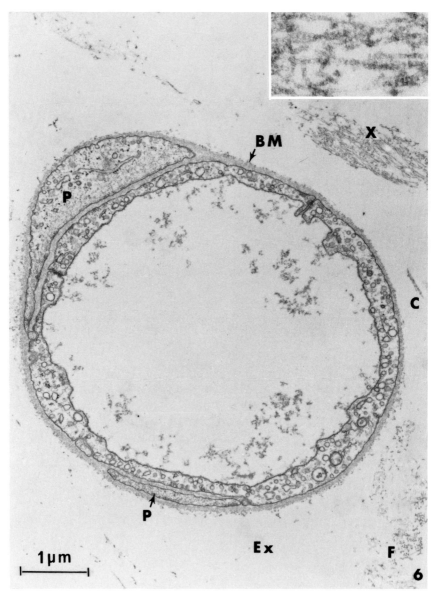

Fig. 6

mucopolysaccharides, such as hyaluronic acid and various chondroitin sulfates (Zugibe, 1963; Gaines, 1960; Mathews, 1967), plus traces of plasma protein and ultrafiltrate. Under the electron microscope, however, only collagen (and occasional elastic) fibers can be seen, together with smaller filaments of uncertain origin. In Figs. 5–7, these are labeled C (for collagen) and F (for filaments). Figure 6 shows a group of rather different filaments (at X) which are further enlarged in the inset. They have a period of approximately 150 Å and may be fibrin which was induced to clot when the tissue was cut away from the animal. The collagen is easily identified by its cross-striation which shows a repeat periodicity of 650–700 Å. This striation is easily seen in Fig. 7, but the presence of many sub-bands within the period tends to obscure the fundamental pattern. All the collagen fibers visible in these four micrographs have a diameter smaller than the period, measuring about 300–400 Å in diameter, and have the distribution associated with reticular fibers when compared with a section prepared with an appropriate silver stain and examined under the light microscope (Fawcett, 1959). They are continuous in one dimension only at dimensions appropriate to molecules, but, in the aggregate, they probably represent barriers to cell- or bacteria-sized particles. They are undoubtedly the prime structural element of the tissues.

Often associated with or interspersed between collagen fibers and visible individually are fine filaments (F in Figs. 5–7). It is difficult to estimate the diameter of such filaments when lightly stained, but intense staining provides sufficient contrast for them to be measured. Many of the filaments are about 100 Å in diameter, but some are as small as 40 Å (Myers *et al.*, 1969). Figure 9 shows such a preparation with a portion of capillary endothelium surrounded by its basement membrane, fibrils, and filaments in the extracellular space. These filaments have been described at intervals over the years without acquiring a permanent name. In 1962, Low clearly described both thick and thin varieties in human heart and lung and termed them "microfibrils." They were described in association with elastic fibers (Greenlee *et al.*, 1966) as "fine fibrils." Bruns and Palade (1968a) clearly describe their distribution in capillaries also as "fine fibrils." Frequently, they seem to be associated

Fig. 6. Capillary composed of two endothelial cells partially enfolded by cytoplasmic processes of two pericytes (P), and with a complete basement membrane (BM). The endothelial cells abut at two junctions, one of which is shown at higher magnification in Fig. 21. The lumen contains a granular material, probably plasma. The edematous extracellular space (Ex) contains collagen (C) in various planes of section, fine filaments (F), and a different type of filament (at X) which shows a periodicity of about 150 Å (inset) and may be fibrin. Mouse diaphragm, stained with uranyl acetate and lead. (× 19,000; inset, × 100,000.)

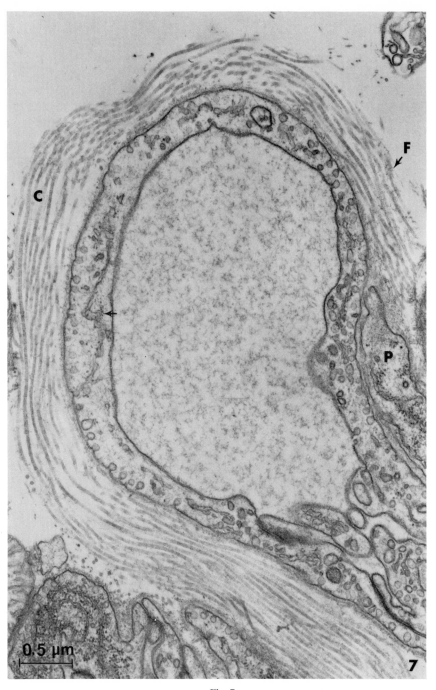

0.5 μm

7

Fig. 7

with the basal lamina or basement membrane. As is the case with collagen fibers, these filaments or microfibrils are rather dispersed and probably do not constitute a significant permeability barrier even to macromolecules, although together with the mucopolysaccharides they contribute to the viscoelasticity of the extracellular space (Laurent, 1970).

An important consideration is the size of the extracellular space. The electron micrograph at low magnification (see Fig. 4) shows the capillary wedged rather tightly between two muscle cells, but displays a larger extracellular space (Ex) on the third side. This space is an artifact: it is edema which developed during the isolation of the strip of diaphragm while it was immersed in mammalian Locke's solution. There are certain advantages to such edematous preparations, but it is important to be aware that had the tissue been fixed as quickly as possible the large space would have been absent, and the capillary would have been confined on three sides at least as tightly as it is between the two lower muscle cells (see Fig. 5).

C. The Barriers and Their Limits by Electron Microscopy

As seen in the previous section, little light is shed on the problem of capillary permeability by an examination of the spaces involved; the most important conclusion is that they exist. The barriers present a different situation; here, there is more complexity and more room for new concepts and considerations.

1. THE ENDOTHELIUM

Vascular endothelium is the cellular component directly facing the blood. This configuration is easy to recognize under the electron microscope and forms the basis of the operational definition of endothelium used by Bennett *et al.* (1959) and which will be used here, namely, the cells lining any blood of lymphatic channel, including sinusoids.

a. THE CYTOPLASM. There are no unique characteristics of the cytoplasm of the endothelial cell, and it is distinguished only by the abundance of "pinocytotic" vesicles and by the usually small mitochondria. The cell con-

Fig. 7. Portion of capillary with evenly dispersed luminal contents. The endothelial cytoplasm shows several strands of endoplasmic reticulum with attached ribosomes (arrow). The capillary is sheathed with a heavy layer of collagen fibers (650-Å period, 300- to 400-Å diameter), but with a very thin basement membrane. Mouse myocardium stained with uranyl acetate and lead. P, Pericyte; C, collagen; F, fine filaments. (× 30,000.)

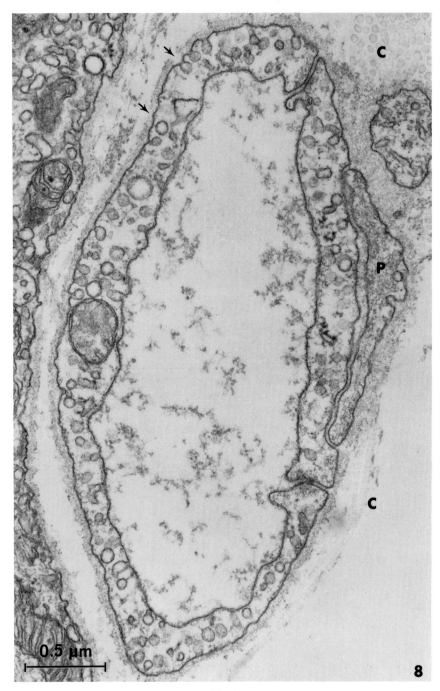

0.5 µm

8

Fig. 8

tains a single, rather flattened nucleus, bulging, but still surrounded by a thin layer of cytoplasm which is limited by a cell membrane. The cell scaled up 10,000 times is reminiscent of an egg about to be fried, the yolk being the nucleus and the surrounding white representing the cytoplasm. The fillet of cytoplasm near the nucleus contains most of the cell's complement of mitochondria, the Golgi apparatus, some cisternae of endoplasmic reticulum (ER) both smooth and studded with ribosomes, free ribosomes, a pair of centrioles, and an occasional multivesicular body. The thin portion of the endothelial cytoplasm contains occasional mitochondria, frequent free ribosomes, sparse elements of the ER both smooth and rough, and occasional intracellular filaments. Microtubules have attracted attention as a recently identified cytoplasmic organelle in a variety of cells (Fawcett, 1966). They are found also in capillary endothelium (Bruns and Palade, 1968a). The marginal extensions of the endothelial cytoplasm approach to within 100–200 Å of the adjacent endothelial cells to which they are joined by structures to be described in the next section (Section III,C,1,b,v). The marginal cytoplasm frequently forms a thin leaf of flap which sometimes overlaps the adjacent cell and, at other times, seems to be involved in an activity suggestive of pinocytosis or phagocytosis (Fawcett, 1963; Majno, 1965, p. 2303). Filaments commonly occur in the marginal cytoplasm in a pattern compatible with the function of reinforcing the intercellular junctions (Fawcett, 1963) (see Figs. 21 and 22). Filaments also suggest the possibility of contractility or at least slow changes of shape (Wessels *et al.*, 1971). Endothelial cells of venules seem to be able to separate from one other and round up when stimulated by histaminelike substances (Majno *et al.*, 1969). Many of these cytoplasmic components are illustrated in Figs. 5–8.

b. THE CELL MEMBRANE AND ITS MODIFICATIONS. These include (1) the cell membrane (or plasma membrane) and its fenestrations and diaphragms, (2) the pinocytotic vesicles (pits, invaginations, or caveolae intracellulares), and (3) the attachments such as the tight junction or zonula occludens and desmosomes.

i. The cell membrane. The structure of the cell membrane is one of the fundamental riddles of biology, and it is not the purpose of this chapter to

Fig. 8. Very thin section (about 300 Å) of capillary showing two endothelial cells and two junctions, the upper one being shown in more detail in Fig. 22. Many vesicles are seen in the cytoplasm and attached to both blood and tissue surfaces of the endothelial cell membrane. The basement membrane is defective in several regions (arrows). Collagen is seen at C. Unit membrane is visible (in the original) in all membrane components of the muscle and endothelial cytoplasm. Mouse diaphragm stained with uranyl acetate and lead. P, Pericyte. ($\times$46,000.)

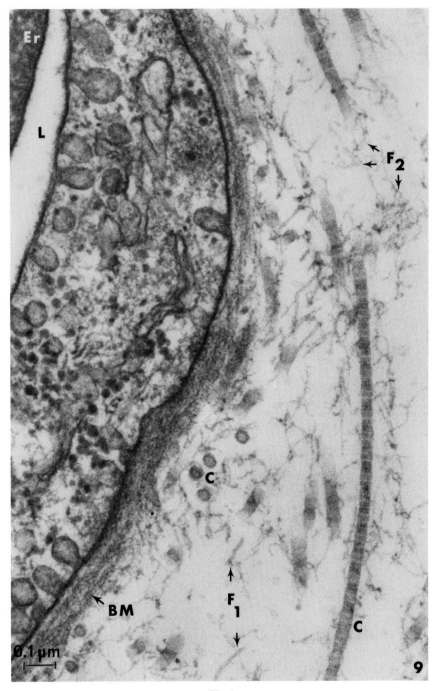

Fig. 9

review this field of reserach, however important it may be to understanding cell permeability. Stoeckenius and Engelman (1969) have reviewed the various models postulated for biological membranes. There are several features of cell membranes, however, which are worth further consideration.

First, the permeability to water of a number of unicellular organisms is normally very low—several orders of magnitude lower than capillaries (Davson and Danielli, 1952). In these cases, the cell membrane appears to be the primary, if not the only, barrier involved. It seems, therefore, that the cell's problem is not so much that of reducing an uncomfortably high permeability to water, but rather of producing a controlled porosity in an otherwise relatively waterproof layer. This normally low permeability is consistent with the behavior of thin films or monolayers of lipid toward penetration by water (Höber, 1945; Davson and Danielli, 1952; Davson, 1962; Mueller and Rudin, 1963; Ti Tien and Diana, 1968; Träuble, 1971). Although water is a "lipid-insoluble molecule," it is so small and the endothelial cell surface is so large in capillaries that a moderate amount of the total water exchange across capillary walls may occur through the cells themselves (across both cell membranes and the cytoplasm of the endothelial cells) and not only at junctions or through pores. The cell membrane is so impermeable to larger lipid-insoluble molecules that.their nonspecific diffusion through the endothelial cell membranes must be virtually nil (Landis and Pappenheimer, 1963; Pappenheimer et al., 1970).

Second, nearly all electron micrographs of cell membranes with adequate resolution show two dark lines separated by a lighter space. This pattern in cell membranes recurs so commonly that Robertson gave it the name "unit membrane" (Robertson, 1960). He found that each of the three layers is about 25 Å thick, giving an overall thickness of about 75 Å. Many of his preparations were fixed by potassium permanganate which shows the two dark layers approximately equal in density or thickness. Recent papers have suggested that the dimensions of the unit may be different in different structures or regions of the same cell (Yamamoto, 1963) and that the two dark layers may not be equivalent after different technical procedures (Sjöstrand, 1962,

Fig. 9. Edge of capillary heavily overstained to emphasize the fibers and filaments of the extracellular space and the basement membrane. The membranes of the cytoplasm are thickened and obscured, but large glycogen granules and a few filaments can be seen therein. An erythrocyte (Er) is seen in the lumen (L). The basement membrane (BM) is distinctly seen as a feltwork of circumferentially oriented filaments of about the same size as the fine branching filaments (F_2) having a diameter of about 50 Å. There is no abrupt edge of the basement membrane, but the filaments become progressively more dispersed. A second, thicker type of filament (F_1) is occasionally seen. The collagen period is 620 Å. Frog sartorius with prolonged uranyl acetate and lead staining. ($\times$ 89,000.)

1963; Farquhar and Palade, 1963). There is evidence that the light central region represents the lipid leaflet and that the two dark lines are polar regions associated with protein or similar hydrated polymeric material such as polysaccharide (Stoeckenius, 1962; Finean, 1962; Stoeckenius and Engelman, 1969).

It is clear that the unit membrane structure appears in electron micrographs of the cell membrane of capillary endothelial cells as well as in other cells. Figure 10 is an electron micrograph of microvilli from mouse intestinal epithelium prepared by conventional EM methods; it was chosen because it is a site where the unit membrane is easily demonstrated. Figure 11 is an electron micrograph of mouse capillary endothelium at the same magnification and prepared in the same way as that in Fig. 10. It is clearly evident that the unit membrane in Fig. 11 is seen only with difficulty, primarily because the density of the outer leaflet of the unit is low and appears to be interrupted at intervals. Palade and Bruns (1968) have developed tissue processing methods that preserve and enhance the outer leaflet so that both leaflets stain strongly, and, in their micrographs, the capillary unit membrane can be seen to be structurally equivalent to that recognized in other cells.

Both Figs. 10 and 11 have another significant feature in common. In Fig. 10 there is an irregular thickening external to the outer leaflet (EL) which is

Fig. 10. Microvillus from mouse intestinal epithelial cell, intestinal lumen at L. The unit membrane is easily seen, the internal layer (IL) being intensely stained, the middle component pale (presumably lipid), and the external layer (EL) less intensely stained and appearing thinner with an attached fuzz layer. A layer of mucus (M) floats over the tips of the microvilli and contacts the fuzz layer. The unit spacing (center-to-center distance of the IL and EL) is about 60 Å. Uranyl acetate and lead staining. (× 160,000.)

Fig. 11. Portion of capillary containing an erythrocyte (Er). The unit membrane is seen in the cell membranes of the erythrocyte, in the endothelial cell (both on the luminal and tissue surfaces), and in the vesicles. The endocapillary layer (ECL) is seen as an irregular, coarsely granular material attached to, or part of, the external layer of the unit. The center-to-center spacing of the unit composing the endothelial cell and the vesicles is about 60 Å, whereas that of the erythrocyte is about 50 Å. Mouse diaphragm stained with uranyl acetate and lead. (× 160,000.)

Fig. 12. Cross section of a capillary from striated muscle tissue exposed to ruthenium red in both glutaraldehyde and osmium fixation stages. The capillary lumen (L) contains two platelets (Pl). The bound ruthenium red produces density which surrounds the capillary and which marks the surface of the muscle cells (M) where the sarcolemma should be. Individual collagen fibrils (C) are also surrounded by material staining intensely with ruthenium red which appears to hold them in a bundle. Ruthenium red normally is confined to the extracellular space (Ex) since it does not penetrate cell membranes significantly and is excluded from the capillary lumen by the endothelial cells. However, it slowly enters the narrow extracellular slit between endothelial cells as indicated at J, and also labels the vesicles (V) or pits which open onto the tissue surface of the endothelium. Mouse diaphragm tissue stained with ruthenium red; section lightly stained with lead. (× 21,500.)

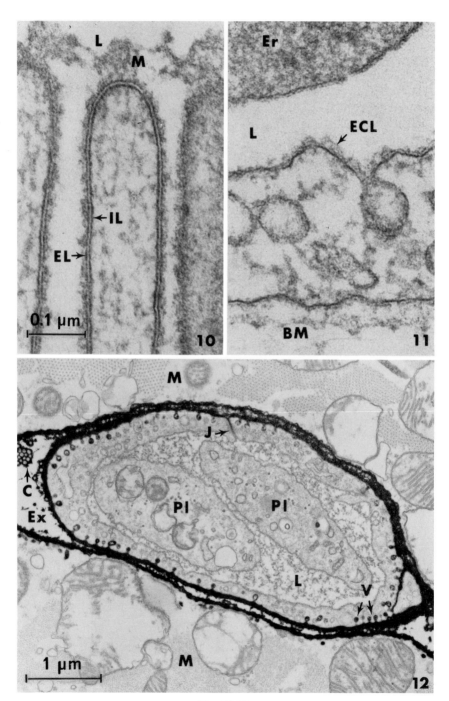

Figs. 10–12

now known, through the work of Ito (1965), as the "fuzz" layer. This layer is present at the free surface of many epithelial cells, but especially those of the gastrointestinal tract. The fuzz layer is luxurious in the intestinal epithelial cells of the bat and cat, and rather thin in the mouse and other animals. Ito's work (1965) strongly suggests that it contains acid mucopolysaccharide and that it tenaciously adheres to and may be an integral part of the plasma membrane of these cells. The fuzz layer of intestinal epithelial cells seems to be similar in several ways to the "extraneous coat" in amebas (Brandt, 1962). In Fig. 11, an irregular thickening (ECL) is also seen external to the fragmentary outer leaflet of the unit membrane of the endothelial cell. There is some resemblance to the fuzz layer in Fig. 10, but not sufficient to establish the equivalence of one to the other. The erythrocyte (Er) in the lumen in Fig. 11 also shows a unit membrane, but there is nothing to suggest a fuzz layer or coat on its surface despite its proximity to the endothelial cell. The coat in Fig. 11 labeled ECL probably represents the endocapillary layer.

ii. The endocapillary layer. The existence of a layer covering the luminal surface of capillary endothelial cells and in direct contact with the blood was deduced by Chambers and Zweifach (1940, 1947) while observing living capillary beds with the circulating blood containing suspended carbon black. The adherence of the carbon pigment to the capillary luminal surface and its release under various conditions were interpreted to indicate a coating on the endothelial cells which they termed the "endocapillary layer" and which seemed to resemble the intercellular cement thought to occur at junctions of endothelial cells. Although electron microscopists have searched for such material in their micrographs, it has not been recognized (Fawcett, 1959, 1963) except for a vague density in an intestinal capillary reported by Bennett *et al.* (1959) and a rather substantial periodic acid-Schiff (PAS) positive layer similar to basement membrane lining the interior of blood vessels of the earthworm (Hama, 1960). The existence of an intercellular cement in capillaries, at least in the sense of the earlier workers, has been explicitly denied (Florey *et al.*, 1959; Stehbens and Florey, 1960; Stehbens, 1963).

In 1964, I found that the dye ruthenium red (RR) could be adapted to electron microscope preparation methods to strongly stain the extraneous coats of cells including the fuzz layers (Luft, 1964b). In 1965, the method had given indications of a recognizable layer in capillaries where the endocapillary layer should have been. The first electron micrographs of such a layer were included in the first edition of this treatise (Luft, 1965a, Figs. 14–17), at which time its occurrence seemed to be infrequent and not characteristic of all capillaries. Later that year (Luft, 1965b), the layer was found in all capillaries into which the dye could penetrate, and the next year, a detailed paper was published (Luft, 1966). The binding of ruthenium red has been examined in a wide variety of tissues (Luft, 1971b), and it is clear that many animal cells possess a cell coat which stains strongly with ruthenium red; so the endo-capillary layer is not unique. As far as can be recognized under the electron microscope, the differences in cell coat among various cells seem to be quantitative rather than qualitative. The extraneous coat surrounding the ameba also stains strongly with ruthenium red and has been examined in detail (Szubinska and Luft, 1971). The chemistry underlying the ruthenium red reaction and the basis for its selectivity for acidic mucopolysaccharides has been published (Luft, 1971a).

Figure 12 illustrates the appearance of muscle tissue exposed to ruthenium red showing the dye confined to the extracellular spaces. A thin mantle of densely staining material completely envelopes the capillary in the center of the micrograph, and also is closely applied to the surface of the muscle cells above and below the capillary. The dye has been unable to penetrate the endothelial cells to reach the capillary lumen, although a small amount has entered the junction (J) between two endothelial cells. The dye has invaded and thus identified a number of vesicles which open onto the tissue surface of the capillary, but has not reached the other vesicle populations. Figure 13 shows a capillary from the same tissue, but where the capillary split open accidentally to extravasate two erythrocytes, and where ruthenium red has been able to enter the capillary lumen through the defect. The dye has stained a layer which appears to line the vacular surface of the endothelial cells completely. It is this layer which faces the blood circulating through the capillary lumen, rather than the plasma membrane of the endothelial cell itself. This luminal coat corresponds in location and, in some respects in chemical properties, to the layer predicted by Chambers and Zweifach (1947) and therefore is designated the endocapillary layer (ECL). Clearly, it is thin-ner than the layer *outside* of the endothelial cells which faces the muscle cells. This outer layer is *not* identical to the basement membrane; rather, it *includes* the basement membrane by interpenetration of its filaments, and continues intact through the space usually found between the basement membrane and its host cell to the outer leaflet of the plasma membrane of the endothelial cell (Luft, 1971b). These features can be seen more clearly in Fig. 14, which is an enlargement of that portion of Fig. 13 marked "X." In Fig. 14, it is apparent that the endocapillary layer, as stained by ruthenium red, has a finely granular texture. It luminal boundary is very irregular and not filamen-tous, but rather is diffuse or fluffy. Conversely, its cellular boundary is abrupt and coincides with the position expected for the external leaflet of the unit membrane of the endothelial cell. The inner leaflet (IL) is visible and can be traced continuously into one of the luminal pits or vesicles (V). The density of the endocapillary layer also fills the lumen of several pits.

An alternative method for staining this layer would be welcomed. A very similar layer has has been shown on endothelium by Behnke and Zelander

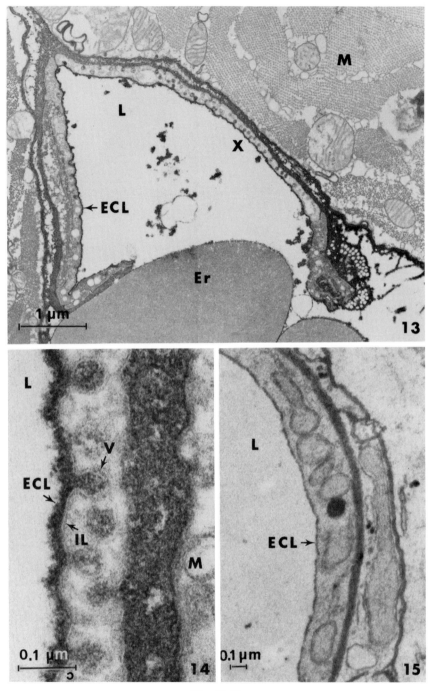

Figs. 13–15

(1970) using glutaraldehyde together with alcian blue, although the mechanism underlying this procedure is not clear. The layer is not visible in freeze-etched preparations (Nickel and Grieshaber, 1969; Weinstein and McNutt, 1970). The layer has been recognized, however, by the method developed by Pease (1966) for staining mucopolysaccharides with phosphotungstic acid. Figure 15 is an electron micrograph of a capillary prepared in this way and kindly provided by Dr. W. J. Meyer. The endocapillary layer is seen as a thin, dense line (ECL) at the luminal surface of the capillary.

iii. The diaphragms. There is an important variation in the structure of the capillary wall which is significant as an apparent exception to the rule of endothelial continuity. These are the fenestrae which are found in the endo-thelimum of certain capillaries; they were first described in detail by Yamada (1955b) in the renal glomerulus. Subsequently, they have been found in capillaries of the intestinal villus, pancreas, adrenal and pituitary, glands corpus luteum (Florey, 1968), tongue (Palade and Bruns, 1968), and other organs (Majno, 1965) as circular holes in the thinner portions of the endothelial cell about 400–500 Å in diameter. It was first thought that these fenestrations, or windows, were perforations with patent openings, but delicate membranes or diaphragms have been seen stretched across most, if not all, of them. Since the diaphragms are thin and difficult to identify positively in oblique sections, morphology alone is insufficient to identify a small population of open fenestrae in a large population of fenestrae closed by diaphragms. Tracer experiments using large molecules, such as ferritin or peroxidase, that

Figs. 13 and 14. Cross sections of another capillary from the same tissue as in Fig. 12 prepared in the same way. The capillary was split open accidentally to extravasate two erythrocytes (Er), thus permitting ruthenium red to gain access to the capillary lumen (L). The dye has stained a layer of material lining the luminal surface of the endothelial cells which corresponds to the endocapillary layer (ECL). The region designated "X" in Fig. 13 is enlarged in Fig. 14. The endocapillary layer has a diffuse luminal boundary, but terminates sharply at the outer leaflet of the unit membrane of the endothelial cell. It also fills the pits on the luminal surface of the endothelium as well as those on the tissue surface. The coats on the tissue surfaces of both muscle (M) and endothelium are confluent at X, but diverge elsewhere in Fig. 13. These coats are thicker than the layer usually designated basement membrane; each coat includes the basement membrane by interpenetration of its filaments and fills the space between the basement membrane and the cell to the outer leaflet of the unit membrane. Both Figs. 13 and 14 are mouse diaphragm fixed in the presence of ruthenium red; sections lightly stained with lead. (Fig. 13, × 18,500; Fig. 14, × 160,000.)

Fig. 15. Electron micrograph of portion of a capillary from rat cerebral cortex, prepared without fixation by inert dehydration and by staining the section with aqueous phosphotungstic acid (Pease, 1966). The endocapillary layer (ECL) appears as a thin line of density against the luminal surface of the capillary endothelial cell. (× 44,000.) (Micrograph courtesy of Dr. W. J. Meyer.)

should be retarded or arrested at the diaphragm are more useful. Although diaphragms have been reported across renal glomerular fenestrae, tracer experiments suggest that most of them are open (Farquhar *et al.*, 1961; Graham and Karnovsky, 1966). In all other tissues, however, morphology suggests that nearly all of the fenestrae are closed by diaphragms. In the case of intestinal capillaries, tracer experiments suggest that a small fraction of the diaghragms across fenestrae are partially or fully open and that this fraction of the population may be transient rather than permanent (Clementi and Palade, 1969a).

The structure of the diaphragms has significant implications with respect to the high permeability of these fenestrated capillaries. Various authors have described the diaphragm as being identical in thickness to the plasma membrane, or thinner and more tenuous than the cell membrane, or as being half the thickness of the cell membrane. Several years ago, Luft (1964a, 1965a) and Elfvin (1965) suggested that the diaphragm might be composed of only the outer leaflet of the plasma membrane of the endothelial cell. Both also suggested that this might be formed by a vesicle within the cytoplasm of the endothelial cell fusing with the plasma membrane, with subsequent re-traction of all other components of the two membranes except for the outer leaflet. Both authors illustrated the concept with pictures of a vesicle closed by a diaphragm. Wolff (1966) also described diaphragms resulting from vesiculation. This hypothesis for the origin of diaphragms had already been suggested by Karrer and Cox (1960). The sequence of stages in this vesicle–plasma membrane fusion hypothesis has been diagramed clearly by Palade and Bruns (1968) and is accompanied by many excellent micrographs illus-trating various stages.

The appearance of diaphragms as seen by conventional electron micro-scopy in the fenestrated capillaries of intestinal villi is illustrated in Figs. 16–18. In cross section, the diaphragms are recognized as a thin gray line

Figs. 16–20. Diaphragms across fenestrae in capillaries of mouse intestine. It can be seen that the diaphragm is similar in density and thickness to the external layer (EL) of the unit membrane and that in several places the diaphragm appears to originate from the material com-prising the external layer. However, the more densely staining internal layer (IL) follows the cytoplasm around the window and does not accompany the outer component. The knobs at the centers of the diaphragms are seen at the arrows. In Fig. 16, a diaphragm is stretched across a vesicle. Figure 18 shows the face view of three fenestrae with diaphragms; the knob is seen as the central density with lines radiating to the rim of the window. The capillaries in Figs. 19 and 20 were exposed to ruthenium red to stain the endocapillary layer (ECL). The layer is seen to be thick, fluffy, and continuous over the endothelial cytoplasm, as well as over the diaphragms. The diaphragms are faintly visible as thin, dark lines in a similar location to Figs. 16 and 17, but the density external to the diaphragms does not coincide with the basement mem-brane seen in Figs. 16 and 17. Figs. 16–18 from sections stained with uranyl acetate and lead; Figs. 19 and 20 from tissue exposed to ruthenium red: sections stained with lead. (× 160,000.)

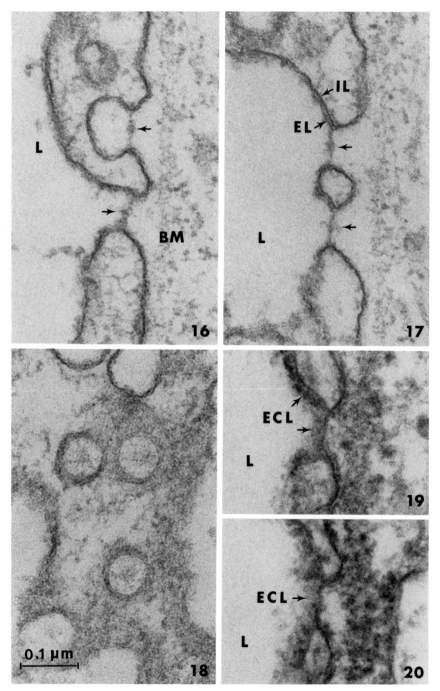

Figs. 16–20

stretched between two portions of endothelial cytoplasm. Frequently, a thickening or knob is seen in the center of the diaphragm (arrows, Figs. 16 and 17). Figures 16 and 17 suggest the continuity and, hence, the origin of the diaphragm with the outer leaflet of the endothelial unit membrane. Figure 18 is a section cut in the plane of three diaphragms showing that they are circular holes in the endothelium. The knob appears as a faint central density, and delicate lines radiate from the knob to the margin of the diaphragm. It has been suggested that these striations represent the trace of the retracting lips of the vesicle after fusion; the outer leaflet material is left stretched across the opening, with the knob being the "umbilicus" left at the point of initial contact of the vesicle with the plasma membrane (Luft, 1965a). Recently, Maul (1971) examined the fenestrations in renal tubular capillaries by the method of freeze-etching, and concludes that the diaphragm consists of two central fibrous rings (the knob) connected to the rim with radiating fibers.

Ruthenium red penetrates intestinal fenestrated capillaries without obvious restriction, in contrast to muscle capillaries (see Fig. 12). The endocapillary layer is present on the luminal surface of these fenestrated capillaries and spreads over the luminal surface of the diaphragms in about the same thickness as over the cytoplasm. This is illustrated in Figs. 19 and 20, where the fluffy substance of the endocapillary layer is seen to be much thicker than the diaphragm itself.

The composition of the diaphragm is unknown, but has been suggested to be similar to the cell coat or outer leaflet by those authors sympathetic to vesicle fusion as the mechanism of origin. Thus, Luft (1965a) implied that it is composed of mucoprotein or mycopolysaccharide because of the results with ruthenium red, while Elfvin (1965) suggested either pure protein or polysaccharide and mucoprotein. Palade and Bruns (1968) proposed that it is a stretched protein film or, possibly, an adsorbed layer of plasma proteins or fibrin, while Clementi and Palade (1969a) suggested that the diaphragm is a protein–polysaccharide film. Clementi and Palade (1969b) showed that the diaphragms are destroyed by EDTA—an observation consistent with an acid mucopolysaccharide as an important structural component. The sensitivity of the diaphragms to histamine is less easily explained. Vesicles may be a convenient, but not essential, mechanism for the formation of such diaphragms; other sources of membrane for fusion of the external leaflets may do as well. The filtration slit membrane extending between the foot processes of glomerular podocytes appears both structurally (Yamada, 1955b) and in its connection to the outer leaflets of the foot processes (Bloom and Fawcett, 1968) to be equivalent to the diaphragm of the fenestrated capillaries (Luft, 1965a). Yamada (1955b) described it as ". . . a very delicate gossamer-like membrane about 30 Å thick—the filtration slit membrane." Each pair of foot processes across which the filtration slit membrane is stretched, arises from two separate cells (Yamada, 1955b); therefore, the general mechanism of a perforation in a continuous cytoplasmic sheet is very improbable. Cell contact followed by controlled separation is the more likely mechanism of formation.

The diaphragms and slits have been clearly demonstrated as to be molecular ultrafilters by means of various large molecular weight tracer molecules. Florey (1961b) and Pappas and Tennyson (1962) demonstrated that the fenestrated capillaries in the colon and in the ciliary body of the eye hold back ferritin and colloidal thorium dioxide. In 1968, Florey surveyed with ferritin and carbon the permeability of fenestrated capillaries in various organs, and concluded that some fenestrae seemed to restrain ferritin in the anterior pituitary, pancreas, and intestine, while the adrenal cortex was very leaky, as was the corpus luteum, to colloidal carbon. The fenestrated intestinal capillaries were carefully tested by Clementi and Palade (1969a) using horseradish peroxidase (50 Å in diameter) and ferritin (110 Å). Most of the diaphragms could sustain a large number of ferritin molecules on one side, with few or none on the other side, i.e., they were more or less impermeable to ferritin. However, they occasionally encountered an isolated fenestra or a group of them with many ferritin molecules on both the luminal and tissue sides of the fenestra, as well as some within it. The smaller peroxidase molecules penetrated the fenestrae more rapidly, but the authors presented several convincing micrographs of fenestrae showing high concentrations of peroxidase reaction product in the lumens with a rapid decrease in concentration through the fenestra fading away in the extracellular tissue space. The diaphragm tends to be obliterated by the reaction product, but can be discerned in several micrographs. This appearance of a gradient in peroxidase is the expected morphological counterpart of restricted diffusion by a membrane.

Corresponding experiments have been done with glomerular capillaries. Farquhar et al. (1961) demonstrated that ferritin quickly penetrated the fenestrae in the endothelium, was retarded in the thick glomerular basement membrane, and was essentially blocked at the filtration slit membrane. Graham and Karnovsky (1966) used horseradish peroxidase (mw 40,000) as well as another peroxidase four times as heavy to investigate glomerular permeability. The light peroxidase rapidly penetrated the fenestrae, basement membrane, and epithelial slits with a slight indication of restriction in the slits. The heavy peroxidase penetrated the same barriers, but was convincingly retained in the slits between the foot processes up to the filtration slit membrane.

iv. The caveolae intracellulares or pits.   One of the first structural features of capillaries to attract the attention of electron microscopists was the large number of vesicles or circular profiles of cytoplasmic membranes, presumably enclosing spherical droplets. They were about 500–700 Å in diameter, and were visible in the endothelial cell cytoplasm (Palade, 1953). Furthermore, it appeared that some of these vesicles were connected to the cell surface, giving the appearance of flasklike invaginations of the endothelial cell membrane. Also, they were seen in roughly equal numbers on both luminal and tissue surface (see Figs. 5, 8, and 11). Similar structures were seen in other tissues; Yamada (1955a) saw them in the gall bladder and labeled them caveolae intracellulares. This discovery prompted the suggestion that they might account, at least partially, for capillary permeability by engulfing fluid in bulk on one side of the capillary endothelial cell, ferrying it through the cytoplasm, and disgorging the fluid contents on the other side (Palade, 1953, 1960, 1961; Bennett, 1956; Moore and Ruska, 1957; Wissing, 1958; Alksne, 1959; Florey, 1961a; Jennings et al., 1962). A new world, "cytopempsis," was coined (Moore and Ruska, 1957) to express the transfer of fluid by vesicles, thus complementing the word pinocytosis introduced by Lewis (1931) to describe the uptake or drinking by macrophages which had frequently assumed to represent the mechanism of fluid uptake by vesicles in capillaries. The vesicles continue as the focus of controversy in morphological contributions to capillary permeability (Crone and Lassen, 1970). It is not so much their structure which is in dispute, but rather their function. By all measures, the most elaborate investigation of the structure of endothelial vesicles is the work of Bruns and Palade (1968a) culminating in the reconstruction by serial sections of a segment of endothelium 1.33 μm long, 0.33 μm wide, and 0.30 μm thick. Of the 82 completely sectioned vesicles within this volume, 23 opened to the blood front of the cell, 35 opened to the tissue front, and 24 were completely enclosed in the cytoplasm. There were five instances of two vesicles fusing to form a pair, but no continuous pathway was found across the endothelium. The vesicles were sparse in the thick regions near the endothelial cell nucleus, and attained the greatest frequency in the thin periphery of the cell (120 vesicles/μm^2 of cell surface) (Bruns and Palade, 1968a).

The function of the vesicles is unknown. In electron micrographs, they often are labeled pinocytotic vesicles or micropinocytotic vesicles—the pinocytotic component implying that the author was convinced that these vesicles were involved in fluid uptake or cell drinking. The original descriptions of pinocytosis and the word itself stem from the work of Lewis (1931), by direct light microscopic observations of cell cultures, and pinocytosis has been clearly documented in amebas (Chapman-Andresen, 1962). The vesicles or pits in capillaries are an order of magnitude smaller than the true pinocytotic vesicles in the original references, so that the vesicles in living capillaries have never been seen. The function imputed to them by the term micropinocytotic vesicle rests with experiments using intravascular injections of small colloidal particles (carbon, mercuric sulfide, thorium dioxide) or large molecules (ferritin, peroxidase). The subject is reviewed by Majno (1965, pp. 2324–2332). The experiments are very difficult technically to carry out in a manner which will yield unambiguous results. In many tracer experiments, a section for the electron microscope shows tracer within pits at the capillary lumen, as well as tracer in vesicles in the cytoplasm, when the tracer is administered intravenously a few minutes before the tissue is fixed. If the interval between the tracer injection and sampling is longer, such as 10–20 minutes, tracer is often found in the pits on the tissue surface of the endothelial cell as well as in the intercellular space. The straightforward interpretation is that the tracer has been transported by vesicles across the endothelium from the blood to the tissue space, and this is certainly one possible explanation of the results. However, the EM section is a two-dimensional sample of tissue, and the validity of this explanation rests on the ability to exclude alternate (extracellular) pathways for the tracer in three dimensions over a radius of perhaps 5–10 μm from the vesicular pathway in question. Serial reconstruction at the EM level of this volume of tissue is a truly heroic venture; it has been reported only once on a very much smaller volume of endothelium (Bruns and Palde, 1968a).

Since the definitive experiment is nearly impossible to carry out and since a statistical approach with the electron microscope is equally appalling (what does one do with 10 m^3 of electron micrographs?), the current approach is to accumulate circumstantial evidence. The team of Bruns and Palade is perhaps the strongest proponent of transcapillary transport of large molecules by vesicles, and they have gone to great effort to provide experimental evidence to support their point of view. This culminates in the paper by Bruns and Palade (1968b) and is supported by other work (Bruns and Palade, 1968a; Palade and Bruns, 1968). They suggest that the vesicular transport mechanism is the morphological equivalent of the large pore capillary permeability which is indicated by physiological experiments with large molecules (Mayerson et al., 1960; Renkin, 1964; Renkin and Garlick, 1970). A great deal of work was also accomplished at Oxford in the laboratory of Sir Howard Florey on vesicular transport in capillaries. In 1962, the results obtained with colloidal tracers prompted the statement that there was little doubt about the role of vesicles in transport through the cytoplasm (Jennings et al., 1962). In 1967, after summarizing this work and that of others, they concluded, however, that only a small number of particles relative to the luminal concentration passed through the vesicle system (Jennings and Florey, 1967).

The introduction of peroxidases in electron microscopy added another tracer with which to test vesicular transport. In an early report, Karnovsky

(1965) was very enthusiastic in support of the vesicular hypothesis; the detailed report (Karnovsky, 1967) qualified, but still supported, vesicles as a secondary transport pathway. No major changes occurred during a recent conference (Karnovsky, 1970). A useful analysis of vesicular transport driven by Brownian motion (Shea and Karnovsky, 1966) did not find any fault or inconsistency in the model. Detailed consideration of vesicular transport raises the question of disposal of vesicular membrane if the vesicles fuse with and thus contribute to the plasma membrane of the endothelial cell; an alternative hypothesis is that the vesicles remain at the surface to unload, refill, and make the reverse trip. There is some support for the latter suggestion from neurophysiologists. Synaptic vesicles in nerve endings are superficially similar to endothelial vesicles, and there is good physiological evidence for their involvement in neurotransmitter release (Katz, 1971). Recent work in estimation of membrane turnover (Bittner and Kennedy, 1970) and electron microscopy with peroxidase (Holtzman et al., 1971) during prolonged stimulation of crayfish or lobster neuromuscular preparations suggests that the vesicles retrieved by the nerve endings are still in the form of vesicles. Thus, there is no doubt as to the existence of the endothelial pits or vesicles, but, as far as their inclusion in, or exclusion from, transcapillary transport is concerned, the evidence is circumstantial and, in my opinion, mutually cancelling.

v. The junctions. For years, physiologists have been interested in the role of the junctions between endothelial cells as the sites of fluid movement across capillaries. Starling (1909) thought "cracks between endothelial cells, containing either lymph of cement substance" were the most probable location for fluid escape. Chambers and Zweifach (1940, 1947) elaborated this point of view, regarding the intercellular cement as a product of the endothelial cell and describing the alterations produced in capillary endothelium by changes in calcium ion concentration and pH. The physiological work on muscle capillaries (Pappenheimer et al., 1951) had drawn attention to the behavior of capillaries in terms of pores, although slits were also mentioned. The electron microscopists did not find pores when they looked for them (Bennett et al., 1959), nor did they find any intercellular cement (Florey et al., 1959), and, in any case, the junctions between endothelial cells were thought to be tight seals or zonulae occludentes (Farquhar and Palade, 1963; Karnovsky, 1967, Footnote 5). The introduction of new methods, however, provided electron micrographs which indicated that in muscle capillaries the cracks between endothelial cells were not as tight as had been supposed (Luft, 1965a,b, 1966; Revel and Karnovsky, 1967; Karnovsky, 1967). The use of peroxidase as a tracer which could slowly penetrate the small pore system under physiological conditions (Karnovsky, 1967) produced results which could not be ignored. By 1969, the endothelial junctions were so firmly established in this role that Crone (1970, p. 29) introduced the Copenhagen conference with a "minimum platform" of agreement which included ". . . that the transport for small hydrophilic molecules takes place through the free space between the endothelial cells. . . ." Thus was Starling vindicated after 60 years.

There is still uncertainty about the precise dimensions of the filtration slits between capillary endothelial cells. Again, the final solution lies in serial reconstruction of a sample of endothelial junctions to provide the three-dimentional structure for a reasonable number of such junctions, but this is tedious work. Karnovsky (1967) provided evidence from small groups of serial sections that the junctions varied in spacing over short distances, and, rather than using "zonulae occludentes" which implied long belts of occlusion, he proposed the term "maculae occludentes" (Farquhar and Palade, 1965) to indicate that they were spots instead. The filtration slits would then be formed at cell interfaces between the occluding spots, and would perhaps be oval or elliptical in projection on the capillary luminal surface, with the minor axis about 40 Å and the major axis indeterminate (Karnovsky, 1967, 1970).

In electron micrographs, the intercellular slits appear as illustrated in Figs. 21 and 22. Figure 21 is one of the junctions from the whole capillary shown in Fig. 6, while Fig. 22 comes from the capillary in Fig. 8. These micrographs confirm that the plasma membranes of the two adjoining endothelial cells run more or less parallel over much of the region of contact, but that the space between them narrows somewhat at one segment (X). At this point, the external layers (EL) of the two unit membranes appear to be confluent as a central gray line. In tissue prepared and stained as these sections were, the central line is never as dense as the internal leaflets of the unit membranes, implying a different composition. The center-to-center distance between the dark, internal leaflets is about 200–250 Å in the wider portions of the junctional region and reduces to about 135–140 Å at the constricted portion X. The constriction here is about 500–600 Å long (radial to the capillary long axis), but in other pictures it often appears shorter.

When muscle tissue (diaphragm) is exposed to ruthenium red during fixation, the dye usually diffuses toward the capillaries from the intercellular tissue spaces, as illustrated in Fig. 12. In fortunate instances, it stains the extracellular contents of the endothelial junctions with sufficient contrast to delineate the morphology of the slits. This is illustrated in Figs. 23–25, showing slits of three different path lengths corresponding to different amounts of endothelial cell overlap. In each case, however, a short constriction is present between the capillary lumen and the tissue space, which is equated with the sieving element that confers the small pore molecular selectivity upon the capillary. The concentration of ruthenium red (as

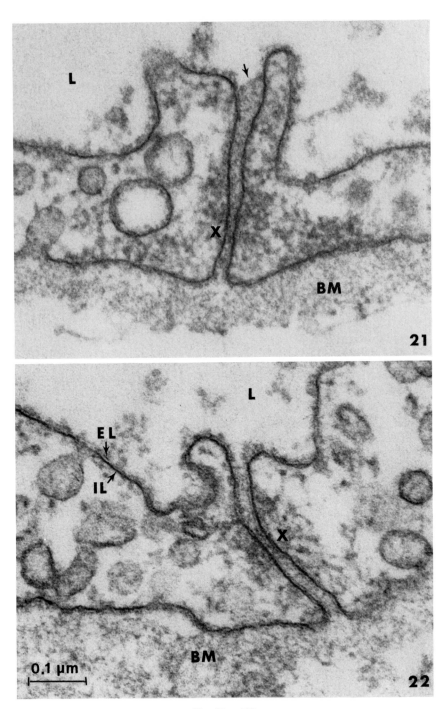

Figs. 21 and 22

indicated by the density in the micrographs) decreases slowly along the intercellular pathway from tissue space toward the lumen, but falls abruptly at the constriction to vanish as the dye is diluted into the capillary lumen. In Fig. 24, there are two constrictions in series, and enough density is retained in the outer of the two to permit an estimate of the dimensions. The gap appears to be about 40- to 45-Å minimum width and has an hourglass configuration as if pressed between two parallel cylinders of about 500- to 1000-Å radius. It is suggested that the constriction is not empty, but rather that it is formed by the confluence of the two external leaflets of the two participating endothelial cells. The endocapillary layer is envisioned as being thinned away at this point leaving only a residue of hydrated acid mucopolysaccharide chains to which the ruthenium red binds (Luft, 1966) and through which the small water-soluble molecules diffuse, as described by Laurent (1970).

This type of open slit at the junction of endothelial cells applies to muscle-type capillaries, and cerebral capillaries are specifically excluded. The use of peroxidase as a tracer has demonstrated conclusively that the endothelial cells in brain make extensive tight junctions or zonulae occludens with one another (Reese and Karnovsky, 1967), so that the mammalian "blood–brain barrier" exists at the level of the cerebral endothelium. In an exception which proves the rule, the choroid plexus of the brain has fenestrated capillaries which pass peroxidase to the tissue space, but it is still prevented from entering the cerebrospinal fluid by tight junctions of the choroidal epithelium (Brightman, 1967; Brightman et al., 1970).

2. THE BASEMENT MEMBRANE

The basement membrane was recognized early on as one of the components of the capillary wall (Palade, 1953) and continues to be routinely assigned an important function, frequently being alluded to as the primary functional barrier controlling capillary permeability. For example, Farquhar (1961) and Fawcett (1963) both agreed that although there was some uncer-

Figs. 21 and 22. Intercellular junctions between pairs of endothelial cells showing the region of constriction (X) which is reinforced by intracellular filaments seen as granular material in the adjacent cytoplasm. In Fig. 22 and, to some extent, in Fig. 21, the unit membrane of the endothelial cell can be seen, with the granular or flocculent material of the endocapillary layer adherent to the external leaflet (EL) and accumulating at the junction (arrow, Fig. 21). The internal layer (IL) is recognized as a dense line that limits the cytoplasm and outlines the junctional region. The basement membrane (BM) appears filamentous or granular and seems to contact the endothelial cells in the vicinity of the junction. Mouse diaphragm section stained with uranyl acetate and lead. (× 160,000.)

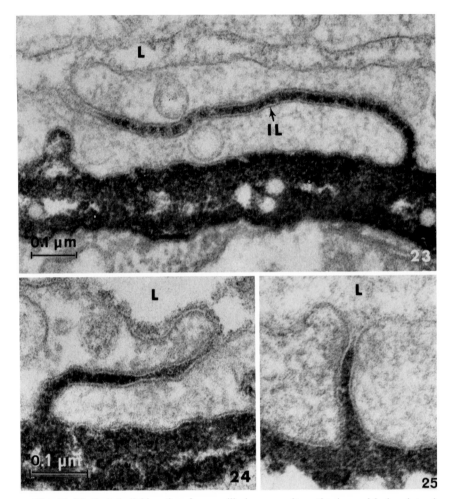

Figs. 23–25. Endothelial junctions from capillaries exposed to ruthenium red during glutaraldehyde and osmium fixation. The dye has heavily stained the cell coat from the tissue space and has penetrated the extracellular region of the junctions down to the level of the constriction. At that point, the density due to the dye falls off abruptly as the dye is diluted into the capillary lumen (L). The cell coat material appears granular with ruthenium red, and its density is continuous to and stops abruptly at the outer leaflet of the endothelial unit membrane. The light (central) leaflet of the unit membrane is easily visible in many regions of each micrograph, and helps to clearly delineate the inner, cytoplasmic leaflet (IL) of the unit membrane. In Fig. 24, there are two constrictions in series along the junction, and sufficient dye is retained on both sides of the external constriction to reveal its structure clearly. Mouse diaphragm tissue exposed to ruthenium red; sections stained with lead. (Fig. 23, × 125,000; Figs. 24 and 25, × 160,000.)

tainty about the diaphragms of fenestrated capillaries the basement membrane must be an important filter, and both also agreed that it constituted the main filtration barrier of the glomerular capillaries of the kidney. Farquhar *et al.* (1961) showed that intravenously injected ferritin accumulated on the basement membrane of the glomerulus of the rat, although some ferritin did go through the basement membrane randomly (i.e., not through any defects or visible channels) to accumulate along the filtration slit membranes and foot processes of the glomerular epithelial cells where it was phagocytized. However, their data can be reinterpreted to suggest that the basement membrane functions as a coarse or prefilter for the glomerulus and that the filtration slit membrane is the significant membrane from the standpoint of permeability characteristics (Luft, 1965a). The use of peroxidase as a test molecule supports this suggestion (Graham and Karnovsky, 1966). Even so, physiological experiments, such as the clearance of various-sized dextrans by the normal human glomerulus, are still interpreted as indicating that the normal glomerular membrane is a gel filter localized in the basement membrane (Arturson, 1970).

The structure of the basement membrane is not easily described even at the level of ultrastructure. Its appearance in Fig. 9 is that of a felt or a brush heap, and it is not continuous everywhere, even in muscle capillaries, as illustrated in Fig. 8 (arrows). Its structure and composition have been reviewed in great detail by Majno (1965, pp. 2303–2308), and this has been updated by Bruns and Palade (1968a).

The function of the basement membrane has also been discussed at length by Majno (1965, pp. 2335–2338). There is no doubt that it behaves as a filter to large particles. This function is illustrated beautifully in its retention of 340-Å (average) carbon particles in fenestrated intestinal capillaries from which the diaphragms were removed with EDTA (Clementi and Palade, 1969a). These same basement membranes permitted the passage of colloidal gold particles smaller than about 200 Å. It is thus apparent that the basement membrane is a filter, but a relatively coarse one which must impose relatively little resistance to the molecules that are used to test the small pore system and even to those probing the large pores. Its contribution to overall capillary permeability must be a minor one for the reasons presented by Perl (1971, p. 246). In the absence of any endothelial permeability barriers, the basement membrane may provide significant restriction, so that it is reassuring to find large gaps in the basement membrane of sinusoids (Bennett *et al.*, 1959; Majno, 1965) and of lymphatics (Leak, 1971).

The basement membrane may be of great importance from a mechanical standpoint. Chambers and Zweifach (1947) cite experiments which indicate that the basement membrane is essential to the structural integrity of the capillary. Pease (1960) called the basement membrane a microskeleton, and suggested that the glomerular basement membrane in various animals may be thickened in proportion to the blood pressure which it is required to sustain. Schoefl (1964) also called attention to the association between the fragility of newly formed capillary sprouts and the incompleteness or absence of their basement membrane, whereas the older and stronger portions of the capillary had acquired a basement membrane.

3. THE PERICAPILLARY CELLS

Early investigators described cells with branching processes outside and enfolding the capillary endothelium. They stain poorly by ordinary histological methods, but are demonstrable in the living animal or by silver impregnation. They came to be known as "Rouget cells" after Rouget (1873) described contractile cells surrounding certain capillaries of the frog's eye. Zimmermann (1923), using silver methods, demonstrated pericapillary cells around a great variety of capillaries, calling them "pericytes." The uncertainty in equating Rouget cells with pericytes and with capillary contractility generally is discussed by Krogh and Vimtrup (1932). The electron microscope, however, has demonstrated that cells of some sort are associated with most, if not all, capillaries and the name pericyte appears to be acceptable. Such cells are shown in Figs. 5–8 (P) where they are seen to be enveloped by the same basement membrane as the endothelial cell, a location which serves to define them at the ultrastructural level. These cells and their processes are discontinuous over spaces of more than 10 μm and, hence, cannot play any direct part as a barrier in capillary permeability. Very probably, they are involved in the long-term maintenance of capillaries. In many experiments using colloidal tracers, the pericytes have been shown to be phagocytic. Their history, structure, and function were reviewed by Majno (1965) and were updated by Bruns and Palade (1968a).

IV. Discussion of Various Mechanisms Proposed for the Control of Capillary Permeability

Factors important to capillary permeability relate to the two components involved—the vascular and tissue spaces and the barriers between them. This chapter concerns capillary permeability in the sense of those agencies directly related to the capillary itself, i.e., to the capillary as a barrier. Factors influencing the spaces are intravascular or tissue pressures, both of which are distant or gross effects, and changes in protein content which are a systemic effect. There is no morphological equivalent for these factors, so they will not be pursued. Local events in the tissue space, however, can have profound effects on capillaries. Capillary here, as well as generally throughout this chapter, has referred to "vessels of capillary thinness," as Majno (1965, p. 2296) grouped them, rather than distinguishing true capillaries from venules (Cotran *et al.*, 1965). It is clear that histamine or serotonin released from mast cells in the connective tissue space can dramatically increase the permeability of the venules in the capillary bed. This special case is treated elsewhere under Tissue Injury or Inflammation.

As to the normal, undisturbed capillary functioning as a barrier, there is much more to be said. One line of argument suggests a strictly passive function for the endothelium (and its associated membranes or layers), and the proponents of this view can duplicate the spectrum of molecular discrimination measured in living capillary beds with artificial membrane models. On the other side are those who support an active and essential role for endothelial cytoplasm in the flow or exchange of solutes across the capillary wall. Then there is a continuum of positions intermediate between these extremes.

A. The Passive Role of Endothelium in Capillary Permeability

When this section was first written, the literature was fragmented; so it was convenient to group the advocates into those who assigned the passive characteristics of capillaries to a system of small and large pores, another group who attached primary importance to the basement membrane, and a third who considered the intercellular cement between the endothelial cells as the filter. It is now quite clear that the introductory statement of Crone (1970) "that the transport for small hydrophilic molecules takes place through the free space between endothelial cells" did not draw a violent protest from any of the participants at that Symposium, as far as muscle-type capillaries were concerned. It is only fair to point out that various degrees of abstraction are apparent in the papers from both that Symposium and elsewhere, in that certain authors preferred to express their results as "equivalent pore radii," whereas others were more willing to fit numbers to a specific model. Nevertheless, there appeared to be no vigorous opposition to Crone's initial statement for the location of the small pore system. As for the location of the large pore system, any unanimity vanishes: in the recent literature, there are implications that the leaks are passive defects in the capillary wall, as well as proposals that vesicular transport may account for the movement of molecules larger than 50-Å diameter.

B. *The Active Role of Endothelium in Capillary Permeability*

The proponents of this hypothesis express the view that the endothelium is necessary for the immediate or short-term passage of fluid across the capillary wall—not merely for the long-term maintenance of otherwise passive structures (such as basement membranes, diaphragms, or cement substrances). The details vary, but the most popular proposal attributes transport to the pinocytotic vesicles. Palade and co-workers have been the strongest proponents of this view, and they have presented their evidence and arguments in a series of elegant papers (Bruns and Palade, 1968a,b; Palade and Bruns, 1968; Clementi and Palade, 1969a). They clearly identified the large pore system with the plasmalemmal vesicles, at least in capillaries of the diaphragm (Bruns and Palade, 1968b), which probably are typical of muscle capillaries in general. The fenestrated capillaries of the intestine are a special case; Clementi and Palade (1969a) concluded that both the large and small pore systems exist in the fenestrated part of the endothelium and that the vesicles do not represent the main pathway followed by the tracer (peroxidase). In these capillaries, they felt that the basement membrane must be a significant filter for large pore molecules (Clementi and Palade, 1969b). As far as the small pore system was concerned, their conviction appeared to be weaker. They occasionally found open intercellular channels between endothelial cells in muscle capillaries, but with low frequency (Bruns and Palade, 1968a). Based on physiological data available to them, they felt that the morphological evidence for pores or slits did not fit the permeability calculations, and thus by exclusion implicated the vesicular system in the small pore system as well as the large. Their subsequent paper (Palade and Bruns, 1968) developed the details of vesicular fusion and movement, and implied fluid movement by vesicles with filtration selectivity by the diaphragms across vesicles.

C. *Intermediate Hypotheses*

Virtually all workers concerned with capillary permeability agree that cells are somehow involved. For those inclined toward the dynamic view, cellular activity is of immediate importance; for the proponents of mechanistic views, it is the long-term role of cells. As more and more evidence accumulates, both experimental, from the fields of morphology and physiology, as well as theoretical, there appears to be a general convergence toward this middle ground. Thus, one finds pure-blooded physiologists not only considering but defending vesicular transport, as well as morphologists advocating a noncellular, mechanistic view of capillary permeability. Under these conditions, all proposals receive vigorous consideration and criticism, which is a healthy state of affairs and which should lead to the rapid refinement of our knowledge of capillary permeability.

V. Summary and Conclusions

It would appear that there is still no single hypothesis of the mechanism of capillary permeability which can account for all of the known facts, although there is now more agreement among those working in this field than there was seven years ago (Luft, 1965a). The "known facts," i.e., the working data, seem to be reproducible in various laboratories by different people using different techniques. It is worth keeping in mind, however, that there may be some snags in the experimental methods. The discussions included in the recent Symposium on capillary permeability (Crone and Lassen, 1970) indicate that the physiological experiments may be complicated or indirect enough so that not all variables are under control or even recognized fully. In electron microscopy, there is a serious problem regarding the speed of the fixation process, which is very slow with respect to most physiological phenomena.

The basic problem is how to reconcile what appears to be a purely passive phenomenon (the molecular selectivity of capillaries) with the indisputable fact that capillaries are composed of living cells which can be disturbed very quickly by mechanical or chemical insults, coincident with drastic alterations in permeability. This apparent paradox is not unique to capillaries or to animal cells. For example, Mees and Weatherley (1957) reported experiments in plants dealing with the mechanism of water absorption by roots and the effect of pressure gradients on water uptake. They concluded that it is striking

that the flux through the root could suffer a 90% reduction due to metabolic inhibition . . . in view of the fact that the movement was surely a passive one in response to gradients of diffusion potential. Aerobic metabolism seemed essential to the maintenance of low resistance in the pathway, indeed, it was evident that the diffusional pathway could be closed completely by drastic metabolic inhibition.

The differences between fluid transport in the vascular plants (Weatherley and Johnson, 1968) and circulation in animals is not as great as might be thought at first. There are parallels between plant physiology and plant microanatomy (Cronshaw and Anderson, 1969) and the subject of this chapter. In the face of conflicts of this sort, it would be helpful to put aside for the moment the necessity of explaining all of the phenomena associated with each of the many variations of capillaries and to attempt to find a unified model of capillary function which could account for much of the morphological data available without violating the physiological evidence of capillary behavior. Occam's Razor dictates that simplicity be an important consideration in the model.

The model proposed here is based primarily on the arguments and conclusions of Chambers and Zweifach (1947) and modified by recent morphological knowledge. It is proposed that most animal cells are provided with outer coats or layers of acid mucopolysaccharide (Luft, 1971b) of which the endocapillary layer of vascular endothelial cells is merely one specialization. This layer, in all cases where it has been examined, seems to be intimately associated with, or attached to, the outer leaflet of the plasma membrane. There is now substantial agreement that the diaphragms of the fenestrated capillaries are formed from this same outer coat material. It is proposed that the material which forms the diaphragm is porous and together with its endocapillary layer constitutes the selective filter of small pore size required by the theory developed by Pappenheimer and that the high permeability of these capillaries is due to the large area and thinness of these diaphragms. It is further proposed that in capillaries of the type found in muscle the fluid movement takes place at the intercellular junctions through the middle lamella of the junction itself at the constriction. This central layer is formed by the confluence of the external leaflets and remnants of the endocapillary layers of the two adjoining endothelial cell membranes, is identical to the material composing the diaphragms of the fenestrated capillaries, and, in fact, can be regarded as a "diaphragm" seen edge-on by the penetrating molecules. The low permeability of these capillaries results from the decreased area and increased path length presented to the capillary lumen. The constrictions at the junctions become the morphological equivalent of the slit in Pappenheimer's model, and the walls of the slit are defined by the lipid layers of the two unit membranes. The minimum dimension of the middle lamella seems to be about 40 Å (Luft, 1965; Karnovsky, 1967), which is close to that suggested originally by Pappenheimer (1953) and as refined recently by Perl (1971). The filtration slit membrane between the foot processes of the glomerular epithelial cells is also considered to be a derivative of the outer leaflet and associated layers of the plasma membranes of the two adjacent foot processes, to have properties similar to those of the diaphragms of the fenestrated capillaries, and also to be associated with material reacting with ruthenium red in a manner similar to the endocapillary layer (Groniowski, *et al.*, 1969). The basement membrane of muscle as well as of glomerular capillaries is regarded primarily as a structural element, a porous feltwork strong in tension and functioning as a coarse filter. It would function as a postfilter in muscle capillaries or a prefilter in glomerular capillaries, but is not envisioned as causing significant molecular discrimination by itself under normal conditions, even in the glomerulus.

So far, the vesicles have been ignored, although there is no question as to their existence; if they agree on nothing else, all morphologists find vesicles in their capillaries. It is proposed here that the vesicles are irrelevant in capillary permeability because they are not necessary to the explanation, even as the large pore equivalent. It is quite possible that all capillaries, except those in brain, create fenestrae with diaphragms from time to time and that occasionally diaphragms break to form the rare large pores, literally as well as those required theoretically. Fenestrae with diaphragms have been reported, but are rare, in cardiac-type muscle (Karrer and Cox, 1960). These large pores derived from fenestrae would be much more under the control of the capillary endothelial cell than would be the occasional defects at three-way endothelial cell junctions postulated earlier (Luft, 1965a). They have a precedent already established on a grand scale in the glomerulus. The vesicles are regarded as a secretory phenomenon common to most cells of the connective tissue, but perhaps specialized to some degree in endothelium. It has been suggested that the vesicles contribute to the formation of the endocapillary layer in a secretory fashion (Luft, 1966). It is quite clear that the turnover time of acid mucopolysaccharides of certain connective tissues is a few days (Schiller et al., 1956; Delaunay and Bazin, 1964; Mankin and Lippiello, 1969), and there is no reason to exclude vascular endothelium. The endocapillary layer is reactive toward ruthenium red in a manner similar to some of these connective tissue acid mucopolysaccharides (Luft, 1971a,b). There is also substantial precedent for the involvement of vesicles of this size and category in secretory processes. Thus, the vesicles are simply assigned a role in the general maintenance of the cell surface and the local cellular environment, rather than in direct molecular transport processes.

This proposal, then, suggests that the primary selection membrane for all capillaries, be they of the muscular, fenestrated, or glomerular type, is the thin external layer of the unit membrane. Capillary permeability in the short run in a passive process, with the cells playing a vital long-term role in terms of synthesis of the required cellular layers, repair, and maintenance. Only time will tell whether this simplification is helpful or further obscures the field of capillary permeability.

Acknowledgments

I am grateful to Dr. Daniel C. Pease and to his colleague, Dr. William J. Meyer, for contributing the micrograph used in Fig. 15.

This work was supported by United States Public Health Service grant GM-16598 and by a grant-in-aid from the American Heart Association, 67-665.

References

Alksne, J. F. (1959). *Quart. J. Exptl. Physiol. Cog. Med. Sci.* **44**, 51.
Arturson, G. (1970). *In* "Capillary Permeability" (C. Crone and N. A. Lassen, eds.), pp. 520–530. Academic Press, New York.
Behnke, O., and Zelander, T. (1970). *J. Ultrastruct. Res.* **31**, 424.
Bennett, H. S. (1956). *J. Biophys. Biochem. Cytol.* **2**, No. 4, Suppl., 99.
Bennett, H. S., Luft, J. H., and Hampton, J. C. (1959). *Amer. J. Physiol.* **196**, 381.
Benninghoff, A. (1930). *In* "Handbuch der mikroskopischen Anatomie des Menschen" (W. von Möllendorff, ed.) Vol. 6, Part 1, pp. 18–49. Springer-verlag, Berlin and New York.
Bittner, G. D., and Kennedy, D. (1970). *J. Cell Biol.* **47**, 585.
Bloom, W., and Fawcett, D. W. (1968). "A Textbook of Histology," 9th ed., pp. 654–655. Saunders, Philadelphia, Pennsylvania.
Brandt, P. W. (1962). *Circulation* **26**, 1075.
Brightman, M. W. (1967). *Progr. Brain Res.* **29**, 19.
Brightman, M. W., Reese, T. S., and Feder, N. (1970). *In* "Capillary Permeability" (C. Crone and N. A. Lassen, eds.), pp. 468–476. Academic Press, New York.
Bruns, R. R., and Palade, G. E. (1968a). *J. Cell. Biol.* **37**, 244.
Bruns, R. R., and Palade, G. E. (1968b). *J. Cell Biol.* **37**, 277.
Chambers, R., and Zweifach, B. W. (1940). *J. Cell. Comp. Physiol.* **15**, 255.
Chambers, R., and Zweifach, B. W. (1947). *Physiol. Rev.* **27**, 436.
Chapman-Andresen, C. (1962). *C. R. Trav. Lab. Carlsberg* **33**, 73.
Clementi, F., and Palade, G. E. (1969a). *J. Cell Biol.* **41**, 33.
Clementi, F., and Palade, G. E. (1969b). *J. Cell Biol.* **42**, 706.
Cotran, R. S., La Gattuta, M., and Majno, G. (1965). *Amer. J. Pathol.* **47**, 1045.
Crone, C. (1970). *In* "Capillary Permeability" (C. Crone and N. A. Lassen, eds.), pp. 15–31. Academic Press, New York.
Crone, C., and Lassen, N. A., eds. (1970). "Capillary Permeability." Academic Press, New York.
Cronshaw, J., and Anderson, R. (1969). *J. Ultrastruct. Res.* **27**, 134.
Danielli, J. F., and Stock, A. (1944). *Biol. Rev. Cambridge Phil. Soc.* **19**, 81.
Davson, H. (1962). *Circulation* **26**, 1022.
Davson, H., and Danielli, J. F. (1952). "The Permeability of Natural Membranes," 2nd ed. Cambridge Univ. Press, London and New York.
Delaunay, A., and Bazin, S. (1964). *Int. Rev. Connect. Tissue Res.* **2**, 301.
Elfvin, L. G. (1965). *J. Ultrastruct. Res.* **12**, 687.
Farquhar, M. G. (1961). *Angiology* **12**, 270.
Farquhar, M. G., and Palade, G. E. (1961). *J. Exp. Med.* **114**, 699.
Farquhar, M. G., and Palade, G. E. (1963). *J. Cell Biol.* **17**, 375.
Farquhar, M. G., and Palade, G. E. (1965). *J. Cell Biol.* **26**, 263.
Farquhar, M. G., Wissig, S. L., and Palade, G. E. (1961). *J. Exp. Med.* **113**, 47.
Fawcett, D. W. (1959). *In* "The Microcirculation" (S. R. M. Reynolds and B. W. Zweifach, eds.), pp. 1–27. Univ. of Illinois Press, Urbana.
Fawcett, D. W. (1963). *In* "The Peripheral Blood Vessels" (J. L. Orbison and D. E. Smith, eds.), Int. Acad. Pathol. Monogr. No. 4, pp. 17–44. Williams & Wilkins, Baltimore, Maryland.
Fawcett, D. W. (1966). "An Atlas of Fine Structure. The Cell. Its Organelles and Inclusions," pp. 219–232. Saunders, Philadelphia, Pennsylvania.
Finean, J. B. (1962). *Circulation* **26**, 1151.
Florey, H. W. (1961a). *Nature (London)* **192**, 908.
Florey, H. W. (1961b). *Quart. J. Exp. Physiol. Cog. Med. Sci.* **46**, 119.

Florey, H. W. (1968). *Quart. J. Exp. Physiol. Cog. Med. Sci.* **53**, 1.
Florey, H. W., Poole, J. C. F., and Meek, G. A. (1959). *J. Pathol. Bacteriol.* **77**, 625.
Gaines, L. M. (1960). *Bull. Johns Hopkins Hosp.* **106**, 195.
Graham, R. C., and Karnovsky, M. J. (1966). *J. Exp. Med.* **124**, 1123.
Greenlee, T. K., Jr., Ross, R., and Hartman, J. L. (1966). *J. Cell Biol.* **30**, 59.
Groniowski, J., Biczyskowa, W., and Walski, M. (1969). *J. Cell Biol.* **40**, 585.
Grotte, G. (1956). *Acta Chir. Scand., Suppl.* **221**, 1.
Hama, K. (1960). *J. Biophys. Biochem. Cytol.* **7**, 717.
Heidenhain, R. (1891). *Arch. Gesamte Physiol. Menschen Tiere* **49**, 209–301.
Höber, R. (1945). "Physical Chemistry of Cells and Tissues." Churchill, London.
Holtzman, E., Freeman, A. R., and Kashner, L. A. (1971). *Science* **173**, 733.
Ito, S. (1965). *J. Cell Biol.* **27**, 475.
Jennings, M. A., and Florey, H. (1967). *Proc. Roy. Soc. Ser. B* **167**, 39.
Jennings, M. A., Marchesi, V. T., and Florey, H. W. (1962). *Proc. Roy. Soc., Ser. B* **156**, 14.
Karnovsky, M. J. (1965). *J. Cell Biol.* **27**, 49A.
Karnovsky, M. J. (1967). *J. Cell Biol.* **35**, 213.
Karnovsky, M. J. (1970). *In* "Capillary Permeability" (C. Crone and N. A. Lassen, eds.), pp. 341–350, 366–370, and 563. Academic Press, New York.
Karrer, H. E., and Cox, J. (1960). *J. Biophys. Biochem. Cytol.* **8**, 135.
Katz, B. (1971). *Science* **173**, 123.
Kölliker, A. (1852). *In* "Manual of Human Microscopical Anatomy" (J. DaCosta, ed.), p. 690. Lippincott, Philadelphia, Pennsylvania (transl. by G. Busk and T. Huxley in 1854).
Krogh, A. (1930). "The Anatomy and Physiology of Capillaries." Hafner, New York. (Reprint 1959 with new Introduction and Preface by E. M. Landis and including a lecture given at Harvard Medical School in 1946. [Reminiscences of work in capillary circulation.])
Krogh, A., and Vimtrup, B. (1932). *In* "Special Cytology" (E. V. Cowdry, ed.), 2nd ed., Vol. I, Sect. XII, pp. 475–503. Harper (Hoeber), New York.
Landis, E. M. (1927). *Amer. J. Physiol.* **82**, 217.
Landis, E. M. (1934). *Physiol. Rev.* **14**, 404.
Landis, E. M., and Pappenheimer, J. R. (1963). *In* "Handbook of Physiology" (Amer. Physiol. Soc., J. Field, ed.), Sect. 2, Vol. II, pp. 961–1034. Williams & Wilkins, Baltimore, Maryland.
Lassen, N. (1970). *In* "Capillary Permeability" (C. Crone and N. A. Lassen, eds.), pp. 549–550. Academic Press, New York.
Laurent, T. C. (1970). *In* "Capillary Permeability" (C. Crone and N. A. Lassen, eds.), pp. 261–277. Academic Press, New York.
Leak, L. V. (1971. *J. Cell Biol.* **50**, 300.
Lewis, W. H. (1931). *Bull. Johns Hopkins Hosp.* **49**, 17.
Low, F. N. (1962). *Anat. Rec.* **142**, 131.
Luft, J. H. (1961). *J. Biophys. Biochem. Cytol.* **9**, 409.
Luft, J. H. (1964a). *Anat. Rec.* **148**, 307.
Luft, J. H. (1964b). *J. Cell Biol.* **23**, 54A.
Luft, J. H. (1965a). *In* "The Inflammatory Process" (B. W. Zweifach, L. Grant, and R. T. McCluskey, eds.), pp. 121–159. Academic Press, New York.
Luft, J. H. (1965b). *J. Cell Biol.* **27**, 61A.
Luft, J. H. (1966). *Fed. Proc., Fed. Amer. Soc. Exp. Biol.* **25**, 1773.
Luft, J. H. (1971a). *Anat. Rec.* **171**, 347.
Luft, J. H. (1971b). *Anat. Rec.* **171**, 369.
Majno, G. (1965). *In* "Handbook of Physiology" (Amer. Physiol. Soc., J. Field, ed.), Sect. 2, Vol. III, pp. 2293–2375. Williams & Wilkins, Baltimore, Maryland.
Majno, G., and Palade, G. E. (1961). *J. Biophys. Biochem. Cytol.* **11**, 571.

Majno, G., Palade, G. E., and Schoefl, G. I. (1961). *J. Biophys. Biochem. Cytol.* **11**, 607.

Majno, G., Shea, S. M., and Leventhal, M. (1969). *J. Cell Biol.* **42**, 647.

Mankin, H. J., and Lippiello, L. (1969). *J. Bone Joint Surg., Amer. Vol.* **51**, 1591.

Mathews, M. B. (1967). *In* "The Connective Tissue" (B. Wagner and D. Smith, eds.), pp. 304–329. Williams & Wilkins, Baltimore, Maryland.

Maul, G. G. (1971). *J. Ultrastruct. Res.* **36**, 768.

Mayerson, H. S., Wolfram, C. G., Shirley, H. H., and Wasserman, K. (1960). *Amer. J. Physiol.* **198**, 155.

Mayor, H. D., Hampton, J. C., and Rosario, B. (1961). *J. Biophys. Biochem. Cytol.* **9**, 909.

Mees, G. C., and Weatherley, P. E. (1957). *Proc. Roy. Soc., Ser. B* **147**, 381.

Moore, D. H., and Ruska, H. (1957). *J. Biophys. Biochem. Cytol.* **3**, 457.

Mueller, P., and Rudin, D. O. (1963). *J. Theor. Biol.* **4**, 268.

Myers, D. B., Highton, T. C., and Rayns, D. G. (1969). *J. Ultrastruct. Res.* **28**, 203.

Nickel, E., and Grieshaber, E. (1969). *Z. Zellforsch. Mikrosk. Anat.* **95**, 445.

Palade, G. E. (1953). *J. Appl. Phys.* **24**, 1424.

Palade, G. E. (1960). *Anat. Rec.* **136**, 254.

Palade, G. E. (1961). *Circulation* **24**, 368.

Palade, G. E., and Bruns, R. R. (1968). *J. Cell Biol.* **37**, 633.

Pappas, G. D., and Tennyson, V. M. (1962). *J. Cell Biol.* **15**, 227.

Pappenheimer, J. R. (1953). *Physiol. Rev.* **33**, 387.

Pappenheimer, J. R., Renkin, E. M., and Borrero, L. M. (1951). *Amer. J. Physiol.* **167**, 13.

Pappenheimer, J. R., Yudilevich, D., Ussing, H., Renkin, E., and Johnson, J. (1970). *In* "Capillary Permeability" (C. Crone and N. A. Lassen, eds.), pp. 287–288. Academic Press, New York.

Pease, D. C. (1960). *Electron Microsc., Proc. Int. Congr., 4th 1958* pp. 139–158.

Pease, D. C. (1966). *J. Ultrastruct. Res.* **15**, 555.

Perl, W. (1971). *Microvasc. Res.* **3**, 233.

Prothero, J., and Burton, A. C. (1961). *Biophys. J.* **1**, 565.

Reese, T. S., and Karnovsky, M. J. (1967). *J. Cell Biol.* **34**, 207.

Renkin, E. M. (1964). *Physiologist* **7**, 13.

Renkin, E. M., and Garlick, D. G. (1970). *In* "Capillary Permeability" (C. Crone and N. A. Lassen, eds.), pp. 553–559 and 564–568. Academic Press, New York.

Revel, J.-P., and Karnovsky, M. J. (1967). *J. Cell Biol.* **33**, C7.

Robertson, J. D. (1960). *Progr. Biophys. Biophys. Chem.* **10**, 343.

Rouget, C. (1873). *C. R. Acad. Sci.* **79**, 559.

Sabatini, D. D., Bensch, K., and Barrnett, R. J. (1963). *J. Cell Biol.* **17**, 19.

Schiller, S., Mathews, M. B., Cifonelli, J. A., and Dorfman, A. (1956). *J. Biol. Chem.* **218**, 139.

Schoefl, G. I. (1964). *Ann. N. Y. Acad. Sci.* **116**, 789.

Shea, S. M., and Karnovsky, M. J. (1966). *Nature (London)* **212**, 353.

Sjöstrand, F. S. (1962). *In* "The Interpretation of Ultrastructure" (R. J. C. Harris, ed.), pp. 47–67. Academic Press, New York.

Sjöstrand, F. S. (1963). *J. Ultrastruct. Res.* **8**, 517.

Starling, E. H. (1896). *J. Physiol. (London)* **19**, 312.

Starling, E. H. (1909). "The Fluids of the Body." Keener, Chicago, Illinois.

Stehbens, W. E. (1963). *Quart. J. Exp. Physiol. Cog. Med. Sci.* **48**, 324.

Stehbens, W. E., and Florey, H. (1960). *Quart. J. Exp. Physiol. Cog. Med. Sci.* **45**, 252.

Stoeckenius, W. (1962). *Circulation* **26**, 1066.

Stoeckenius, W., and Engelman, D. M. (1969). *J. Cell Biol.* **42**, 613.

Szubinska, B., and Luft, J. H. (1971). *Anat. Rec.* **171**, 417.

Ti Tien, H., and Diana, A. L. (1968). *Chem. Phys. Lipids* **2**, 55.

Träuble, H. (1971). *J. Membrane Biol.* **4**, 193.

Weatherley, P. E., and Johnson, R. P. (1968). *Int. Rev. Cytol.* **24**, 149.

Weinstein, R. S., and McNutt, N. S. (1970). *In* "Microcirculation, Perfusion and Transplantation of Organs" (T. Malinin, *et al.*, eds.), pp. 23–38. Academic Press, New York.

Wessells, N. K., Spooner, B. S., Ash, J. F., Bradley, M. O., Luduena, M. A., Taylor, E. L., Wrenn, J. T., and Yamada, K. M. (1971). *Science* **171**, 135.

Wissig, S. L. (1958). *Anat. Rec.* **130**, 467.

Wolff, J. (1966). *Z. Zellforsch. Mikrosk. Anat.* **73**, 143.

Yamada, E. (1955a). *J. Biophys. Biochem. Cytol.* **1**, 445.

Yamada, E. (1955b). *J. Biophys. Biochem. Cytol.* **1**, 551.

Yamamoto, T. (1963). *J. Cell Biol.* **17**, 413.

Zimmermann, K. W. (1923). *Z. Anat. Entwicklungsgesch.* **68**, 29.

Zugibe, F. T. (1963). *J. Histochem. Cytochem.* **11**, 35.

Chapter 3

CAPILLARY PERMEABILITY

II. Physiological Considerations

CHRISTIAN CRONE

I. Introduction

The function of the capillaries is to permit intimate contact between the two compartments of the extracellular space: a stirred compartment, the plasma, and an unstirred compartment, the interstitial fluid. The system must be designed to make this contact as efficient as possible, while at the same time securing a constant partition of the extracellular spaces between the two sides of the capillary membrane. A great many influences contribute to the net transfer of fluid between the two compartments, and it has become clear that pressure-regulating mechanisms operate at the level of the small vessels (arterioles and venules) to ensure constant fractional distribution of the extracellular fluid (Mellander and Folkow, 1960).

The general concept is that the capillaries *sensu strictu* behave passively under all circumstances, but the issue is not definitely settled. Recently, filamentous structures have been demonstrated in capillary endothelium which might give the cell power to change shape (Bensch *et al.*, 1964).

In any case, it is the net transcapillary pressure gradient which determines bulk fluid movement across the capillary wall, while the transcapillary concentration gradient determines net transport of solutes. It is one of the goals of capillary physiology to obtain reliable measurements of these parameters in various tissues under physiological circumstances. A difficulty arises because of major experimental shortcomings when one attempts to describe events in capillaries in strict physicochemical terms. First, the structure is extremely delicate, and only in a few instances has it been possible to perform experiments on single capillaries, although considerable progress is being made. Second, even when information is obtained from single capillaries, this knowledge is not easily translated into useful information with respect to transport in a whole organ under physiological circumstances.

The mental trick we use to translate events in single capillaries into events in whole organs is the concept of a "single capillary" model. This is an abstraction which states that the capillary bed of an organ is composed of a multitude of equally sized and spaced capillaries with equal pressures and permeabilities which is surrounded by similar "tissue cylinders." How far this picture is from reality is not known, but everyone who has examined living capillaries under a microscope has a vivid impression of obvious heterogeneities with respect to the above-mentioned parameters.

Studies on either single capillaries or whole organs over the last 20–30 years have provided us with a wealth of quantitative data. These data have led to a general understanding of capillary transport processes.

In order not to let this general useful picture vanish among the many problems and unsolved details which intrigue the capillary physiologist, a rough outline of present day concepts of capillary permeability will be given first.

II. General Outline of Capillary Permeability

Because of the nature of the capillary wall, i.e., a structure composed of cells and cellular interspaces (interendothelial clefts), transport can take place either through the endothelial cells or through the interspaces. Bulk transport of fluid due to hydrostatic and osmotic forces probably occurs mainly through the interspaces because of the small hydraulic conductivity of the cell surfaces as compared to the clefts. If fluid transfer takes place as Poiseuille flow, the resistance would be small in the interspaces because of their large dimensions (40- to 100-Å diameter) as compared to the dimensions (6- to 8-Å diameter) of the hydrophilic pathways (pores) in the endothelial cell membranes themselves.

The forces determining net fluid transfer are the hydrostatic pressure difference across the capillary wall and the osmotic pressure difference. Only the first parameter can change rapidly, and, therefore, the intracapillary hydrostatic pressure is by far the most important factor influencing transcapillary fluid movements. The intracapillary hydrostatic pressure is, under most physiological circumstances, mainly dependent on the venous pressure which is transmitted passively to the capillary. There is no mechanism which can "protect" a capillary from changes in venous hydrostatic pressure. At the entrance of the capillary, a precapillary sphincter (Zweifach, 1961) governs the fraction of arterial pressure which is transmitted to the capillary (Fig. 1). This sphincter is under influence of the sympathetic nervous system, but it is also affected by several, mostly unknown, local chemi-

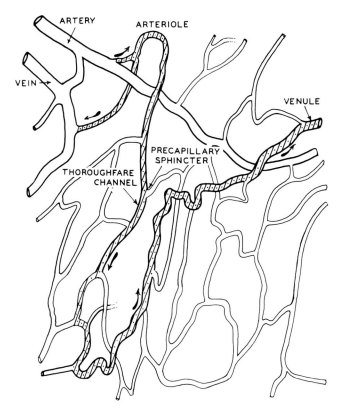

Fig. 1. Schematic tracing of capillary bed indicating terminology for different structural components. The preferential pathway for the microcirculation is shaded. Also indicated is a direct anastomosis between a small arteriole and its adjacent venule—a so-called arteriovenous anastomosis. (From Zweifach, 1961.)

cal substances (see Chapters 8 and 9). The sympathetic innervation is responsible for the adjustment of the microcirculation to the general blood pressure regulating mechanisms. The local factors serve the immediate interests of the tissue.

Osmotic pressure differences across the capillary wall are due not only to proteins, but also to small hydrophilic solutes which transiently affect transcapillary fluid distribution. This latter feature is especially relevant during muscular work when the production of lactic acid in the tissue leads to fluid movement into working muscles at the same time that fluid is being dragged out of organs with less permeable capillaries (Lundvall *et al.*, 1970).

In a general description of transcapillary transport processes, the emphasis should be laid upon *transport by diffusion*, in contrast to the above-described convective transport due to pressure differences.

It was shown by Kruhøffer (1946) that diffusion is by far the most important mode of transporting the substances which are really relevant in capillary physiology: small hydrophilic molecules and gases. The paracapillary circulation plays virtually no role in either nutrition of tissue or in removing cellular waste products.

When considering the diffusion processes taking place across the capillary wall, it is again useful to distinguish between the endothelial cell moiety of the wall and the intercellular gaps. The hydrophilic solutes (glucose, amino acids, lipoproteins, polypeptides, proteins) appear to pass through these gaps to and from the parenchymal cells. The lipophilic substances, first and foremost the respiratory gases, O_2 and CO_2, use the entire capillary surface and, thus, have an enormous advantage over the hydrophilic substances. By some curious freak of nature, the most hydrophilic molecule, water (H_2O), shares with the lipophilic gases the ability to diffuse via the entire endothelial surface. This is probably because of the extremely small size of the water molecule which allows it to sneak in between the lipids in the cell membrane. It is interesting to note that the two end products of oxidative metabolism, CO_2 and water, meet virtually no hindrance on their way back to plasma and red cells (the bicarbonate moiety, of course, does).

The passage of proteins across the capillary wall via the interendothelial gaps is severely restricted, and current investigations leave unknown the extent to which the intraendothelial vesicles contribute to the transport of large molecules.

III. Modes of Transport through Capillary Walls

Transport across capillaries appears to be a purely passive process. The following modes of transport must be considered: (a) diffusion; (b) filtration and osmosis; and (c) vesicular transport.

A. Diffusion

The energy that moves solutes in diffusion processes is the inherent kinetic energy which allows molecules and ions in solution move randomly. Whenever concentration differences exist, there is a mass transfer toward regions with lower concentrations. The force which is responsible for the net transfer is the concentration gradient, and the flux of solutes is proportional to the negative concentration gradient as expressed in Fick's first law of diffusion,

$$J_D = -D \frac{dc}{dx} \tag{1}$$

where J_D equals flux is the mass which passes through a unit of area in a unit of time (moles per cm^2 per second); dc/dx is the concentration gradient; and D is the diffusion coefficient (cm^2 per second).

Equation (1) is applicable only under time-invariant steady state conditions. If the concentration gradient varies with time, the diffusion process is described by a second order differential equation, Fick's second law of diffusion;

$$\frac{\partial c}{\partial t} = D\left(\frac{\partial^2 c}{\partial x^2}\right) \tag{2}$$

where c is a function of both length (x) and time (t). There are numerous solutions to Eq. (2) according to specific boundary conditions.

Several important papers have been published which analyze diffusion processes in tissue. Krogh, in 1919, conceived the idea of what was later called the Krogh cylinder. This concept makes it possible to establish a mathematical model, the consequences of which can be compared with experiments. In this way, Krogh managed to submit capillary–tissue exchange processes to numerical treatment—an enormous step forward toward making capillary physiology quantitative. Since I do not intend to consider diffusion in tissues, but only transcapillary transport, I shall only refer to the most important contributions in this area: Hill (1928), Blum (1960), Thews (1960), Johnson and Wilson (1966), and Reneau *et al.* (1967).

In regard to diffusion processes, Einstein (1905) from first principles deduced that the average displacement is equal to $\sqrt{2Dt}$. It is well known that diffusion processes are very efficient over short distances (of the order of microns). Table I gives examples of mean displacements of sucrose molecules diffusing from a finite source.

Table II contains selected values for diffusion coefficients and molecular weights of substances which are often considered in investigations on capillary permeability.

TABLE I

DISTRIBUTION AFTER 1 HOUR OF DIFFUSION OF
1,000,000 SUCROSE MOLECULES DIFFUSING FROM
A VERY THIN LAYER AT THE BOTTOM OF A
CYLINDRICAL VESSEL[a]

Distance from the bottom of the vessel (mm)	Number of Molecules
0–1	453,500
1–2	318,700
2–3	157,350
3–4	54,590
4–5	13,290
5–6	2,280
6–7	170
over 7	20

[a]After Jacobs (1935).

Experiments on capillary transport can sometimes be carried out under near steady state conditions; i.e., the concentration gradient across the capillary wall can be considered constant in time. This is especially permissible when dealing with substances which meet a significant hindrance in the capillary wall. The system can, under these circumstances, be treated as a two-compartment system, where the concentration drop lies within the membrane, while the two compartments behave as well-stirred pools. Under these conditions, it is permissible to assume that the concentration gradient is zero or near zero in the compartments (capillary blood and tissue), while

TABLE II

FREE DIFFUSION COEFFICIENTS IN WATER AT 25°C $(D_{25}^{0})^{a}$

Molecule	$D_{25}^{0} \times 10^{5}$ (cm^{2} sec^{-1})	Reference
THO	2.44	Wang et al. (1953)
Urea	1.38	Longsworth (1954)
Glycerol	0.97	Thovert (1914)
Glucose	0.67	Longsworth (1954)
Sucrose	0.52	Gosting and Morris (1949)
Inulin	0.16	Bunim et al. (1937)

[a]After Kampp (1970).

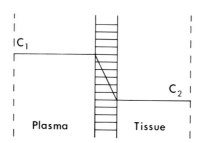

Fig. 2. Quasistationary flow through membrane (capillary wall) separating two stirred compartments (plasma and tissue). Constant gradient within membrane.

it is significant within the capillary membrane. Figure 2 illustrates this situation. It is permissible to express the gradient, the driving force, as the concentration difference across the membrane divided by the thickness of the membrane. This approximation was used by Krogh and Krogh (1910), in an analysis of the oxygen capacity of lungs, by Pappenheimer *et al.* (1951), in their analysis of transcapillary diffusion, and by Crone (1961, 1963), in an analysis of data obtained by means of the "indicator diffusion" technique.

When analyzing transcapillary transport by means of Fick's first law of diffusion, the basic equation is

$$J_D = PA\,\Delta c \tag{3}$$

where $P(= D/\Delta x)$ is the permeability coefficient (cm sec^{-1}), and A is the capillary surface area.

This equation makes it possible to calculate the permeability coefficient if the unidirectional flux across the capillary membrane can be determined and if the surface area and concentration difference across the membrane are known. If the area is included in P, this figure changes dimension from cm

TABLE III

ESTIMATED CAPILLARY SURFACE AREA PER GRAM OF TISSUE

Organ	Capillary surface area (cm²/gm)	Reference
Brain	240	Crone (1963)
Muscle (resting)	70	Crone (1963)
Myocardium	500	Schafer and Johnson (1964)
Lung	250	Crone (1963)
Kidney (cortex)	350	Crone (1963)

$\sec^{-1}$ to $\mathrm{cm^3\ sec^{-1}}$, and it now expresses the capillary diffusion capacity of a whole organ. This application of Fick's law is basic to the study of alveolar gas exchange. Although capillary surface areas are not known with any degree of certainty, it is nevertheless of interest to know the order of magnitude with which one is dealing, and Table III is a collection of figures mainly from anatomical studies. As a rule of thumb, the capillary surface area is about 100–400 $\mathrm{cm^2}$ per gram of tissue.

In experiments which are designed to determine the capillary permeability for a given molecular species, the real difficulty lies in the estimation of the concentration difference across the capillary membrane. The reason for this is that it is not possible to sample fluid from the immediate vicinity outside the capillary. Three separate solutions to this experimental dilemma have been proposed:

1. Application of a gas, the tension of which is extremely small due to its extremely high affinity for blood. Such a gas, CO, was proposed by Bohr (1909) for determination of permeability of the alveolar membrane.

2. The single injection technique (Crone, 1963) takes advantage of the initial, steeply rising intracapillary concentration after a fast intra-arterial injection. During this phase, the transcapillary concentration can, with some safety, be disregarded when substances with a comparatively low permeability are studied.

3. Pappenheimer et al. (1951) calculated the transcapillary concentration difference (Δc) via its osmotic equivalent ($\Delta \pi$) using van't Hoff's law.

$$\Delta \pi = RT\ \Delta c \qquad (4)$$

Once a method is available for determination of the transcapillary concentration difference, it becomes possible to obtain capillary permeability coefficients experimentally.

Before proceding with experimental methods for studying diffusion through capillaries, an account of filtration and osmosis in capillaries is given.

B. Filtration and Osmosis

Why does fluid remain within capillaries when the walls are permeable to water and a hydrostatic pressure is present? This enigma was solved by Starling (1896), seemingly once and forever. He realized that the only explanation was the presence of another force of similar magnitude acting in the opposite direction. The intracapillary pressure in most tissues lies between 10 and 30 mm Hg, and the osmotic pressure exerted by plasma proteins is about 25 mm Hg, so the two forces are of the same order of magnitude.

Starling's concept of fluid balance in the capillaries is formulated in Eq. (5),

$$J_w = K_f [(P_c - P_T) - (\pi_c - \pi_T)] \qquad (5)$$

where J_w is the filtration flow; K_f is the filtration coefficient; P_c is intra-capillary hydrostatic pressure; P_T is tissue fluid hydrostatic pressure; π_c is colloid osmotic pressure of capillary plasma; and π_T is colloid osmotic pressure of tissue fluid.

Only when the value of the bracketed material is zero is there no net flow across the capillary wall. However, since the pressure drops along the length of the capillary, the value of the material may be positive at the arterial end of the capillary and below zero on the venous end. There is, therefore, a con-tinuous flow of fluid out of and into capillaries, despite the fact that the net flow may be quite small.

Landis (1927) was the first to put Starling's idea to an experimental test in experiments carried out on single capillaries in frog mesentery. Landis determined the intracapillary hydrostatic pressure and the colloid osmotic pressure of frog plasma. The intracapillary hydrostatic pressure varied over a wide range, and the resultant fluid movement out of or into the capillary was quantified by observing the linear velocity of blood corpuscles. This linear velocity was transformed into volume flow, and it appeared that within a short time there was a linear relationship between movement of corpuscles and capillary pressure. The slope of the line relating fluid passage to capil-lary pressure gave the filtration coefficient.

Pappenheimer and Soto-Rivera (1948) took the theme up again in experi-ments on cats and verified Starling's concepts in an elegant series of experi-ments in which they indirectly determined the intracapillary pressure at which no net movement at fluid occurred (where the weight of the prepara-tion remained constant). When the colloid osmotic pressure in the perfusate was varied over a wide range, it was found that there was a linear relationship between isogravimetric capillary pressure and colloid osmotic pressure of the perfusate. The osmotic pressure of the plasma proteins was about 2 mm Hg higher than the isogravimetric pressure, which was taken as evidence that the tissue fluid proteins exerted a slight colloid osmotic effect. The hydrostatic pressure of the tissue fluid was disregarded.

In other experiments, intracapillary pressure was increased. The filtration coefficient thus determined was found to be of the order of 0.01 ml/minute per 100 gm of tissue at a net pressure difference of 1 mm Hg. Figure 3 shows values from Pappenheimer and Soto-Rivera's filtration experiments.

It has been frequently suggested that outward filtration at the arterial end of a capillary is important for transport of low molecular weight solutes to the tissues. Such an assumption is basically incorrect, as indicated by the following simple quantitative example. If the intracapillary pressure in

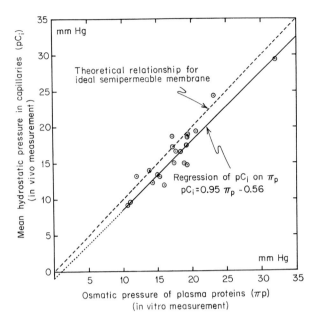

Fig. 3. The effective osmotic pressure of the plasma proteins in the hindlimb capillaries of cats and dogs. The mean hydrostatic pressure in the capillaries required to prevent net transfer of fluid is slightly less than the (*in vitro*) osmotic pressure of the plasma proteins. The mean difference between the two quantities is 1.7 mm Hg. (From Pappenheimer and Soto-Rivera, 1948.)

muscle falls from 35 to 15 mm Hg, then the average pressure driving fluid out of the capillary in the arterial half of the capillary is $(35 - 25)/2$ or 5 mm Hg. With a filtration coefficient of 0.01, this gives an outward filtration at the arterial end of the capillary which is $0.5 \times 0.01 \times 5$ ml/minute $= 0.025$ ml/minute per 100 gm. The plasma flow under resting conditions is about 2 ml/minute per 100 gm, so that only about 1% of the plasma with dissolved solutes is delivered to the tissue in this manner, which is, of course, quite insufficient for transport of nutrients.

However, if the venous pressure in the organism is increased by 10 mm Hg, about 1% of the plasma water (or 35 ml) can be transferred to the interstitial space per minute (initially). The two phases of the extracellular space are in a state of dynamic equilibrium, and rather extensive displacements can occur quite rapidly.

In recent years, basic assumptions in the Starling–Landis concept have been questioned. The assumptions which are open to contention are (1) that the permeability to water and solutes is uniform along the length of the capillary, (2) that the surface areas of the arterial and venous ends of the capillary are identical, (3) that the hydrostatic and colloid osmotic pressures of tissue fluid are negligible when compared to corresponding blood values.

Wiederhielm (1967) determined the filtration permeability of single capillaries in three locations: at the arterial end, in the middle, and at the venous end of the bed and found that the filtration coefficient at the venous end is twice that of the arterial or middle portion. Quite similar results were obtained by Intaglietta (1967). Such a gradient of permeability favors fluid reabsorption into the capillary. Careful anatomical studies indicate that the surface area of the so-called postcapillary venules are six times as large as that of the capillary itself (Wiedemann, 1963). Furthermore, the oncotic pressure of the tissue fluid is probably not insignificant, being, in many organs, about 2–5 mm Hg. This is sufficient to upset the equilibrium conditions of the classic Starling model. If to this is added the finding that the interstitial pressure may be slightly negative (Guyton, 1963), it may become somewhat of a problem to reach an equilibrium state. Wiederhielm has proposed a two-segment model (1967) in which two specific features prevent net loss of fluid. These are the larger surface areas available for reabsorption and the higher water permeability of the venous segment. The fact that the concentration of protein in the interstitial spaces is not inconsequential provides a type of buffering effect in states of increased outward filtration, because the subsequent dilution of proteins will increase the reabsorptive power at the venous ends of the system.

It should be emphasized in this context that the Starling model is a general description which should be carefully studied according to the special characteristics of each capillary area, but it must be admitted that the available knowledge is still far too limited to permit a complete quantitative treatment of even the most important capillary beds. The intracapillary pressure is lower than the above-stated values in liver sinusoids and in pulmonary capillaries in which the pressure is about 5–8 mm Hg. In kidney, in contrast, the capillary pressure is at least about 50 mm Hg. In brain, special conditions exist, as reflected in the extremely low filtration permeability in this organ (the blood–brain barrier). According to Fenstermacher and Johnson's (1966) measurement the filtration coefficient is about 0.0003 ml/minute per 100 gm of brain. Net outward filtration in the brain is further prevented by the virtually protein-free interstitial fluid.

C. Vesicular Transport

The endothelial vesicles discovered by Palade in 1953 represent a particularly interesting feature of the endothelial cell interior. These vesicles measure about 700 Å (outside diameter). They are surrounded by a membrane identical in appearance to the plasma membrane surrounding the endothelial cell. Some vesicles open onto the blood or tissue side of the cell, and, in such cases, the vesicular membrane is continuous with the endothelial plasma membrane. The number of vesicles varies with the cell region. They are most numerous at the periphery of the cell where they can occupy 25–35% of the nonnuclear volume. In a given vesicle, 55% of the volume is occupied by membrane. About 125 vesicles are found attached per square micron of surface, while the cytoplasm contains up to 600–800 vesicles per cubic micron. It has been speculated that the vesicles might form continuous tubes passing through the endothelial cell, connecting plasma with interstitial fluid. Reconstructed models of serial sections (Bruns and Palade, 1968a) do not support this contention (see Fig. 4).

The function of the vesicles remains unknown; it is, however, tempting to attribute to them the transport of large molecules from plasma to interstitial fluid. Considerable evidence favors such a role for them (Florey, 1961; Bruns and Palade, 1968b). Casley-Smith (1969) calculated that a vesicle may be attached to the endothelial cell membrane for about 2.5 seconds. The average free time of a vesicle is 1.5 seconds. It is convincingly argued that Brownian movements could account for the release of the vesicles and their movement within the cytoplasm. Vesicular transport cannot be classified, therefore, as active transport in any sense. Florey (1964), for example, found

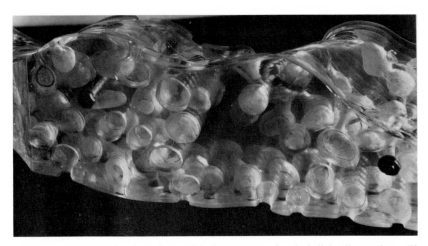

Fig. 4. Three-dimensional Lucite model of a segment of endothelial cell cytoplasm. The model represents a segment of endothelium 1.33 μm long, 0.33 μm wide, and 0.30 μm thick. It contains 98 vesicles, of which 23 open onto the blood front of the cell, 35 open on the tissue front, and 24 are completely enclosed within the cytoplasm. In the original model, this sector of endothelium was magnified × 200,000; in this figure, × 129,600. (From Bruns and Palade, 1968a.)

that neither cyanide, dinitrophenol, cooling, nor anoxia affects the speed with which vesicles take up tracer particles.

The intracellular vesicles do not contain granules as do vesicles concerned with transmitter or storage functions. They are most abundant in muscle capillaries, including heart, but are particularly scanty in lung and brain capillaries.

Bruns and Palade (1968b) found that injected ferritin molecules could be found within the endothelial cytoplasm only in vesicles. Ferritin-labeled vesicles are empty, with the particulate material accumulated along the basement membrane 10 minutes after injection.

Garlick and Renkin (1970) recently reinvestigated the transport of large molecules from blood to lymph. By establishing a constant concentration of dextrans of different molecular sizes and by subsequent collection of lymph from the hindlimb of dogs, a steady state lymph–plasma ratio could be determined. It was found that the lymph–plasma ratio drops rather sharply in the range of molecular weights between 10,000 and 40,000. The lymph–plasma ratio was essentially constant for dextrans with a molecular weight above 100,000. This is in agreement with the findings of Grotte (1956) and Mayerson (1963) who interpreted them as reflecting a double mode of transport of large molecules, in which the very large molecules pass only via special pathways, presumably by vesicular transport. It should be noted that brain endothelium contains remarkably few vesicles (Brightman and Reese, 1969), consonant with the inability of proteins to pass into brain interstitial fluid.

In the following, methods developed for studying diffusion of solutes in capillaries will be dealt with at some length because the limitations of the procedures need to be known in order to evaluate the findings.

IV. Methods for Studying Diffusion Permeability of Capillaries

A. Arterial Disappearance Curves

When various solutes are injected into the vascular system of an animal or a human subject, each disappears from the blood at different velocity. It is reasonable to expect that this velocity bears some relationship to the ease with which each permeates through the capillaries. In the 1940's, such arterial disappearance curves were studied as a means of quantifying capillary exchange processes (Flexner et al., 1942, 1948). These attempts at making capillary physiology a quantitative discipline should not be forgotten because they established that labeled, low molecular weight substances disappear from the plasma at an extremely rapid rate.

TABLE IV

EXCHANGE RATES OF VARIOUS TEST SUBSTANCES BETWEEN BLOOD AND TISSUE
DETERMINED FROM ANALYSIS OF ARTERIAL DISAPPEARANCE CURVES

Substance	Exchange rate[a] (%/minute)	Animal	Reference
D_2O	73	Guinea pig	Flexner et al. (1942)
D_2O	140	Guinea pig	Flexner et al. (1948)
^{24}Na	60	Guinea pig	Flexner et al. (1948)
^{24}Na	46–49	Rabbit	Morel (1950)
^{42}K	225	Rabbit	Walker and Wilde (1952)
^{38}Cl	64	Guinea pig	Cowie et al. (1949)
SCN^-	75	Dog	Sapirstein et al. (1955)
Mannitol	7.3	Dog	Halpern and Fritel (1952)
Inulin	3.0	Dog	Halpern and Fritel (1952)
Ferriglobulin	0.3	Guinea pig	Flexner et al. (1948)

[a]Fraction (expressed as percent) of amount in plasma exchanging with extravascular amount per minute.

Table IV compiles various estimates of transcapillary exchange rates determined from arterial disappearance curves. Early workers realized that water exchanges extremely rapidly, so that in effect all of the water in the plasma exchanges every minute. In 1940, Hevesy and Jacobsen found in experiments on rabbits that D_2O equilibrated with the total extracellular space (as they expressed it) in less than a minute. The results from arterial disappearance curves must be taken with a grain of salt today, but they express the essence of a basic fact which frequently gets lost in all too refined and sophisticated studies.

B. Osmotic Transient Technique

If material is not introduced into the blood in tracer amounts, a disturbance of the osmotic conditions arises, and water is drawn into the blood. The time course of this osmotic effect will, among other factors, depend on the rate with which the molecular species passes from blood into interstitial tissue. Hence, if the time course of blood dilution is followed, some information concerning transcapillary diffusion should be gained. This method was actually used by Keys (1937), but the results were quite imprecise. Out of these early studies, there arose, as a kind of hybrid, the osmotic transient technique which, in the hands of Pappenheimer and colleagues (1951), served as a very powerful tool. It once and for all transformed the study of transcapillary diffusion processes into a quantitative discipline. A thorough account of the theory has been given in several articles (Pappenheimer *et al.*, 1951; Pappenheimer, 1953, 1970; Renkin and Pappenheimer, 1957; Landis and Pappenheimer, 1963). Only a short version is presented here.

Once it was recognized that a weakness in the study of arterial disappearance curves was the fact that the average intracapillary concentration was unknown (at any rate, not identical with the arterial concentration because material is being lost during the passage through the capillary), Pappenheimer attacked this problem. He was able to measure the transcapillary concentration gradient due to added solutes by counteracting the osmotic force with an increased intracapillary hydrostatic pressure so that the weight of the preparation remained constant. In cases where the reflection coefficient of the solute is unity (i.e., the membrane acts as a perfect semipermeable membrane toward the test solute), van't Hoff's law applies, and, via the equivalence of osmotic pressure and an increment in hydrostatic pressure, the average concentration difference across the capillaries in the organ (muscle) can be calculated.

The following equations give the main points of the formal description of the transient osmotic technique,

$$J_D = F\,(c_a - c_v) \tag{6}$$

where F is flow of perfusate through the organ; J_D is the net transport of solute out of the capillaries; c_a is concentration of test solute at the entrance; and c_v is concentration of test solute at the outlet.

By combining Eqs. (3), (4), and (6), the following expression is obtained.

$$P = \frac{F(c_a - c_v)\,RT}{A\Delta\pi} \tag{7}$$

The actual rise in intracapillary mean pressure was calculated from the rise in venous pressure necessary to counteract fluid movement from extravascular regions to blood (isogravimetric conditions). No account seems to have been given of how to correct for the changes in blood volume (and, therefore, weight of the preparation) which occur when outflow resistance is increased. The venous pressure had to be readjusted during the experiment when the test solutes diffused out of the capillaries. One snag in the experiments is obvious: to exert its full osmotic pressure, the test substance must not be able to pass through the capillary membrane, which it, of course, does. It was tacitly assumed that the reflection coefficient was close to 1. This point in the methodology has been criticized several times (Ussing, 1953; Grim, 1953; Kedem and Katchalsky, 1958; Johnson, 1970). Very important equations dealing with the situation when the test solutes are not totally reflected by the capillary membranes (reflection coefficient below 1) have been derived by Lifson (1970).

TABLE V
PERMEABILITY OF MAMMALIAN MUSCLE CAPILLARIES TO LIPID-INSOLUBLE
MOLECULES[a]

Substance	Approximate molecular radius (cm × 10^8)	Permeability coefficient (cm sec^{-1} × 10^5)
H_2O	1.5	28
NaCl	2.3	15
Urea	2.6	14
Glucose	3.7	6
Sucrose	4.8	4
Raffinose	5.7	3
Inulin	12–15	0.3
Myoglobin	19	0.1
Serum albumin	36	0.001

[a] After Landis and Pappenheimer (1963).

The results obtained by Pappenheimer and co-workers are tabulated in Table V. An important feature of the Table is the fact that the permeability decreases faster than the free diffusion coefficient, which suggests that diffusion is partly restricted in the capillary wall. Not only is the passage via the interendothelial clefts not analgous to free diffusion, but the effective pore area for free diffusion decreases with the increasing molecular size. The total pore area which permits passage of hydrophilic molecules is obtained by extrapolating the data to a fictitious molecule the size of water. When this area is inserted into Eq. (8), a so-called pore radius is obtained,

$$\text{pore radius} = \sqrt{\frac{K_f(8\eta)}{A_p/\Delta x}} \tag{8}$$

where K_f is the filtration coefficient of the preparation; η is the viscosity of isotonic saline; A_p is the calculated total pore area (for water); and Δx is the thickness of the capillary wall. Values of about 30–60 Å were calculated.

Further calculation led to an estimated pore number of 10^9 per square centimeter. The fractional pore area was about 0.1% of the whole surface.

The interesting conclusion from Pappenheimer's experiments was that diffusion of hydrophilic solutes across a very small fraction of the capillary surface is sufficient for the nourishment of tissues.

What do the endothelial cells contribute? Very little is known about this, but, at the very least, they give the capillaries a length dimension which is necessary in order to allow the blood flow through the tissue to establish contact with a reasonable number of tissue cells. The permeability characteristics of the endothelial membrane per se is, for the most, part unknown.

C. Osmotic Determination of Reflection Coefficient

Vargas and Johnson (1964) determined the reflection coefficient (σ) for various hydrophilic molecules in heart capillaries. They followed the weight change of a perfused heart suspended on a force transducer after a step change of osmolality of the perfusion fluid. The addition of osmotically active solutes leads to a flow of water from tissue to perfusate, which can be expressed by the following equation,

$$J_w = K_f(\Delta P - \Delta \pi) \tag{9}$$

where J_w is flow of water across capillary, and the other symbols have their usual meanings. Introducing the reflection coefficient, σ, the equation can be written,

$$J_w = K_f(\Delta P - \sigma RT \Delta c) \tag{10}$$

from which follows

$$\sigma = \frac{J_w}{K_f \Delta c RT} \tag{11}$$

The filtration coefficient, K_f, was determined in experiments with albumin as the osmotic agent. Albumin has a reflection coefficient of 1. The concentration difference of solute across the capillary wall, Δc, was, in this case, made equal to the arterial concentration of the test substance at the start of the experiment. This is permissible because the perfusate flow was extremely high, i.e., the concentration on the tissue side of the capillary of the test

TABLE VI

REFLECTION COEFFICIENTS OF FOUR
NONELECTROLYTES IN HEART CAPILLARIES[a]

Molecule	Reflection coefficient, σ, $\pm$ SEM
Urea	0.10 ± 0.01
Sucrose	0.30 ± 0.01
Raffinose	0.38 ± 0.02
Inulin	0.69 ± 0.03

[a]From Vargas and Johnson (1964).

solute is thought to be zero during the initial phase of the experiment. Table VI lists results from this kind of experiment.

Through the use of curve-fitting procedures, values for pore size in heart capillaries could be obtained from the measured values of reflection coefficients. An equivalent pore radius was 35 Å, essentially in agreement with Pappenheimer's figures, the fact notwithstanding that the two authors used different reflection coefficients. It is not at all clear why methods which involve quite different reflection coefficients can yield the same pore radii. An approach to the problem is seen in a discussion between Pappenheimer and Johnson in the book "Capillary Permeability" (Crone and Lassen, 1970).

D. Indicator Diffusion Technique

The theory for this methodology was originally worked out by Crone (1961, 1963) and was later dealt with by Martin and Yudilevich (1964), Goresky et al. (1970), and Levitt (1970). The method analyzes the outflow curves from an organ in response to a unit input into the artery leading to the organ. The injectate contains a nondiffusible reference substance and a diffusible test solute.

A starting point in modeling was a material balance stating that the rate of loss of material from a whole capillary from inflow to outflow will equal the product of flow and the arteriovenous concentration difference, or, equivalent, the product of the flow, arterial concentration, and extraction, i.e.,

$$J_D = F(c_a - c_v) = Fc_a E \qquad (12)$$

where J_D equals rate of transcapillary loss of material; F is capillary flow rate; c_a is arterial concentration; c_v is venous concentration; and E equals $(c_a - c_v)/c_a$.

The rate of loss may be expressed as the product of the permeability (P), the capillary surface area (A), and the average transcapillary concentration difference (Δc), i.e.,

$$J_D = PA \, \Delta C \qquad (13)$$

One of the main assumptions of the single injection technique is that there is no back-diffusion during the initial phase of the passage of the injected bolus. Under these circumstances, the rate of loss from the capillary is proportional to the concentration remaining inside the capillary at each point along the length. If the velocity is uniform, the corresponding intracapillary concentration profile is one of exponential decline along the length. In the time domain, the expression for the venous concentration becomes $c_v =$

$c_a e^{-\alpha\tau}$, where α is an assumed rate constant describing the exponential decline in concentration, and τ is the transit time through the capillary. The average concentration inside the vessel, $\bar{c}$, is then

$$\bar{c} = \frac{1}{\tau} \int_0^\tau c_a \, \exp(-\alpha\tau) \, dt \tag{14}$$

$\bar{c}$ is then put equal to Δc, and the equations are solved for α and the product, $\alpha\tau$. The following result is obtained

$$c_v = c_a e^{-PA/F} \tag{15}$$

$$P = -\frac{F}{A} \ln(1 - E) \tag{16}$$

This equation, which combines the most important parameters that influence capillary undirectional extraction (tracer experiments), requires that several conditions be fulfilled for it to be used properly. The main condition deals with the above-mentioned assumption of no back-diffusion during the early passage of the test bolus. Stated differently, permeability can only be calculated for those substances to which the capillary membrane offers a resonable degree of resistance.

In effect, the wall shows a graded increase in permeability from large protein molecules, to small hydrophilic molecules, to lipid-soluble gases. Lipid-soluble gases and similar substances meet so little resistance in the capillary membrane that the blood leaving the capillary is in "equilibrium" with the tissue. "Equilibrium" means that there is a maximal degree of back-diffusion from tissue to capillary during a single passage. The single injection method is not applicable for such substances (including water). These substances are commonly denoted "flow-limited," because the rate of delivery of material to the tissue is wholly dependent on the flow rate. It is not possible to measure the capillary permeability to such substances; rather, the tissue uptake serves as an expression of flow (Kety, 1949; Lassen, 1967).

The indicator diffusion technique or single injection technique is applicable to the exchange of substances with a moderate permeability. It is, of course, not possible to state in absolute terms what is meant by moderate permeability, but the dimensionless parameter PA/F is a valuable means for classifying test molecules under given experimental conditions. This statement will become clear if one inspects Eq. (15). When PA/F is zero, then c_v equals c_a, i.e., there is no loss during the capillary transit. The substance in question is totally barrier limited. If, on the other hand, PA/F is very large, c_v becomes very low relative to c_a, and back-diffusion is large. Table VII compiles the drop in intracapillary concentration at four values of PA/F. The corresponding values for the extraction (E) are also calculated. As a rule

TABLE VII

CORRESPONDING VALUES OF PA/F, E, AND c_v/c_a [a,b]

PA/F	E	c_v/c_a
0.1	0.1	0.9
0.3	0.25	0.75
1.0	0.6	0.4
5.0	0.99	0.01

[a] See text for explanation.
[b] All figures are dimensionless.

of thumb, only when the extraction is 0.3 or less is it permissible to use the indicator diffusion technique to obtain capillary permeabilities quantitatively.

This restriction probably applies to all known quantitative methods of determining capillary permeability, but it is rarely stated explicitly. The above-mentioned studies by Goresky *et al.* (1970) and Levitt (1970) are particularly informative, but the reader is also referred to the study of Renkin (1955) in which the dependence of the PA product on flow was investigated.

What happens in a single injection experiment when the indicator bolus has traveled through the vascular network and has delivered its content to

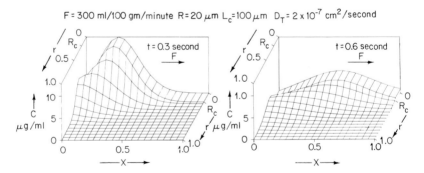

Fig. 5. Concentration profiles in capillary and tissue when exchange is diffusion limited. Three-dimensional picture of computer-simulated model of capillary–tissue exchange. Left figure represents the concentration matrix 0.3 second after introduction of a brief pulse at the input of a capillary. Right figure shows situation 0.6 seconds after input. The intracapillary concentration is represented by the hindmost squares, the "tissue" is seen in front of that. (After Bassingthwaighte *et al.*, 1970.)

the tissue? This has been studied by Bassingthwaighte *et al.* (1970) in computer simulation experiments with single Krogh cylinders. Figure 5 shows that the concentration map is much more complicated than generally recognized.

The figure stresses the fact that tissue exchange at the capillary level is a multitude of events distributed in time and space. Inasmuch as a full description of the events can be obtained only by using partial differential equations to formulate the problems, the formalism soon goes beyond the domain of the ordinary physiologist or clinician. The reader is referred to the earlier mentioned authors for further reading.

A wealth of quantitative data have appeared over the last 10 years from studies with the single injection technique, and Table VIII contains data collected from various sources. Notice how very much smaller the permeability of brain capillaries is when compared with muscle or myocardial capillaries (about ten times smaller). The simplest explanation for this difference is that the interendothelial cleft in muscle capillaries is about 40–60 Å, while, in brain capillaries, it is 10–15 Å (with circumferential tight junctions between the endothelial cells). Such interendothelial pathways do not always permit solutes with a molecular weight as low as 2000 to pass, which is another indication of the special design of the cerebral capillaries (Brightman and Reese, 1969).

Comparison of the permeability data in Tables V and VIII, as to permeability of capillaries in muscle tissue, discloses some interesting differences. The calculated permeabilities obtained with osmotic transient technique are definitely higher than those obtained with indicator diffusion technique. This is particularly obvious for the smaller hydrophilic molecules where the values are five to ten times higher. The explanation probably lies in the fact that the osmotic transient technique determines P/σ, rather than the true P (Perl, 1971). As σ approaches zero, for the small molecules, the effect can be quite large.

E. Inhomogeneity Problems

As mentioned earlier, most, if not all, studies of capillary permeability performed on whole organs—and also model studies—are based on the concept of an organ composed of a multitude of equally spaced and perfused capillaries with similar permeability characteristics. This idealization is used because of the almost insurmountable difficulties which arise when attempts are made to describe inhomogeneous conditions. A step in surmounting this difficulty may be studies of exchange between neighboring capillaries, a feature which is not contained in the single capillary organ.

TABLE VIII

PERMEABILITY COEFFICIENTS (P) AND INITIAL EXTRACTIONS (E) IN CAPILLARIES IN
MUSCLE, MYOCARDIUM, AND BRAIN[a]

Organ	Substance	P (cm sec^{-1} × 10^5)	E	References
Muscle	Inulin	0.09	0.02	Trap-Jensen and Lassen (1970)
	Inulin	0.26	0.10	Crone (1963)
	Sucrose	0.86	0.30	Trap-Jensen and Lassen (1970)
	Sucrose	0.74	0.33	Crone (1963)
	Fructose	1.3	0.38	Trap-Jensen and Lassen (1970)
	Urea	2.9	0.4	Trap-Jensen and Lassen (1970)
	^{24}Na	3.5	0.6	Trap-Jensen and Lassen (1970)
Myocardium	Inulin	0.27	0.26	Alvarez and Yudilevich (1969)
	Sucrose	0.8	0.51	Alvarez and Yudilevich (1969)
	Glucose	1.0	0.57	Alvarez and Yudilevich (1969)
	Urea	3.1	—	Alvarez and Yudilevich (1969)
	^{24}Na	>3.8	0.77	Alvarez and Yudilevich (1969)
Brain	Inulin	0	0	Crone (1965)
	Sucrose	~0	0.004	Crone (1965)
	^{36}Cl	0.04	0.01	Crone and Thompson (1970)
	^{42}K	0.08	0.02	Crone and Thompson (1970)
	Mannitol	0.12	0.03	Crone and Thompson (1970)
	Fructose	0.16	0.04	Crone (1965)
	^{24}Na	0.21	0.05	Crone and Thompson (1970)
	Glycerol	0.21	0.05	Crone (1965)
	Urea	0.44	0.11	Crone (1965)
	Antipyrin	3.3	0.56	Crone (1965)
	Ethanol	>10	0.93	Crone (1965)

[a]The values are calculated from results obtained with indicator diffusion technique in various laboratories.

Crone and Garlick (1970) studied inhomogeneity problems in a perfused gastrocnemius preparation which was equilibrated with several extracellular tracers—inulin, sucrose, and mannitol. After equilibration, perfusion with tracer-free medium was begun so that the tracers were removed progressively from the organ. Since the exchange of these substances was completely passive, it was anticipated that the fraction of material which was removed per unit of time would occur at a constant rate during the wash-out. In actual fact, this fractional rate of removal fell continuously. It was proposed that concentration gradients in the tissue might be responsible for the observation. Computer simulations by J. B. Bassingthwaighte, T. Knopp and C. Crone (unpublished) pointed, however, toward inhomogeneity as the feature responsible for the observed wash-out pattern. Inasmuch as the experimental studies dealt with barrier-limited substances, flow inhomogeneities could not be responsible. The permeability inhomogeneities and inhomogeneities of distribution volume (Krogh cylinder inhomogeneity) were most probably responsible for the experimental results. Recently, Levick and Michel (1970) obtained evidence for permeability inhomogeneities in mesenteric capillaries of the frog.

Pulmonary physiology has for a long time been plagued by inhomogeneity problems. Only time will show whether or not capillary physiology in general will also be forced to accept deviation from ideality as being physiologically important.

References

Alvarez, O. A., and Yudilevich, D. L. (1969). *J. Physiol.* (*London*) **202**, 45.

Bassingthwaighte, J. B., Knopp, T., and Hazelrig, J. B. (1970). *In* "Capillary Permeability" (C. Crone and N. A. Lassen, eds.), pp. 60–80. Academic Press, New York.

Bensch, K. G., Gordon, G. B., and Miller, L. (1964). *Z. Zellforsch. Mikrosk. Anat.* **63**, 759.

Blum, J. J. (1960). *Amer. J. Physiol.* **198**, 991.

Bohr, C. (1909). *Skand. Arch. Physiol.* **22**, 221.

Brightman, M. W., and Reese, T. S. (1969). *J. Cell. Biol.* **40**, 648.

Bruns, R. R., and Palade, G. E. (1968a). *J. Cell Biol.* **37**, 244.

Bruns, R. R., and Palade, G. E. (1968b). *J. Cell Biol.* **37**, 277.

Bunim, J. J., Smith, W. W., and Smith, H. W. (1937). *J. Biol. Chem.* **118**, 667.

Casley-Smith, J. R. (1969). *J. Microsc.* (*Oxford*) **90**, 251.

Cowie, D. B., Flexner, L. B., and Wilde, W. S. (1949). *Amer. J. Physiol.* **158**, 231.

Crone, C. (1961). "On the Diffusion of Some Non-electrolytes from Blood into Brain." Munksgaard, Copenhagen (in Danish).

Crone, C. (1963). *Acta Physiol. Scand.* **58**, 292.

Crone, C. (1965). *Acta Physiol. Scand.* **64**, 407.

Crone, C., and Garlick, D. (1970). *J. Physiol (London)* **210**, 387.

Crone, C., and Lassen, N. A., eds. (1970). "Capillary Permeability." Academic Press, New York.

Crone, C., and Thompson, A. M. (1970). *In* "Capillary Permeability" (C. Crone and N. A. Lassen, eds.), pp. 447–453. Academic Press, New York.

Einstein, A. (1905). *Ann. Phys. (Leipzig)* [4] **17**, 549.

Fenstermacher, J. D., and Johnson, J. A. (1966). *Amer. J. Physiol.* **211**, 341.

Flexner, L. B., Gellhorn, A., and Merrell, M. (1942). *J. Biol. Chem.* **144**, 35.

Flexner, L. B., Cowie, D. B., and Vosburgh, G. J. (1948). *Cold Spring Harbor Sympo. Quant. Biol.* **13**, 88.

Florey, H. W. (1961). *Proc. Roy. Soc., Ser. A* **265**, 1.

Florey, H. W. (1964). *Quart. J. Exp. Physiol. cog. Med. Sci.* **49**, 117.

Garlick, D. G., and Renkin, E. M. (1970). *Amer. J. Physiol.* **219**, 1595.

Goresky, C. A., Ziegler, W. H., and Bach, G. G. (1970). *Circ. Res.* **27**, 739.

Gosting, L. J., and Morris, M. S. (1949). *J. Amer. Chem. Soc.* **74**, 4155.

Grim, E. (1953). *Proc. Soc. Exp. Biol. Med.* **83**, 195.

Grotte, G. (1956). *Acta Chir. Scand., Suppl.* **211**, 1–84.

Guyton, A. C. (1963). *Circ. Res.* **12**, 399.

Halpern, B. N., and Fritel, D. (1952). *Acta Med. Scand.* **144**, 15.

Hevesy, G., and Jacobsen, C. F. (1940). *Acta Physiol. Scand.* **1**, 11.

Hill, A. V. (1928). *Proc. Roy. Soc. Ser. B* **104**, 39.

Intaglietta, M. (1967). *Bibl. Anat.* **9**, 465.

Jacobs, M. H. (1935). *Ergeb. Biol.* **12**, 1.

Johnson, J. A. (1970). *In* "Capillary Permeability" (C. Crone and N. A. Lassen, eds.), pp. 293–301. Academic Press, New York.

Johnson, J. A., and Wilson, T. A. (1966). *Amer. J. Physiol.* **210**, 1261.

Kampp, M. (1970). *In* "Capillary Permeability" (C. Crone and N. A. Lassen, eds.), pp. 163–170. Academic Press, New York.

Kedem, O., and Katchalsky, A. (1958). *Biochim. Biophys. Acta* **27**, 229.

Kety, S. S. (1949). *Amer. Heart J.* **38**, 321.

Keys, A. (1937). *Trans. Faraday. Soc.* **33**, 930.

Krogh, A. (1919). *J. Physiol. (London).* **52**, 409.

Krogh, A., and Krogh, M. (1910). *Skand. Arch. Physiol.* **23**, 236.

Kruhøffer, P. (1946). *Acta Physiol. Scand.* **11**, 37.

Landis, E. M. (1927). *Amer. J. Physiol.* **75**, 548.

Landis, E. M., and Pappenheimer, J. R. (1963). *In* "Handbook of Physiology" (Amer. Physiol. Soc., J. Field, ed.), Sect. 2, Vol. II, pp. 961–1034. Williams & Wilkins, Baltimore, Maryland.

Lassen, N. A. (1967). *Acta Med. Scand., Suppl.* **136**, 471.

Levick, J. R., and Michel, C. C. (1970). *J. Physiol. (London)* **211**, 37P.

Levitt, D. G. (1970). *Circ. Res.* **27**, 81.

Lifson, N. (1970). *In* "Capillary Permeability" (C. Crone and N. A. Lassen, eds.), pp. 302–305. Academic Press, New York.

Longsworth, L. G. (1954). *J. Phys. Chem.* **58**, 770.

Lundvall, J., Mellander, S., Westling, H., and White, T. (1970). *Acta Physiol. Scand.* **80**, 31A.

Martin, J. P., and Yudilevich, D. L. (1964). *Amer. J. Physiol.* **207**, 162.

Mayerson, H. S. (1963). *In* "Handbook of Physiology" (Amer. Physiol. Soc., J. Field, ed.), Sect. 2, Vol. II, pp. 1035–1073. Williams & Wilkins, Baltimore. Maryland.

Mellander, S., and Folkow, B. (1960). *Acta Physiol. Scand.* **75**, Suppl. **50**, 52.

Morel, F. F. (1950). *Helv. Physiol. Pharmacol. Acta* **8**, 146.

Palade, G. E. (1953). *J. Appl. Phys.* **24**, 1424.

Pappenheimer, J. R. (1953). *Physiol. Rev.* **33**, 387.

Pappenheimer, J. R. (1970). *In* "Capillary Permeability" (C. Crone and N. A. Lassen, eds.), pp. 278–286. Academic Press, New York.

Pappenheimr, J. R., and Soto-Rivera, A. (1948). *Amer. J. Physiol.* **152**, 471.

Pappenheimer, J. R., Renkin, E. M., and Borrero, L. M. (1951). *Amer. J. Physiol.* **167**, 13.

Perl, W. (1971). *Microvasc. Res.* **3**, 233.

Reneau, D. D., Bruley, D. F., and Knisely, M. H. (1967). *In* "Chemical Engineering in Medicine and Biology" (D. Hershey, ed.), pp. 135–341. Plenum, New York.

Renkin, E. M. (1955). *Amer. J. Physiol.* **183**, 125.

Renkin, E. M., and Pappenheimer, J. R. (1957). *Ergeb. Physiol., Biol. Chem. Exp. Pharmakol.* **49**, 59.

Sapirstein, L. O., Buckley, N. M., and Ogden, E. (1955). *Amer. J. Physiol.* **183**, 178.

Schafer, D. E., and Johnson, J. A. (1964). *Amer. J. Physiol.* **206**, 985.

Starling, E. H. (1896). *J. Physiol. (London)* **19**, 312.

Thews, G. (1960). *Pflügers Arch. Gesamte Physiol. Menschen Tiere* **268**, 197.

Thovert, M. J. (1914). *Ann. Chim. Phys.* [9] **2**, 369.

Trap-Jensen, J., and Lassen, N. A. (1970). *In* "Capillary Permeability" (C. Crone and N. A. Lassen, eds.), pp. 135–152. Academic Press, New York.

Ussing, H. H. (1953). *Annu. Rev. Physiol.* **15**, 1.

Vargas, F., and Johnson, J. A. (1964). *J. Gen. Physiol.* **47**, 667.

Walker, W. G., and Wilde, W. S. (1952). *Amer. J. Physiol.* **170**, 401.

Wang, J. H. Robinson C. V. and Edelman I. S. (1953). *J. Amer. Chem. Soc.* **75**, 466.

Wiedeman, M. P. (1963). *Circ. Res.* **12**, 375.

Wiederhielm, C. A. (1967). *In* "Physical Bases of Circulatory Transport" (E. B. Reeve and A. C. Guyton, eds.), pp. 307–326. Saunders, Philadelphia, Pennsylvania.

Zweifach, B. W. (1961). "Functional Behavior of the Microcirculation." Thomas, Springfield, Illinois.

Chapter 4

CAPILLARY PERMEABILITY
III. Connective Tissue

HUBERT R. CATCHPOLE

I. Historical Perspective

The concept of the extracellular, extravascular environment as a matrix involved in vascular transport is recent. As late as 1963, an authoritative physiological text recognized that collagen and elastic fibers and mucopolysaccharides were components of the vascular wall and possessed viscoelastic properties which were important in the stretching of the wall (Bader, 1963). However, this was the extent of their official physiological function, and they have rarely been incorporated into considerations of vascular exchange. The Starling formulation envisions the extravascular compartment as a fluid with hydrostatic and osmotic pressures. Prior to 1932, the interstitial tissue was indeed viewed as a kind of swamp occupied by a brushwork of fibers and fibrils and by interstitial fluid. However, these water-filled spaces gradually were recognized as histological shrinkage artifacts (Manery, 1954). The existence of a ground substance, which had been proposed much earlier (Flemming, 1876), gained acceptance, particularly after the ingenious experiments of Bensley (1934). She observed microscopically that flagellates (paramecia) injected subcutaneously appeared to be curiously restricted in their movement by invisible barriers. Explicit extracellular compounds were isolated from connective tissues by Karl Meyer beginning in 1934 (Meyer, 1970). The idea of a tissue matrix had meanwhile received support after the discovery of the spreading factors by Duran Reynals (1928, 1942). For if the spread of particles in the skin was enhanced by a "spreading factor," then evidently something was present which obstructed their movement in the first place.

II. Morphology and Composition of Connective Tissue

A. Cells

Cells of the connective tissue are lineal descendants of the primitive mesenchyme, and they include fixed and wandering cells (macrophages) first differentiated by the classic use of vital dyes (Evans and Scott, 1921). The fibroblast is the characteristic cell, but in specific tissues it appears in the guise of a chondroblast, an osteoblast, an odontoblast, or a synovioblast. These cells have in common the secretion of collagen, reticulin, elastin, various mucopolysaccharides, and glycoproteins. They are the proximate source of the fibrillar and nonfibrillar components of the connective tissue which are formed locally. However, they may not be the sole source of such products. Cells differentiated along different lines of ontology may contribute similar products to their own environment, e.g., lens epithelium (Dische and Zelmenis, 1966), corneal epithelium (Dodson and Hay, 1970), and skin epithelium, kidney epithelium and endothelium, and several epithelial tumors (Pierce, 1970).

B. Fibers

1. COLLAGEN FIBERS

Collagen fibers, the principal structural components of connective tissue, occur in the body as coarse bundles a few millimeters in diameter and can be seen under the electron microscope as fine fibrils with a diameter of 600 Å or less showing a banded structure with 640-Å periodicity. The fundamental chemical unit of collagen which is shared with reticulin is the tropocollagen molecule which consists of three helically wound polypeptide chains (Ramachandran, 1967). Aggregations of tropocollagen molecules "in phase" lead first to various forms of soluble collagen and finally to the relatively insoluble fibrillar collagen. The tropocollagen molecule is a rodlike structure 3000 Å long and 15 Å wide; hydrogen bonding is responsible for both its internal stability and its capacity to react externally to form bundles (cross linking). Cross links increase in number with age. Soluble forms of collagen are not visualized ultrastructurally and, for our purposes, are classified as components of the ground substance. Other compounds, particularly saccharides, may participate in fiber formation; the amount of carbohydrate forming part of the intrinsic structure of collagen may be low (0.5–1.0% in tendon collagen) or quite high (10% or more in basement membrane collagen). Collagens differ in composition from species to species, and differences become large across zoological lines. Collagens have a high content of glycine (~25%) and low amounts of the aromatic amino acids. Additionally, they contain two amino acids unique to this class of protein, hydroxyproline and hydroxylysine; extensive reviews have appeared (Gustavson, 1956; Bailey, 1968).

Native collagen is crystalline and birefringent and shows a transition point at 59°–62°C (melting point) when birefringence disappears (Engel and Catchpole, 1970).

2. RETICULAR FIBERS

About 15 years ago, the relationship of reticular to collagen fibers (the "reticulin riddle") was examined in masterly fashion (Robb-Smith, 1957). Accumulating information suggests that the riddle is a hardy perennial. Reticular fibrils do not differ from collagen ultrastructurally, but, unlike them, they tend to be branched and to remain microscopically fine. Moreover, they have a characteristic distribution. Reticular fibers show a strong but treacherous affinity for silver stains; this led to the idea that they are formed by the aggregation of tropocollagen molecules in a carbohydrate-rich matrix that is responsible for the argyrophilia. Analyses of reticulin isolated from kidney cortex showed 85% of a collagenlike protein, 4.2% carbohydrate, and 11% bound fatty acid (Windrum *et al.*, 1955). Reticular fibrils are observed in close association with basement membrane, which also contains collagen–glycoprotein components, thereby compounding the problems of separation and analysis of these entities.

3. ELASTIC FIBERS

The major component of elastic fibers is the protein elastin, characterized by the presence of two amino acids specific to it: desmosine and isodesmosine (Partridge *et al.*, 1965). These have ring structures which form bridges in a three-dimensional network. The resulting infinitely cross-linked structures are reminiscent of rubberlike polymers whose behavior they mimic. The unstretched elastic fiber is molecularly disorganized (high entropy), and the stretched fiber becomes molecularly oriented (low entropy). Elastin is the most important component of large blood vessel walls where its configurational energy is probably recovered at close to 100% efficiency.

Under the electron microscope, elastic fibers appeared amorphous at less than 15-Å resolution, but, at higher resolution, nonbanded elements arranged randomly in three dimensions appeared (Cox and O'Dell, 1966). A soluble precursor protein, tropoelastin, has been described (Smith *et al.*, 1968).

C. Ground Substance

1. MORPHOLOGY

The ground substance of connective tissue was described as a "place name" for a large, incompletely known variety of chemical substances, which arise locally or from the blood plasma or from either source (Gersh and Catchpole, 1960). The ground substance is heterogeneous (Table I). It is convenient to divide the components into macromolecules and smaller molecular entities. The macromolecular group includes mucopolysaccharides* (Meyer and Palmer, 1934; Meyer and Rapport, 1951); glycoproteins first recognized histochemically as major components of the ground

---

*The nomenclature of this class of substance has shifted to the general designation "glycosaminoglycan" plus derivatives related to its two roots, e.g., glycoprotein, proteoglycan (Balazs, 1970).

TABLE I

ORGANIZATION AND COMPOSITION OF CONNECTIVE TISSUE[a]

Cells: Fibroblasts, chondroblasts, osteoblasts, etc.
Fibers: Collagen fibers—collagen
             Reticular fibers—reticulin
             Elastic fibers—elastin

Ground substance:

Glycosaminoglycans[b] (acid mucopolysaccharides)	Hyaluronic acid	
	Chondroitin 4-sulfate	(ChS-A)[b]
	Chondroitin 6-sulfate	(ChS-C)[b]
	Dermatan sulfate	(ChS-B)[b]
	Keratan sulfate	(keratosulfate)[b]
Some or all present as proteoglycans[b] (protein polysaccharides)	Heparan sulfate	(heparitin sulfate)[b]
	Chondroitin	
	Heparin	

Local origin

Glycoproteins
Soluble collagens
Soluble elastins

Water
Gases
Immune bodies
Metabolites   } Plasma origin

Plasma proteins
Vitamins
Hormones
Ions

[a]Modified from Gersh and Catchpole (1960).
[b]Balazs (1970).

substance and basement membranes (Gersh and Catchpole, 1949; Leblond, 1950); soluble tropocollagens and elastins not yet polymerized to fibrils; and, finally, serum proteins. In tissues, the acid mucopolysaccharides are complexed with proteins to different degrees (proteoglycans) and may be, like the fibrils, relatively water insoluble (Section III,A). The class of smaller molecular components of ground substance includes metabolites, vitamins, hormones, gases (CO_2, O_2, N_2), ions, and water.

Table I also indicates a second classification of components based on origin, i.e., whether derived locally or more closely related to the blood plasma (Gersh and Catchpole, 1949). The connective tissue consists partly

of structural units of local origin, forming an enduring organization (within
biological limits), and partly of materials in transit between the blood and
cells of the region. The latter consists in general of smaller molecular species,
but may include molecules of the dimensions of blood proteins.

2. Morphology

The ground substance is commonly visualized in light microscopic studies
of tissues, preferably using freeze-dried or cryostat vacuum-dried sections
combined with alcohol postfixation, as a homogeneous matrix which stains
metachromatically with toluidine blue and pink to red with the periodic
acid–leucofuchsin (PAS) reaction (McManus, 1946). The ground substance
is contiguous with the basement membrane of endothelial, epithelial,
muscle, fat, and other cells.

Ultrastructural study of the ground substance has been unsatisfactory.
Solution in the fixatives and poor resolution with commonly used electron
microscope "stains" may be responsible for clear resolution of only collagen
and reticulin fibrils. A study of the distribution of intravenously injected ferrocyanide, which was recognized by subsequent formation of the electron
dense product, prussian blue, gave some important information. If the
ground substance were a homogeneous colloidal solution, ferrocyanide
should be distributed homogeneously in it. To the contrary, ferrocyanide was
shown to be present in discrete vacuoles of 1000 Å or less (Chase, 1959;
Dennis, 1959). The findings support the hypothesis of a two-phase, vacuolar
structure of ground substance (Section VII,A).

D. Basement Membrane

1. Histology

The position of the basement membrane frequently earns it the label
"strategic." It stains with the periodic acid–leucofuchsin reaction more
deeply than does the contiguous ground substance, and the staining indicates, with reasonable certainty, the presence of glycoproteins. The basement membrane was considered to be closely related to the ground substance
anatomically, chemically, and functionally (Gersh and Catchpole, 1949).
Characteristically, it appears as a dense-staining line or sheet interposed between connective tissue and (a) ectoderm (skin; membrana preforma of the
tooth germ); (b) entoderm (intestinal mucosa, thyroid gland, bronchi); (c)
highly differentiated mesodermal structures (kidney, muscle, capillaries).
All studies with the light microscope, including those based on the use of
fluorescein-labeled antibodies to basement membrane antigens, presumably
refer to a basement membrane in the above sense.

2. ULTRASTRUCTURE

It is usual to distinguish between the classic basement membrane (above) and the basal lamina of the electron microscopist (Hodges, 1969; Martínez-Palomo, 1970). The latter is an electron dense layer, the lamina densa, present at dermoepithelial and endothelial boundaries, which is continuous and separated from the cell membrane by a less dense layer, the lamina rara, of about the same width. The lamina densa is generally 300–500 Å wide, but may reach 3000 Å or more in the kidney glomerulus.

The relationship between the structures defined by light and electron microscopy, respectively, is not entirely settled. Certainly, in part, the different apparent thickness (1 or 2 μm in the former; a few hundred angstroms in the latter) is attributable to overlay in the much thicker sections used in light microscopic studies (Gersh and Catchpole, 1960). Using a periodic acid–silver method, Swift and Saxton (1967) found that the laminas rara and densa in the dermoepithelial junction were negative, and they inferred that these membranes are not the periodic acid–leucofuchsin-positive structures seen with the light microscope. However, this conclusion appears to be inherently unlikely because of the known chemical composition of these and related membranes.

3. COMPOSITION

Most of our knowledge of basement membrane composition is based on glomerular basement membrane which was first isolated by Krakower and Greenspon (1954). In this cell-free material, obtained by differential centrifugation and sonication, fibrils were absent, but analyses showed a collagenlike protein together with associated carbohydrate. Subsequent studies of similarly isolated membrane have shown the presence of a nonfibrillar collagenous protein containing about 7–10% of neutral sugars present as glycoprotein (Kefalides, 1970; Spiro, 1968; Mahieu and Winand, 1970).

4. ORIGIN

In highly specific instances, e.g., in the absence of mesenchymal cells, epithelial cells may contribute their own environment (Section II,A). In the more usual situation, mesenchyme is present, and it is commonly thought that basement membrane arises through some kind of epithelial–mesenchymal interaction (cf. Fleischmajer and Billingham, 1968). Thus, in the experiments of Kallman and Grobstein (1965), epithelial and mesenchymal cells were grown on either side of a Millipore filter. A soluble, hydroxyproline-rich precursor diffused from the mesenchyme to the epithelial cell base where it aggregated. However, other cells appear to derive the basement membrane (or basal lamina) from the epithelial cell *in toto* (Pierce, 1970;

Ross, 1970). In view of the chemical and antigenic complexity of the basement membrane (Krakower and Greenspon, 1967), a dogmatic statement covering the origin of all forms of basement membrane is currently risky.

E. Cell Coats

Phylogenetically, the ground substance is broadly distributed throughout the flora and fauna (Gersh and Catchpole, 1960; Mathews, 1967). In the simplest animals, it may appear as a soft shell (tectin) that may calcify. Carbohydrate coats are characteristic of bacteria and of many unicellular animals, and mesenchyme (mesoglia) appears in the simplest metazoans, the sponges. When the latter are disaggregated (Moscona, 1963), the cells spontaneously reaggregate through stereospecific interactions. In the older literature, mammalian cells were thought to be joined by an intercellular cement (e.g., for endothelia, Zweifach, 1940; Chambers and Zweifach, 1947). Ultrastructural studies tended to throw these views into temporary eclipse, although theories of cell agglutination and specificity relied largely on the assumption of glycoprotein cell coatings present in continuous or patchy distribution. The pendulum has now swung to the acceptance of extracellular investments of animal cells, possessing "unique immunological, cementing and other properties" (Rambourg and Leblond, 1967; Martínez-Palomo, 1970). Cell coats appear to be macromolecular polyelectrolytes of carbohydrate nature. They may be arbitrarily included with the basal laminas and ground substance when considering some aspects of vascular and cellular exchange.

III. Organization and Functions of Connective Tissues

Major directions of chemical work on connective tissue over the past few years include (1) characterization of the collagen component which is highly ordered ultrastructurally and which forms a relatively coarse supporting network, (2) comparable studies on elastin, (3) isolation of nonfibrillar macromolecules such as soluble collagens, glycosaminoglycans, and glycoproteins, and (4) description of the association of these components in tissues.

A. Interrelationships of Connective Tissue Components

The glycosaminoglycans are associated with proteins as the side chains of protein cores linked rather specifically to serine, threonine, and certain other residues (Spiro, 1970; Marshall and Neuberger, 1970) to give proteoglycans with molecular weights running into the millions. The resulting compounds are spidery or myriapodal structures. Proteoglycans are associated with proteins and glycoproteins as nonfibrillar sols and gels, and these components are, in turn, associated with collagen and other fibrils (Serafini-Fracassini *et al.*, 1970). Day (1952) suggested that the gel was attached to the fiber as a kind of "waterproofing." A related view was that the optically homogeneous ground substance, of fluid to gel-like consistency, infiltrates and encloses a network of oriented fibrils and fibers (Gersh and Catchpole, 1949). Descriptions of the molecular associations between collagen and other major macromolecules remain somewhat speculative (Mathews, 1965; Jackson, 1970).

A portion of the glycoproteins is extractable with buffers and may represent plasma components with which the connective tissue is in equilibrium. This treatment leaves behind the bulk of stainable glycoprotein which is normally insoluble, but which may become soluble in certain physiological and pathological states (disaggregation or depolymerization, Gersh and Catchpole, 1960). Such glycoprotein is thought to be the part which is bound or organized as described above.

B. Adaptive Evolution and Function

The "connective" function of connective tissue ranges from the type of inextensible joining represented by the collagen-rich tendon to the elastic recoil of an arterial wall in which elastin is the major connective component. Cartilage is a semirigid tissue marked by the presence of the strongly acidic, ion-binding, but feebly hydrophilic chondroitin sulfate (its protein complex, on the other hand, is strongly hydrophilic). Umbilical cord (Wharton's jelly) is composed of a network of collagen fibers embedded in a hydrophilic hyaluronic acid gel and is flexible and rubbery in texture. Its properties may be approximated by synthetic models of collagen solutions gelled at 37°C and neutral pH in the presence of hyaluronic acid (Fessler, 1960). Skin connective tissue, containing roughly equivalent amounts of hyaluronic acid and chondroitin sulfate, shows considerable water-holding capacity, and primate skin (sex skin) may show this property to an exaggerated degree. The limit, in an organized tissue, is reached in the vitreous body, being 99% or more water and dissolved substances, 0.1% collagen as an extremely fine network, and 0.15% hyaluronic acid. The structure is nevertheless self-supporting when physically intact. In the vitreous body, the *sine qua non* is transparency. The same holds for the cornea, but here an external protective function is also required. It is composed of highly oriented collagen lamellae in a matrix of keratan and chondroitin sulfates.

In all of the above instances, one senses the theme of adaptive evolution where form, including composition,* and function are equivalent. Other examples of connective tissue adaptation are bulk accomodation (uterus), relaxation (symphysis pubis), lubrication (joint interfaces), and capacity to accumulate and release ions (cartilage, osteoid, bone).

Ogston (1970) expressed the opinion that there was little of biological interest in the work of chemists on the glycosaminoglycans. He believed that the varied composition and distribution must mean something, but that the major biological interest lay in systems rather than in substances. From the foregoing observations, one would not entirely concur with the first proposition because some tentative generalizations seem possible; however, the second is well taken. Several parameters of the connective tissue can be considered independently of a detailed analysis of composition: for example, the colloidal charge density, the equivalent weight of the matrix, and the ionic partition between blood and tissue (Joseph et al., 1952, 1959). Other possibilities suggested by Ogston were osmotic pressure and hydration properties of the matrix, dynamic filtration effects, solute partition and excluded volume relations. The physical chemistry of the connective tissue or ground substances to be described (Section IV) will generally refer to measurable tissue properties, rather than to the behavior of isolated pure substances or models.

IV. Physical Chemistry of Connective Tissue

A. Hydration and Exclusion Effects

Considered as a class, the nonfibrillar molecules of connective tissue are long flexible chains of indefinite or random configuration, branched or linear, more or less highly charged and occupying large domains in solution. Hyaluronic acid is one of the best-studied molecules. It has a molecular weight of 1×10^7, and, with a diameter of about 1 μm, its potential volume is 5 l/gm. A solution at a concentration of 0.2 mg/ml would contain packed, hydrated molecules, and, at a concentration of 1.0 mg/ml, there would be an 80% molecular overlap. It may be noted that 0.2 mg/ml is approximately the concentration of hyaluronic acid in human vitreous body. Such solutions are networks of entangled molecular chains, the nature of which depends very little on the linear or branching nature of individual molecules (this aspect

*The term "chemical morphology" best expresses this idea.

being abundantly provided already by molecular entanglement), on the molecular size (provided it is large), or on cross linking (Ogston, 1970).

When such solutions were equilibrated with large molecular solutes such as inulin, polyglucose, amylose, serum albumin, or CO-hemoglobin, only about one-third of the molecules penetrated the hyaluronic acid, while two-thirds remained in the buffer (Ogston and Phelps, 1960). The authors concluded that the concentration of serum proteins in lymph cannot be assumed to be the same as in the extracellular water, which contains hyaluronic acid. This, therefore, is evidence that the distribution of large molecular solutes, at least, depends upon the molecular organization of the connective tissue. The phenomenon, known as the excluded volume effect, holds also for the proteoglycans of cartilage, which exclude serum albumin and chondroitin sulfate from 50 to 98% of their volume, depending on the concentration (Gerber and Schubert, 1954). These authors compared the exclusion effect to the exclusion of large molecules by Sephardex,* a polyanion commonly used in laboratories for sieving molecules of different sizes.

B. Osmotic Effects

Tissue osmotic pressure is a function of the macromolecular composition. The extravascular osmotic pressure is not due solely to the presence of plasma proteins, but to all large molecular species. The osmotic pressure of polymers behaves nonideally and increases with concentration more rapidly than predicted; hyaluronic acid solutions at physiological concentrations have osmotic pressures many times the ideal values and may approximate actual values for plasma. Similar considerations apply to cartilage in which the high concentration of polysaccharides contributes a high internal osmotic (swelling) pressure to which the ions contribute even more. The total effect is maintenance of the tissue in an "inflated" state (Ogston, 1970). Linn (1968) showed that cartilage under mechanical loading acts as a deformable, self-pressurized bearing surface.

C. Colloidal Charge

The major fibers of connective tissue contribute little to colloidal charge. Collagen is an isoelectric or electrically neutral type of ampholyte, and the colloidal charge of tendon, which is composed largely of collagen, is low. Elastin is also an essentially neutral molecule.

*Sephardex, Pharmacia, Uppsala, Sweden.

TABLE II

Colloidal Charge of Connective Tissues[a]

Tissue	Species	Charge density (negative; Eq/kg tissue water)
Symphysis pubis, unrelaxed	Guinea pig	0.170
Symphysis pubis, relaxed	Guinea pig	0.035
Costal cartilage	Rabbit	0.150–0.170
Comb, control	Capon	0.066
Comb, testosterone	Capon	0.020
Cornea (stroma)	Rabbit	0.070
Dermis	Rat, rabbit, macaque	0.050
Tendon	Rat, rabbit	0.030–0.035
Sex skin (estrogenized)	Macaque	0.020
Synovial fluid	Man	~0.010

[a]Values obtained in numerous determinations, 1952–1970, slightly modified from time to time (cf. Joseph et al., 1954; Gersh and Catchpole, 1960).

The major carriers of colloidal charge in connective tissue are the glycosaminoglycans and the acidic glycoproteins. The colloidal charge, x^-, may be estimated as the difference between the total diffusible cations and the total diffusible anions (Joseph, 1971). Such total measures of ions for tissues are few, apart from the almost unique studies of tendon and cartilage by Eichelberger et al. (1951).

With a method of NaCl dilution potentials, direct measurements were made on a variety of connective tissues (Table II). Values range from a maximum of 0.16–0.20 Eq per liter of tissue water for cartilage (agreeing with analytical values) to 0.02 for sex skin (estrogenized) and 0.035 for relaxed symphysis pubis. Other tissues show intermediate values. Tissue colloidal charge is always negative, owing to the relative preponderance of acidic polyelectrolytes in both cells and connective tissues.

Highly variable connective tissues, in which water content varies with the physiological state, show a wide range of colloidal charge. Examples are the sex skin of primates and the symphysis pubis of guinea pig and mouse.

D. Equivalent Weight

The mean equivalent weight of connective tissue polyelectrolytes is given by W/x^-, where weight, W, and charge density, x^-, are both expressed per kilogram of tissue water. Values are about 1000 for cartilage, 7000 for dermis, and 18,000 for tendon (Joseph et al., 1959). These figures reflect tissue composition: cartilage rich in chondroitin sulfate has a low equivalent weight, and tendon rich in collagen has a very high equivalent weight. Between fetal and adult stages, the equivalent weight of pig skin increases tenfold, from 830 to 7000, indicating changing relationships with age between collagen and glycosaminoglycans of this tissue (Joseph, 1971).

E. Cation Distribution

With increasing colloidal charge, the total ionic content of a tissue increases. The distribution of the different ions is determined by a number of factors, one of which is the configuration of the ion in a given tissue milieu. This relationship is expressed by the standard chemical potential of the ion. The property becomes very important in most cells in which, for example, the standard chemical potential of the sodium ion is high compared with that of potassium; this determines the distribution of sodium and potassium between cells and the blood (Joseph et al., 1965).

In connective tissues, the dielectric constant of water is high and approximates that of the blood (Joseph, 1971), in contrast to cells in which the dielectric constant of water is low. The ionic distribution tends to be related more strongly to binding by connective tissue macromolecules. Maximal effects are observed in cartilage where the colloidal charge is high, and approximate ionic values for blood and cartilage are given in Table III. The concentration of sodium is about double that of blood, and ionic Ca^{2+} and Mg^{2+} have about 3–3.5 times their blood values, as might be expected from

TABLE III

IONIC CONCENTRATIONS IN BLOOD AND CARTILAGE[a]

Ion	Blood (mEq/kg water)	Cartilage (mEq/kg water)	Donnan ratio (r)
Colloid	10	160–170	—
Na^+	150	280	1.86
K^+	5	70	14.0
Ca^{2+} ionic	2.5	7.2	3.0
Ca^{2+} total	5	37	—
Mg^{2+} ionic	1	3.5	3.5
Mg^{2+} total	2	22	—

[a]Values obtained in numerous determinations, 1952–1970, slightly modified from time to time (cf. Engel et al., 1960).

Donnan relationships. However, cartilage K^+ concentration is fourteen times that of blood, suggesting strong binding of this ion. Note that both calcium and magnesium are bound in nonionic forms. Ionic relationships in connective tissues are thus marked by selectivity and by the existence of an extracellular ionic reservoir.

Nomograms describing ionic blood–tissue relationships have been published in some detail for the physiological ions, Na^+, K^+, Ca^{2+}, Mg^{2+}, and for two "foreign" ions of interest, Sr^{2+} and Pb^{2+} (Engel *et al.*, 1954; Joseph *et al.*, 1954; Catchpole *et al.*, 1956).

It is not surprising that organic cations, including the important class of biological amines, also bind to connective tissue, and do so with rather large changes of free energy ranging from 1.5 to 4.8 kcal/mole (Joseph *et al.*, 1959). Among compounds tested using rat dermis were lysine, arginine, histidine, histamine, thiamine chloride, epinephrine, procaine hydrochloride, and glucosamine (Table IV).

F. Anion Binding

The macromolecules of the connective tissue are amphoteric and can. therefore, bind to negative charges. This type of reaction is described extensively in the literature relating to the fibrous proteins, wool and collagen (Steinhardt, 1941; Gustavson, 1956). Thus, as opposed to cation binding, tissue collagen and elastin would be fully reactive. Among anions that react

TABLE IV

REACTION OF BIOLOGICAL AMINES WITH CONNECTIVE TISSUE (RAT DERMIS)[a]

Reagent	Concentration (M)	Equilibrium constant	Change of free energy (kcal/mole)
Lysine	0.001	360	3.6
Arginine	0.001	320	3.6
Histidine	0.001	370	3.6
Histamine	0.001	320	3.6
Thiamine chloride	0.001	440	3.8
β-Propionitrile	0.001	610	4.0
Epinephrine	0.0016	220	3.3
Procaine·HCl	0.0365	10.6	1.4
Glucosamine	0.001	310	3.5
$MgCl_2$	0.01	75.5	2.7
$CaCl_2$	0.01	35.0	2.2

[a]From Joseph *et al.* (1959).

are biochemical metabolites and inhibitors, dyes, vitamins, inorganic anions such as fluoride, bicarbonate, and uncharged organic molecules which are polar (Engel *et al.*, 1961).

Substances in the above categories which were studied were succinic acid, fluoride, alizarin red, and three dihydroxybenzoic acids. All produced a greater or lesser lowering of the colloidal charge of rabbit dermis and costal cartilage. This result implies a binding of the nucleophilic anion to tissue colloid, with simultaneous uptake of protons (Engel *et al.*, 1961). Important physiological consequences may be derived from this type of reaction. Among them is a homeostatic role of extracellular colloids in buffering pH changes in the blood. During intense cellular activity, large amounts of lactic or carbonic acids would be bound extracellularly together with hydrogen ions, and a smaller fraction of the latter would therefore enter the circulation. Such reactions might also provide a basis for cell secretion of hydrochloric and other acids.

V. Role of the Connective Tissue in Vascular Exchange

A. General Considerations

Materials crossing the endothelial wall of small vessels enter a complex environment including the cell coats, basal lamina (basement membrane), and ground substance. The diffusing substances may reenter the blood, pass into cells of the region, or reach the lymphatic system. This constant flux of substances is reflected in the composition of the ground substance as summarized in Table I. In a resting state, i.e., in the absence of overt muscular activity, and in a postdigestive period (conditions traditionally described as basal), the situation approaches an equilibrium or steady state. Among other reactions, oxygen is transported quantitatively to tissues, and CO_2 is transferred quantitatively to the blood. The heat of reactions is also transferred quantitatively to the blood and is dissipated externally. In these circumstances, the tissues and connective tissues would yield values for a given component which would qualify as a biological constant for the given tissue. This, in fact, is a definition of homeostasis.

B. Diffusion in Gels

An early model of diffusion through a matrix was provided by Friedman and Kraemer (1930) who studied diffusion through gelatin gels of different concentrations. The gels were "fine grained" on the basis of the Tyndall effect and showed no "ultrastructure" as defined in 1930; nor would they show a definite ultrastructure by today's methods. The distance between "threads" in very dilute gels was estimated to be 100 mμ (1000 Å). Kraemer had already measured the Brownian movement of mercury droplets suspended in gelatins at different concentrations and found movement at 3% but not at 5%, although, at the latter strength, motion appeared upon warming due to gel breakdown. These ingenious studies gave an insight into the nature of the gel as a three-dimensional semisolid lattice containing fluid. From the diffusion of sucrose, glycerine, and urea into gels, they inferred the presence of "pores" with a diameter of 100 Å at 5%, 30 Å at 10%, and 14 Å at 15% concentration of gel.* Diffusion of nonelectrolytes was slowed in the denser gels and decreased as the molecular weight increased.

The transport properties of artificially cast collagen membranes 25 μm thick composed of tropocollagen molecules was studied by Gliozzi et al. (1969). The fibrils tended to align in two main directions at right angles, thus structurally resembling some biological structures. The filtration of the salts KSCN, KCl, and CaCl$_2$ at increasing molarities from 0.1 to 5.0 M was studied. At low molarity collagen is crystalline, while at higher ionic strengths it becomes amorphous and finally "melts." For KSCN and CaCl$_2$, the filtration coefficient decreased with increasing molarity, while for KCl it increased. All salts showed increased filtration upon melting. A theory of varying pore size was advanced, with a range of diameters 40–80 mμ. In these experiments, pore size was controlled essentially by salt and water, and the overall change was conformational.

Biologically, these collagenous meshworks are filled not with an aqueous fluid, but with a charged macromolecular gel. The behavior of these "simple" models should put us on guard against facile assumptions regarding molecular diffusion in gels, particularly when the diffusing molecular species are large, heterogeneous, asymmetric in shape, and charged.

In the body, the most massively diffusing substance is water. Diffusion of tritiated water (^{3}H^{1}HO) showed an appreciable decrement in agar gels even at 1% concentration, with reduction of the diffusion constant from 2.41 to 2.15 × 10^{-5} cm^2/second (Nakayama and Jackson, 1963).

C. Diffusion in Tissues

In actual tissues, it is well known that the diffusion of very large particles may be prevented almost completely. Examples are the movement of carbon particles in a skin tattoo (the precision as well as the charm of these artistic

---

*The authors use "equivalent pore radius" which has been arbitrarily multiplied by 2 to bring values into line with biological custom.

creations may fade somewhat with the years) and the permanent lodging of silver grains in basement membrane in argyria. The striking effect of the depolymerizing enzyme, hyaluronidase, in facilitating the spread of india ink particles in skin was the basis of Duran Reynal's experiments on spreading factors. In cornea, the flow of water was increased 50-fold after removing polysaccharide (Hedbys and Mishima, 1962). Laurent and Ogston (1963) observed the retarded sedimentation of large solute molecules through solutions of hyaluronic acid, and compared this to the steady state distribution of plasma proteins in connective tissue.

Some interesting experiments were done on the conducting properties of Wharton's jelly (Davies *et al.*, 1944) in which a colloidal dye related to trypan blue, both free and linked to serum albumin by diazotization, was injected under low pressure into Wharton's jelly of sheep fetuses maintained through placental connections. In 3 hours, dye extended throughout the cord substance and into tissues on the fetal side, indicating that molecules as large as albumin could diffuse and pass from cord to embryo.

The use of tracers such as peroxidase (particle size 30–50 Å) and ferritin (particle size 110 Å) is beginning to give some information on protein transport across the blood–tissue–lymph interface. Peroxidase appeared in the interstitium 1 minute after intravenous injection in mice, and in lymphatic lumina in 30 minutes (Leak, 1970).

Probably in most locations in the body, diffusion occurs over distances measured in microns, depending on the nature and distribution of the microvasculature. However, in relatively or completely avascular tissues, such

TABLE V

DIFFUSION IN CALF NUCLEUS PULPOSUS[a]

Substance	Tissue/water ratio (k_1)
NaCl	0.39
CaCl$_2$	0.41
Na$_2$SO$_4$	0.55
Urea	0.52
Glycine	0.42
Acetamide	0.49
Glucose ($C_6H_{12}O_6$)	0.60
Sucrose ($C_{12}H_{22}O_{11}$)	0.58
Raffinose ($C_{18}H_{32}O_{16}$)	0.28
Glucosamine	0.09

[a] From Paulson and Snellman (1950).

as cartilage, nucleus pulposus, and lens, the distances to be traversed by nutrients and metabolites may be large, i.e., millimeters. As an example of diffusion in such tissues, the nucleus pulposus was studied by Paulson and Snellman (1950). Diffusion of salts and organic compounds (maximum mw 500) was determined interferometrically using 40-μm sections of fresh calf nucleus (Table V). Diffusion rates of several compounds listed are about half that in water, and, by comparing with the results of Friedman and Kraemer, a pore size of 30 Å was inferred. Glucose and sucrose diffused faster than raffinose, indicating that the nucleus contains pores permeable to the smaller, but not to the larger, molecules, i.e., there is a heterogeneity of pore sizes.

VI. Reaction of Connective Tissues to Certain Agents

A. Growth, Differentiation, Remodeling

Changes in connective tissue occur with growth and differentiation. Apart from the manifold phenomena of embryonic induction, the remodeling of tissues as they increase in size implies lability of the extracellular elements (Gersh and Catchpole, 1949; Gersh, 1949–1950). In development of the metanephros of the fetal pig, the reticular fibrils, ground substance, and basement membrane of glomeruli and tubules are constantly modified. Similarly, the basement membrane of rat skin appears to organize shortly after birth and becomes progressively more prominent. Basement membranes tend to disappear after injury and are later regenerated. Striking connective tissue changes occur in the uterus during pregnancy. This process includes an increase in muscle mass, collagen content (Harkness and Harkness, 1954), and ground substance (Maibenco, 1960). Conversely, during involution all these tissue elements are progressively and rapidly lost.

B. Hormonal Action

Hormonal actions may produce an increase in organ size and vascularity and seem to include, as an integral part of their activity, effects on connective tissue morphology, water content, and ion distribution (Ihnen and Pérez-Tamayo, 1953; Gersh and Catchpole, 1949, 1960). Only a small sampling of such reactions will be discussed.

1. ESTROGENS AND PROGESTERONE

One of the first events in the action of estrogen on the uterus of an immature or castrate animal is a prompt uptake of water (Astwood, 1938). This may be related to a change in uterine ground substance (Somlyo, 1956; Friederici, 1967). Estrogen increases the extractable glycoprotein fraction of rabbit uterus, cervix, and vagina (Moses and Catchpole, 1955).

A group of physiological swellings or edemas* is expressed in the menstrual cycle of macaques and baboons, and is related to the action of estrogen on the connective tissue of skin and sex skin. The hormone stimulates the synthesis of hyaluronic acid and its protein complexes, and produces a swollen and tense tissue which on cutting oozes a mucinous fluid (Ogston *et al.*, 1939).

In the course of normal pregnancy, an extrauterine accumulation of fluid occurs which must be regarded as a physiological edema (Robertson, 1969). It is very likely that the process involves a new formation of extracellular macromolecules under the influence of anabolic pregnancy hormones, together with a possible change in molecular aggregation. The skin seems to be the most likely site of accumulation of additional fluid.

2. MALE SEX HORMONE

Androgens are responsible for the growth and maintenance of the skin appendages (comb, wattles) of the common fowl, and, in their absence, the appendages atrophy. In the capon, male hormones produce extensive growth of the comb, with synthesis of fibrillar and ground substance components, the most important of which is hyaluronic acid. The comb is hyperemic and, on section, appears glistening and mucinous. An observed increase in water content may be attributed to the strongly hydrophilic hyaluronic acid and to expansion of the water-rich phase (Section VII,A).

3. CONNECTIVE TISSUE-DIRECTED HORMONES

Several hormones have a predominantly direct action on connective tissues. The primary target of the parathyroid hormone is bone. The hormone effects the dissolution (disaggregation) of bone matrix with release of calcium salts and soluble glycoproteins (Engel, 1952). A major action of growth hormone is to widen the cartilagenous plate, and is the basis for a method of

---

*There is some reluctance to concede this term to normal events.

biological assay of the hormone. Relaxin, a polypeptide hormone of the ovary, acts on the fibrocartilagenous matrix of the symphysis pubis. The symphysis, particularly after estrogen "priming," promptly relaxes when relaxin is given. The basic process is a disaggregation and solubilization of symphyseal ground substance accompanied by water uptake (Perl and Catchpole, 1950). The mode of action of the hormone is thought to be via the characteristic connective tissue cells of the region (chondrocytes) with release of depolymerizing enzymes.

C. Action of Enzymes on Connective Tissues

The discovery of the spreading factors triggered much modern work on the nature of the ground substance. These enzymes are present in testis, many microorganisms, cercariae, snake venoms, and leech digestive juices. By 1940, the substrates of the spreading factors had been recognized to be hyaluronic acid and chondroitin sulfates (Chain and Duthie, 1939). Another type of action of these enzymes was the prompt "deflation" of swollen primate sex skin after local injection (Duran Reynals et al., 1950). While the role of the exogenous hyaluronidases seems clear, as in the elegant experiments of Lewert and Lee (1954) on skin penetration by enzyme-bearing cercariae, their physiological role is less certain even when they are known to be present. Thus, testicular hyaluronidase is generally associated with dispersion of cells of the cumulus oophorus as a prelude to successful fertilization, although correlations have been hard to obtain. It might be more fruitful to suggest the enzyme as the agent which enables the sperm themselves to separate from the testicular matrix and to rid themselves of materials which could cause subsequent agglutination, a fatal handicap for a sperm cell.

It has seemed a valid hypothesis that depolymerizing enzymes might be secreted by connective tissue or other cells as a part of the mechanism of turnover of glycosaminoglycans and glycoproteins, and might be triggered by hormones in situations calling for their synthesis or disaggregation. The role of such enzymes in the spread of tumors was also widely canvassed in the earlier literature (cf. Weiss, 1967). Experimental demonstration has, on the whole, lagged in spite of interest in the role of a multiplicity of hydrolytic enzymes contained in and released by lysosomes.

The additional presence of collagenases in tumors related to a role in the breakdown of fibrillar components of connective tissue was also the subject of early studies. Convincing evidence of a tissue action of collagenase has been provided by work on the resorption of the tadpole tail (Gross and Lapiere, 1962; Gross, 1970).

A systemic action of enzymes on connective tissue was shown by Thomas (1964) who injected papain intravenously into rabbits and obtained the "flop-eared" syndrome of cartilage collapse. The enzyme causes apparent breakdown of chondroitin sulfate–protein linkages, with solubilization and release of chondroitin sulfate into the blood and urine.

VII. Connective Tissue Homeostasis

In a review of structure, conformation, and mechanism in the formation of polysaccharide gels and networks (Rees, 1970), the author expressed the opinion that

> if polysaccharides are ever again to make major contributions to molecular theory and molecular biology they can do so only after their behavior in gels has been understood in molecular terms. The gel is the state most typical for carbohydrates both in biological and artificial systems.

Connective tissues possess both a solid and a semisolid character (Joseph, 1971), and their properties must be considered in relation to their water content which may vary from between 15 and 45% for bone to nearly 100% for vitreous body. A representative "soft tissue" value would be 70%. The fluid properties are restricted by the coexistent solid phases, one of which is represented by the organized fibrils. These form a continuous meshwork having certain properties of tensile strength and elasticity. This lattice is permeated by the semifluid ground substance. Models of connective tissue filtration provided by several authors (Section V) would conform to this, with the ground substance consisting of a solution of entangled chains of proteoglycans, glycoproteins, etc. This phase appears to be regarded as locally homogeneous.

We have given reasons (Joseph *et al.*, 1952) why the assumption of a homogeneous ground substance raises problems with respect to its equilibrium with blood plasma. Blood is invariant with respect to the chemical potentials of water and ions, as shown by its constant freezing point and constant ionic composition. On the other hand, the water content of connective tissues is highly variable. This may be partly explained on the basis of composition. However, the same connective tissue can exist in different hydrated states at different times. The rate of hydration may be rapid and difficult to explain on the basis of a compositional change, e.g., water uptake by the uterus after estrogen administration or by the symphysis pubis after a treatment with relaxin. Swelling of the sex skin also appears to involve considerations additional to synthesis of matrix alone (Bentley, 1970).

A. Two-Phase System

The hypothesis of a two-phase system was adopted (Joseph *et al.*, 1952) and a diagrammatic representation is given (Fig. 1). A colloid-rich, water-poor phase is shown in equilibrium with a water-rich, colloid-poor phase. As in physical models of two-phase systems or complex coacervates, the amount of either phase can be changed without disturbing the thermodynamic relations of the whole. Vertical lines define the relative amounts of the two phases as explained in the figure legend; the composition of vitreous body, for example, would be given by a vertical line far to the right. The extracellular matrix of a tissue is described by a given distribution of colloid-rich and water-rich phases which, in turn, is determined by the chemical morphology of the tissue. When this is changed by hormonal or other means the relative amounts of the phases will change. Such a tissue can change its water, electrolyte, and overall macromolecular composition under reversible homeostatic conditions because it remains in equilibrium with the blood in respect of the intensive properties of the system (osmotic pressure, vapor pressure, ionic equilibrium). At the same time, the physical state can

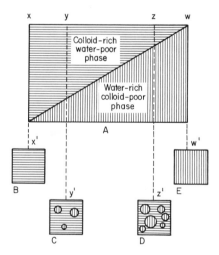

Fig. 1. Schematic diagram representing two phases of ground substance in equilibrium with each other and with blood. Colloid-rich phase is represented by small inset, B. Water-rich phase is represented by small inset, E. Tissue C (vertical line y–y') has a large amount of colloid-rich phase and a small amount of water-rich phase. C represents dense ground substance. Tissue D (vertical line z–z') has a large amount of water-rich phase and a small amount of colloid-rich phase. D represents a loose ground substance. Tissues C and D are in osmotic equilibrium with blood and with each other, despite the difference in water content. (From Gersh and Catchpole, 1960.)

change widely in respect of extensive properties such as total bulk, tensile strength, deformability, consistency, etc. Hormonal actions involving rapid water shifts, reversible physiological edemas, and some enzymic effects may be interpreted on this basis. Two mechanisms are available: over the short term, disaggregation of insoluble macromolecules with solubilization and osmotic uptake of water will shift the balance toward the water-rich type of tissue; over the long run, synthesis of additional glycosaminoglycans and their complexes, with or without disaggregation, will increase the overall amount of ground substance. The essentially homeostatic nature of these reactions is illustrated by the very large and rapid shift of water from sex skin to blood and then to urine during sex skin involution in the baboon, occurring at constant plasma water concentration (Clarke, 1940).

The morphological counterpart of the two-phase system in ground substance is the submicroscopic vacuolar appearance already described (Section II,C,2). It should be stressed that strict morphological "permanency" is not implied. The turnover of ground substance components in itself indicates a dynamic equilibrium of the phases.

B. Edema

In the physiological edemas, the two-phase system remains fully reversible; the water-rich vacuoles expand in an orderly way at the expense of the continuous phase, and, when the hormonal or metabolic stress is removed, the system reverts to its "physiological standard state" (Joseph et al., 1965).

In pathological states where the influx of water becomes excessive through the operation of hemodynamic factors, by vascular damage, by excessive degradation of the matrix, or by a combination of these, the vacuoles may become confluent (Gersh and Catchpole, 1960). This would lead to the formation of actual macroscopic pools of extracellular fluid which can no longer maintain reversible equilibrium with the colloid-rich phase. Correction of the pathological state is not automatic and depends on measures taken to remove excess fluid as a first step in treatment.

C. Inflammation

Many aspects of the foregoing discussion have a bearing on inflammation, although in few of them has a detailed attack on the nature of connective tissue reactions in inflammation become explicit. The problems of reepithelialization, granulation tissue formation, and collagen synthesis and maturation are all intimately tied up with mesenchymal cell reactions and the nature of the matrix. It was shown early on that profound changes occur in epithelial and vascular basement membranes and in the ground substance of a wound. One aspect of this was dissolution and solubilization of macromolecular components of these structures (Gersh and Catchpole, 1949). This would lead to swelling and to modifications of vascular exchange throughout the affected region.

Changes in the gel properties of connective tissue may be related to the different phases of cell migration and multiplication, including the arrival of macrophages, slippage of epithelial cells, and mitosis in endothelial cells. The increased lability of the matrix may facilitate (or initiate) these reactions, since after injury local conditions may be likened to a kind of tissue culture media in which some of the normal constraints on cell movements are removed.

Ionic and other binding properties of the matrix are changed during disaggregation. This introduces many new relationships, not all of them "for the best of all possible worlds." An immediate or early effect of injury is the release of biological amines, not only from cells, but from binding sites on extracellular matrix (Section IV,E). These would exercise their characteristic pharmacological actions on blood vessels, locally and systemically.

A common observation is an increase in vital dye uptake of a region after injury or hormonal stimulation. Since this reaction is also produced by histamine, it has come to be generally regarded as indicative of a change in vascular permeability in accordance with the neat tautology: more permeable vessels leak dye; thus the appearance of dye means that the vessels are more permeable. We have considered dye accumulation to be diagnostic of ground substance change: a reasonable explanation is that more binding sites become available to the dye through partial disaggregation of ground substance complexes (Gersh and Catchpole, 1949, 1960).

The concept of vascular permeability in the sense of a more or less leaky blood vessel is not adequate to describe the continuum of exchange reactions across the connective tissue. The idea of morphological "barriers" also may not be a particularly useful one, since the function of connective tissue is to mediate exchanges in the broadest sense. Very large molecules can, in fact, be transported from blood to cells and from cells to blood.

Among the major themes touched upon in this chapter was the concept of connective tissue in terms of its chemical morphology with emphasis on its macromolecules and polyelectrolytes (sometimes, but not always equivalent). From the macromolecules are derived properties of molecular sieving; from the polyelectrolytes those of ionic binding and exchange; from both the properties of water binding and sol–gel states of aggregation. These are just now being elucidated for the normal state. Their evaluation in inflammation is a program for the future.

References

Astwood, E. B. (1938). *Endocrinology* **23**, 25.
Bader, H. (1963). *In* "Handbook of Physiology" (Amer. Physiol. Soc., J. Field, ed.), Sect. 2, Vol. II, pp. 865–889. Williams & Wilkins, Baltimore, Maryland.
Bailey, A. J. (1968). *Compr. Biochem.* **26**, Part B, 297–423.
Balazs, E. A. (1970). *In* "Chemistry and Molecular Biology of the Intercellular Matrix" (E. A. Balazs, ed.), Vol. 1, pp. xxix-xxxi. Academic Press, New York.
Bensley, S. H. (1934). *Anat. Rec.* **60**, 93.
Bentley, J. P. (1970). *Advan. Biol. Skin,* **10**, 103–121.
Catchpole, H. R., Joseph, N. R., and Engel, M. B. (1956). *AMA Arch. Pathol.* **61**, 503.
Chain, E., and Duthie, E. S. (1939). *Nature (London)* **144**, 977.
Chambers, R., and Zweifach, B. W. (1947). *Physiol. Rev.* **27**, 436.
Chase, W. H. (1959). *AMA Arch. Pathol.* **67**, 525.
Clarke, R. W. (1940). *Amer. J. Physiol.* **131**, 325.
Cox, R. W., and O'Dell, B. L. (1966). *J. Roy. Microsc. Soc.* [3] **85**, 401.
Davies, F., Barcroft, J., Danielli, J. F., Harper, W. F., and Mitchell, P. D. (1944). *Nature (London)* **154**, 667.
Day, T. D. (1952). *J. Physiol. (London)* **117**, 1.
Dennis, J. B. (1959). *AMA Arch. Pathol.* **67**, 533.
Dische, Z., and Zelmenis, G. (1966). *Doc. Ophthalmol.* **20**, 54.
Dodson, J. W., and Hay, E. D. (1970). *J. Cell Biol.* **47**, Abstr. 129, 51a.
Duran-Reynals, F. (1928). *C. R. Soc. Biol. (Paris)* **99**, 6.
Duran-Reynals, F. (1942). *Bacteriol. Rev.* **6**, 197.
Duran-Reynals, F., Bunting, H., and van Wagenen, G. (1950). *Ann N. Y. Acad. Sci.* **52**, 1006.
Eichelberger, L., Brower, T. D., and Roma, M. (1951). *Amer. J. Physiol.* **166**, 328.
Engel, M. B. (1952). *AMA Arch. Pathol.* **53**, 339.
Engel, M. B., and Catchpole, H. R. (1970). *Proc. Soc. Exp. Biol. Med.* **133**, 260.
Engel, M. B., Joseph, N. R., and Catchpole, H. R. (1954). *AMA Arch. Pathol.* **58**, 26.
Engel, M. B., Joseph, N. R., Laskin, D. M., and Catchpole, H. R. (1960). *Ann. N. Y. Acad. Sci.* **85**, 399.
Engel, M. B., Joseph, N. R., Laskin, D. M., and Catchpole, H. R. (1961). *Amer. J. Physiol.* **201**, 621.
Evans, H. M., and Scott, K. J. (1921). *Contrib. Embryol. Carnegie Inst.* **10**, 1.
Fessler, J. H. (1960). *Biochem. J.* **76**, 124.
Fleischmajer, R., and Billingham, R. E., eds. (1968). "Epithelial-Mesenchymal Interactions." Williams & Wilkins, Baltimore, Maryland.
Flemming, W. (1876). *Arch. Microsk. Anat.* **12**, 391.
Friederici, H. H. R. (1967). *Lab. Invest.* **17**, 322.
Friedman, L., and Kraemer, E. O. (1930). *J. Amer. Chem. Soc.* **52**, 1295.
Gerber, B. R., and Schubert, M. (1954). *Biopolymers* **2**, 259.
Gersh, I. (1949–1950) *Harvey Lect.* **45**, 211.
Gersh, I., and Catchpole, H. R. (1949). *Amer. J. Anat.* **85**, 457.
Gersh, I., and Catchpole, H. R. (1960). *Perspect. Biol. Med.* **3**, 282.
Gliozzi, A., Morchio, R., and Ciferri, A. (1969). *J. Phys. Chem.* **73**, 3063.
Gross, J. (1970). *In* "Chemistry and Molecular Biology of the Intercellular Matrix" (E. A. Balazs, ed.), New York.
Gross, J., and Lapiere, C. M. (1962). *Proc. Nat. Acad. Sci. U. S.* **48**, 1014.

Gustavson, K. H., ed. (1956). "The Chemistry and Reactivity of Collagen." Academic Press, New York.

Harkness, M. L. R., and Harkness, R. D. (1954). *J. Physiol. (London)* **123**, 492.

Hedbys, B. O., and Mishima, S. (1962). *Exp. Eye Res.* **1**, 262.

Hodges, G. M. (1969). *In* "Biology of the Periodontium" (A. R. Melcher and W. H. Bowen, eds.), pp. 27–52. Academic Press, New York.

Ihnen, M., and Pérez-Tamayo, R. (1953). *AMA Arch. Pathol.* **56**, 46.

Jackson, D. M. (1970). *Advan. Biol. Skin* **10**, 39–48.

Joseph, N. R. (1971). "Physical Chemistry of Aging," pp. 90–107. Karger, Basel.

Joseph, N. R., Engel, M. B. and Catchpole, H. R. (1952). *Biochim. Biophys. Acta* **8**, 575.

Joseph, N. R., Engel, M. B., and Catchpole, H. R. (1954). *AMA Arch. Pathol.* **58**, 40.

Joseph, N. R., Catchpole, H. R., Laskin, D. M., and Engel, M. B. (1959). *Arch. Biochem. Biophys.* **84**, 224.

Joseph, N. R., Engel, M. B., and Catchpole, H. R. (1965). *Nature (London)* **206**, 6.

Kallman, F., and Grobstein, C. (1965). *Develop. Biol.* **11**, 169.

Kefalides, N. A. (1970). *In* "Chemistry and Molecular Biology of the Intercellular Matrix" (E. A. Balazs, ed.), Vol. 1, pp. 535–573. Academic Press, New York.

Krakower, C. A., and Greenspon, S. A. (1954). *AMA Arch. Pathol.* **58**, 401.

Krakower, C. A., and Greenspon, S. A. (1967). *Proc. 6th Cong. Int. Diabetes Ass. 1967*, p. 595.

Laurent, T. C., and Ogston, A. G. (1963). *Biochem. J.* **89**, 249.

Leak, L. V. (1970). *J. Cell Biol.* **47**, 117a.

Leblond, C. P. (1950). *Amer. J. Anat.* **86**, 1.

Lewert, R. M., and Lee, C. L. (1954). *J. Infec. Dis.* **95**, 13.

Linn, F. C. (1968). *J. Biomech.* **1**, 193.

McManus, J. F. A. (1946). *Nature (London)* **158**, 202.

Mahieu, P., and Winand, R. J. (1970). *Eur. J. Biochem.* **12**, 410.

Maibenco, H. C. (1960). *Anat. Rec.* **136**, 59.

Manery, J. F. (1954). *Physiol. Rev.* **34**, 334.

Marshall, R. D., and Neuberger, A. (1970). *Advan. Carbohyd. Chem.* **25**, 407.

Martínez-Palomo, A. (1970). *Int. Rev. Cytol.* **29**, 29.

Mathews, M. B. (1965). *Biochem. J.* **96**, 710.

Mathews, M. B. (1967). *Biol. Rev. Cambridge Phil. Soc.* **42**, 499.

Meyer, K. (1970). *In* "Chemistry and Molecular Biology of the Intercellular Matrix" (E. A. Balazs, ed.), Vol. 1, pp. 5–24. Academic Press, New York.

Meyer, K., and Palmer, J. W. (1934). *J. Biol. Chem.* **107**, 629.

Meyer, K., and Rapport, M. (1951). *Science* **113**, 596.

Moscona, A. A. (1963). *Proc. Nat. Acad. Sci. U. S.* **49**, 742.

Moses, L., and Catchpole, H. R. (1955). *Fed. Proc., Fed. Amer. Soc. Exp. Biol.* **14**, 104.

Nakayama, F. S., and Jackson, R. D. (1963). *J. Phys. Chem.* **67**, 932.

Ogston, A. G. (1970). *In* "Chemistry and Molecular Biology of the Intercellular Matrix" (E. A. Balazs, ed.), Vol. 3, pp. 1231–1240. Academic Press, New York.

Ogston, A. G., and Phelps, C. F. (1960). *Biochem. J.* **78**, 827.

Ogston, A. G., Philpot, J. St. L., and Zuckerman, S. (1939) *J. Endocrinol.* **1**, 231.

Partridge, S. M., Thomas, J., and Elsden, D. F. (1965). *In* "Structure and Function of Connective and Skeletal Tissue" (S. Fitton Jackson *et al.*, eds.), pp. 88–92. Butterworth, London.

Paulson, S., and Snellman, O. (1950). *Biochim. Bioph. Acta* **6**, 48.

Perl, E., and Catchpole, H. R. (1950). *AMA Arch. Pathol.* **50**, 233.

Pierce, G. B. (1970). *In* "Chemistry and Molecular Biology of the Intercellular Matrix" (E. A. Balazs, ed.), Vol. 1, pp. 471–506. Academic Press, New York.

Ramachandran, G. N. (1967). "Treatise on Collagen," Vol. 1, Chapter 3. Academic Press, New York.

Rambourg, A., and Leblond, C. P. (1967). *J. Cell Biol.* **32**, 27.

Rees, D. A. (1970). *Advan. Carbohyd. Chem. Biochem.* **24**, 267.

Robb-Smith, A. H. T. (1957). *J. Mt. Sinai Hosp. New York* **24**, 1155.

Robertson, E. G. (1969). *J. Reprod. Fert., Suppl.* **9**, 27.

Ross, R. (1970). *In* "Chemistry and Molecular Biology of the Intercellular Matrix" (E. A. Balazs, ed.), Vol. 3, pp. 1739–1751. Academic Press, New York.

Serafini-Fracassini, A., Wells, P. J., and Smith, J. W. (1970). *In* "Chemistry and Molecular Biology of the Intercellular Matrix" (E. A. Balazs, ed.), Vol. 2, pp. 1201–1215. Academic Press, New York.

Smith, D. W., Weissman, N., and Carnes, W. H. (1968). *Biochem. Biophys. Res. Commun.* **31**, 309.

Somlyo, A. P. (1956). (MS) Thesis, University of Illinois at the Medical Center, Chicago, Illinois.

Spiro, R. G. (1968). *N. Engl. J. Med.* **281**, 1043.

Spiro, R. G. (1970). *Annu. Rev. Biochem.* **39**, 599.

Steinhardt, J. (1941). *Ann. N. Y. Acad. Sci.* **41**, 287.

Swift, J. A., and Saxton, C. A. (1967). *J. Ultrastruct. Res.* **17**, 23.

Thomas, L. (1964). *Biophys. J.* **4**, No. 1, Part 2, Suppl., 207.

Weiss, L. (1967). *Proc. Can. Cancer Res. Conf.* **7**, 292.

Windrum, G. M., Kent, P. W., and Eastoe, J. E. (1955). *Brit. J. Exp. Pathol.* **36**, 49.

Zweifach, B. W. (1940). *Cold Spring Harbor Symp. Quant. Biol.* **8**, 216.

Chapter 5

RHEOLOGIC FACTORS IN INFLAMMATION

ROE WELLS

I. Introduction

The rheologic changes of blood and tissue fluid in inflammation are at the heart of the manner by which the inflammatory process attains its ultimate goal. In its broadest sense, inflammation may be regarded as a process that either increases some flow process, e.g., a histamine reaction, or brings flow to a static state, e.g., abscess formation. Rheology is simply the study or science of the flow process. The flow process in inflammation primarily concerns the blood. The reactions involving lymph, white cells, serum, etc., are secondary to or depend upon the initial reactions of blood and its flow. A résumé of normal blood rheology is therefore an appropriate preface to a discussion of its changes in inflammation.

II. Rheology of Normal Blood

The flow properties of blood are determined by both its physical characteristics (cells and plasma proteins) and the dynamics of their interactions during flow.

A. *Influence of Red Cell Volume*

The flow properties or viscosity of blood are greatly influenced by the total volume of cells in suspension (Wells and Merrill, 1962). Plasma has a viscosity of 1.3 centipoise (cp) at 37° C as compared to water, whose viscosity is 0.74 cp at the same temperature. Whole blood with 45% cells and 55% plasma has a viscosity of about 5 cp under steady flow in the major arteries. Clinically, viscosity is influenced more by the volume concentration of cells (hematocrit) than any other variable. This relationship is illustrated in Fig. 1. White cells, which make up less than 0.2% of the total hematocrit, have no apparent rheologic effect upon whole blood viscosity unless they exceed more than half of the total normal red cell mass, i.e., a white cell hematocrit of over 20%, as may be seen in certain leukemic states. As noted below, the rheology or flow behavior of the individual white cell is quite different from that of the red cell. The white cell is a more viscous plastic cell that deforms more slowly than the red cell. Platelets, while twenty or more times more numerous than white cells, represent such a relatively small mass or volume compared to the red cells that they do not influence whole blood viscosity. Their aggregation onto a vessel wall in a thrombotic mass is another matter of major rheologic importance and is often an integral part of the inflammatory process.

B. *Influence of Relative Rates of Flow (Velocity Gradients)*

The qualification of viscosity in major arteries and the value of inverse seconds (sec⁻¹) in Fig. 1 relate to the fact that viscosity is an expression of a relationship between a stress, i.e., the force of one fluid element or layer rubbing or shearing across its neighbor, and a rate of change of strain or the relative motion of the layers with respect to the distance between them. The

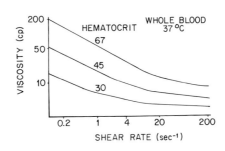

Fig. 1. Viscosity shear rate relationships for three samples of whole blood with different hematocrits.

proportionality of shearing stresses to rate of shear strain defines the quantity of viscosity. Shear strain rate or simply shear rate is an expression of the gradient of velocity of the fluid elements between the stationary wall or sides of the container and the most distant fluid element from the wall. Since this is an expression of velocity (cm/second) per increment of distance from the wall or between elements (cm) the ratio of cm/second/cm resolves to 1/second or inverse seconds (sec^{-1}). The resistance or drag at the wall retards the adjacent layer more than its inner or axial neighbor. Hence, the change of rate of strain or difference in relative motion between one and other fluid lamellae is greatest near the wall and least at the central axis. Viscosity is most commonly quantified by measuring shearing stresses at a given or fixed velocity gradient. The slope of the plot of shear stress to strain rate change yields the viscosity of the tested fluid. Most simple fluids have a constant proportionality of these two variables, and such fluids are described as Newtonian. Newton originally described viscosity as a lack of slipperiness between adjacent fluid layers. Fluids that contain suspensions of particles which are more viscous than the suspending fluid exhibit a changing or inconstant proportionality when caused to flow at changing rates of shear. The majority of complex fluids such as paint, ink, mayonnaise, or blood demonstrates decreasing shear stresses as rate of shearing is increasing. Such fluids are characterized as shear-thinning fluids. Plasma, while not a simple fluid because of its macromolecular proteins, exhibits Newtonian flow properties, i.e., a viscosity independent of changing rate of strain or rate of shear. The analysis of plasma viscosity is treacherous because of its reaction to an air surface in which it develops an invisible but tough film (Wells *et al.*, 1964). It may also react with glass or metal walls where the contact angle may be changed by this surface film reaction. This is not so much a problem at high shear, such as in an Oswald pipette, but in instruments where shear rate or shear stress is very low the film effects may produce pseudo-non-Newtonian flows in Newtonian fluids.

C. Influence of Plasma Proteins

The viscosity of whole blood is greatly influenced by the total concentrations of the plasma proteins, the relative concentrations of each of the major protein fractions, and their individual physical properties (Wells *et al.*, 1962). These effects develop through the interactions of the plasma proteins with the red cells. Red cells in saline have a lower viscosity than the same number of red cells in plasma, and the former are significantly less dependent upon the rate of shear. This is due principally to the effects of globulin and fibrinogen which act as cohesive materials that enhance the attraction of

one red cell for another. Increasing either globulin or fibrinogen levels increases red cell aggregation and the viscosity of the whole blood, especially
under creep flow conditions, i.e., at low rates of shear. Fibrinogen and many
of the globulins are high in molecular weight and are anisometric in form.
Synthetic colloids of similar weight and shape will produce the same effects.
Albumin—which is more globular in shape, lower in molecular weight, and
has a stronger negative charge—reduces aggregation and lowers blood viscosity (Wells, 1965). A loss of albumin with retention of fibrinogen and
globulin will increase viscosity just as if globuin or fibrinogen had been increased per se. Consider the red cell aggregation seen in multiple myeloma
or macroglobulinemia. Microvascular flow due to severe red cell aggregation
is considerably slowed. Aggregation of red cells is not a *sine qua non* of
disease. It can be seen in normal blood under static conditions both *in vivo*
and *in vitro*. When disease, via plasma protein changes, enhances the magnitude of the intercell attractions, then cell aggregation becomes part of
the disease process. When widespread in disease, the title of "sludging"
may be appropriately applied. Hydration, increased albumin, and improved
hydrostatics to increase flow may disperse the aggregates. One of the primary
responses in disease and especially in infection is an alteration of the quality
and quantity of the globulin fractions and, to a lesser extent, fibrinogen. The
oldest test of disease, the sedimentation rate, is simply a measure of red cell
aggregation and settling—both functions of fibrinogen and globulin concentrations.

D Influence of Rheology of Individual Cells

1. RED CELLS

In addition to cell numbers or volume concentration of cells, the rheologic
character of the suspended cells is also an important factor in the overall
flow properties of whole blood. As noted, the viscosity of blood falls or thins
as the velocity gradient increases. Beginning with stasis, red cells are attracted to one another to form chains of cells or rouleaux. This process
also permits more rapid settling or sedimentation of the cell masses. As
flow begins, the flow or shearing forces tend to separate these cell masses
until they are fully dispersed. This reduces the flocculated state and, thereby,
the resistance to flow, i.e., the shearing stress is reduced. In disease the
forces of attraction, via plasma protein alterations, are greatly increased,
and the point at which total dispersion develops is elevated. As the velocity
gradient rises, the cells begin to align themselves in streamlines, further
reducing the resistance to flow, and viscosity falls further. Finally at high
rates of shear, normal red cells have been observed to undergo an ellipsoid
type of deformation (football shaped) so that drag or resistance is further

reduced (Wells and Schmid-Schönbein, 1969). A "school of fish" alignment and shape changes produce minimization of bulk viscosity of blood at high rates of shear. All of this is predicted on the basis that the red cell is normally deformable. Any event or environment which alters normal deformability will restrict the degree to which viscosity falls with high rates of shear. In fact, if one crenates cells by hyperosmolar environments so that little deformability remains, the viscosity may actually rise rather than fall when rate of shear rises (Schmid-Schönbein et al., 1969). Such fluids are described as shear thickening and demonstrate the rheologic quality of dilatancy.

The deformability of red cells while pertinent to bulk viscosity is actually a more critical variable with respect to capillary flow; without some degree of flexibility, a red cell would be incapable of passing through the normal capillary. It has been well demonstrated that the normal red cell is highly deformable much as a partly filled plastic beachball, but, unlike the plastic, the red cell membrane tolerates relatively little stretching (Rand, 1964; Weed et al., 1969). Red cell deformability has been evaluated by viscometry of packed cells (hematocrit 98% +) (Dintenfass, 1964), by filtration of very dilute suspensions through various filter systems (Teitel, 1967), and by aspiration of cells into micropipettes (Rand and Burton, 1964). Each of these methods has certain technological qualifications, but all support the concept that the normal red cell can squeeze through a pore about 3 μm in diameter at physiological pressures without injury (Chien et al., 1971). Changes in pH and osmolality alter this capability by reducing the amount of free membrane for flexion, by concentration of the contained hemoglobin, or by crystallization or fixation of the intracellular hemoglobin (Murphy, 1967; Schmid-Schönbein and Wells, 1971). More than a few workers have invoked these responses to explain the manner in which the spleen and other reticuloendothelial systems remove old or damaged red cells (Usami et al., 1970). The splenic pores are about 3 μm in diameter. The hemoglobinopathies obviously represent the ultimate expression of abnormal red cell deformability of which sicklemia is the most common and clinically the most devastating. Infection and inflammation are often the precipitating factors in a sickle cell crisis. Recent interest in and federal funding for the hemopathology of sicklemia will most likely involve considerable research into the mechanism by which inflammation and/or infection bring on such clinical crises in sickle cell disease. Research into therapy with cyanate is now underway.

2. WHITE CELLS

Quantification of rheology has been carried out considerably less often for the white cell than for the red cell. However, the many direct observations of white cells under flow and viscometric studies in vitro indicate that the normal white cell is considerably more viscous than the red cell. Tests of individual white cell deformation also indicate an increased cell viscosity, as white cells in a 2% suspension will not pass either a 5- or 8-μm pore size filter at physiological pressures, while normal red cells will do so completely in 10 seconds (R. Wells, unpublished observations, 1970). Direct microscopic observations of white cells flowing *in vivo* are perhaps most illustrative of the role of their rheology in the inflammatory response. First, in the capillaries where the red cell is deformed into a bulletlike shape and appears to flow with ease, the white cell moves more as an elongated cylinder with slightly less velocity than the red cell. White cells, which are most easily observed in venules and veins, are usually seen near the wall with more of a rolling motion rather than as a simple particle in streamline flow. Red cells when crenated by hypertonic fluids also exhibit this type of rolling motion. White cell deformability has been used as an explanation of the mechanism of release of cells from the bone marrow when they are adequately matured (Lichtman, 1970). Polymorphonuclear leukocytes are considerably more sticky than lymphocytes as determined by filtration through glass, wool, or glass bead columns (Garvin, 1961). It becomes apparent that the rheologic differences between these white cells result from the biochemical, humoral, and biophysical differences of cell membranes and of endothelial reactions to them. These details are discussed in the other chapters of this treatise.

3. PLATELETS

As noted above, the size and numbers of platelets in normal blood have no apparent effect upon the flow properties or viscosity of blood. Any injury to any vessel wall, whether physical or chemical, will usually result in the accretion of platelets at the site of injury. Similar to white cells, platelets, once activated by some injury or inflammatory stimulus, are extremely sticky and undergo a fissionlike reaction of activating adjacent platelets to form a platelet mass or thrombus (Mustard *et al.*, 1962).

E. *Influence of Vascular Geometry*

As has been well demonstrated, the inflammatory response primarily involves the microcirculation (see Chapter 1 by Zweifach). The hemodynamics and anatomy of the arterioles are different than the venules which are different than the capillaries. Accordingly, the rheology of blood is different in each of these vascular units. The small arteries and arterioles, in general, represent a bulk flow condition with rates of shear at the wall of 20 sec^{-1} and higher. When the precapillary arterioles decrease to an internal diameter of about 25–30 μm, there can be no more than five red cells across the diameter. The total cross-sectional area would therefore include about fifteen cells. Below this point, the blood cannot be considered a hetero-genous mixture of small particles, but rather a collection of relatively large (relative to the size of the vessel) deformable masses. It is the rheology or flow properties of the masses (cells) and their suspending medium that now determine the rheologic resistance. Finally, at the level of the single cell flowing through the capillary, we deal with a pluglike flow in which these two factors are the primary rheologic variables. Hematocrit and cell numbers are not rheologic variables in the capillary. It is the rheology of the individual cell that dominates. If it is stiff or oddly shaped, its passage will be compromised. Beyond the capillary, the cells begin to gather in the progressively larger venous system where flow is considerably slower than in the arterioles, and the walls diverge. Here, the creep flow or low rate of shear is the dominant variable. There are many more venules than arterioles (Wiedeman, 1963). The normal creep flow leads to red cell aggregation which, as rate of shear rises in the larger veins, gradually disperses. Red cell aggregation can be observed in the venules *in vivo* of normal man (Wells, 1967). The changing rheologic conditions between bulk viscosity in the artery, the plug flow in the capillaries, and the creep flow in the postcapillary venules are altered and are directly related to the hydromechanical events seen in the inflammatory process. An understanding of these rheologic changes are at the foundation of understanding the inflammatory process itself.

III. Rheology of Inflammation

The various descriptions of the inflammatory process clearly indicate that no one sequence of events applies to all examples of the process. Vasodilation or constriction may occur early or late; flow stasis may vary from area to area; and cell accumulations, while predominantly made up of white cells, may also involve large concentrations of red cells and/or platelets. These and other qualifications notwithstanding, there is a reasonably common sequence of events which can be analyzed with respect to the rheology of the process. The sequence of arterial vasodilation, increased capillary flow, leakage of plasma through venular walls, reduced venous and capillary flow, white cell and platelet adhesion to the wall and to one other, stasis, diapedesis of white and red cells, and loss of all vascular reactivity comprise a generalized summary of the process. When considered from the rheologic standpoint, there is first a *high flow phase*, with vasodilation and increased volume flow; second, a *low flow phase*, with fluid loss through postcapillary venules, red cell aggregation, white cell sticking, slowing of arteriolar and capillary flow, plus development of shunt flow near the edge of the lesion; and then a *static phase*, with almost complete cessation of flow, diapedesis of

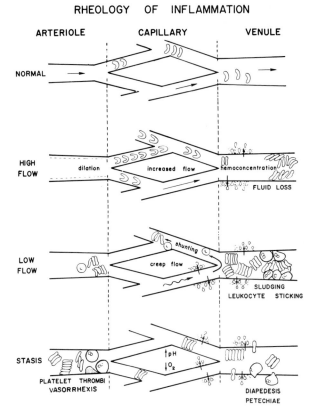

Fig. 2. The rheologic phases of the inflammatory process.

white and/or red cells, profound cell aggregation in all vessels, and leakage of fluid through the capillary wall as well as through the venular walls (Fig. 2).

A. High Flow Phase

Whatever the teleological reason for the arterial vasodilation, increasing the radius of a vessel has a profound effect upon the volume flow. Volume flow is directly proportional to the fourth power of the radius according to the Poiseuillean formula $Q = \Delta P \pi r^4 / 8 \eta L$, where Q is volume flow in cm³/minute, and η is viscosity of fluid in units of poise. This is to say that a 6% increase in radius results in a doubling of the volume flow. The degree of vessel involvement in the area of the inflammatory response is such a small fraction of the total bed that it can be assumed there is no change in the pressure head. The amount of fluid or blood traversing the capillaries and venules can, therefore, be assumed to be greatly increased in this initial part of the reaction. During this high flow phase, viscosity and red cell aggregation would be reduced and venous outflow increased. The fluid loss across venular walls follows and apparently dominates the next phase.

B. Low Flow Phase

Of all the reactions of the inflammatory process, the leakage of plasma through the postcapillary venules is the apparent keystone. Were this prevented, it would be possible that most of the other reactions would be considerably less apparent. It is noteworthy that in all treatments of the Starling Laws we think only in terms of transfer across the capillary wall, but it is becoming increasingly apparent that the postcapillary venule is as dynamic in disease reactions as is the capillary in normal transfer processes. The earliest changes in diabetes are seen in the postcapillary venules (Siperstein et al., 1968). The recent work of Wiederhielm also points to fluid transfer across the normal venular wall as well as greater transfer across the venular end of the capillary than across the arteriolar end (Wiederhielm, 1968).

The leakage of plasma across the walls might well involve more albumin than fibrinogen or globulin, resulting in a relative increased concentration of these components in the vascular compartment. But the simple loss of plasma itself will result in hemoconcentration and a rising viscosity. If globulin and fibrinogen are retained at the expense of albumin, the cell aggregation or sludging will be even more profound. Both hemoconcentration and aggregation will lead to a critical outflow resistance for the capillaries, where, with high inflow, leakage and stasis will soon follow. Shunting, which will often occur during the low flow phase, never completely corrects the problem. It does play a small role in maintaining tissue perfusion at the edge of the lesion.

C. Static Phase

The progressive slowing of flow sets up a viscious cycle of rheologic events. As can be seen in Fig. 1, creep or prestatic flow (shear rates $< 1 \sec^{-1}$) is associated with a rapidly rising viscosity which further impedes in- or outflow of the inflammatory lesion. Stasis leads to further loss of tone; wall leaks are probably further aggravated with subsequent fluid loss; and, in the final state, vasoreactivity to neural or humoral stimuli is lost. Even if the area is artificially reperfused, filling and normal flow will return only to certain areas. Rarely can the morbid tissue ever be fully reperfused. In the static phase, red cell diapedesis to the point of petechiae may be seen. The normal red cell as noted is quite deformable and can pass through very small pores. How it gets through the vessel wall where pores are less than the critical size of 3 μm is an enigma. Perhaps the red cell, given time, can ooze through pores less than 3 μm in diameter. It is hard to imagine that pores of this size develop in the vascular wall. Most studies on the red cell pore passage have been of relatively short duration. It is likely that this phenomenon has been observed *in vivo*.

IV. Summary

The rheology of blood is one of the fundamental biophysical variables in the inflammatory process. The primary site of action and reaction in inflammation is at the microvascular level, which is the site of the greatest rheologic changes that occur with respect to blood.

The rheology of inflammation has been considered in three sequential phases; high flow, low flow, and stasis. As has been shown, slowing of flow results in an almost exponential increase in viscous resistance especially in the postcapillary venules. The loss of fluid through the post-capillary venules results in hemoconcentration, red cell aggregation, and eventual stasis. Blood is most viscous when it is static. Shunting, also at the microvascular level, occurs during the low flow and static phases and must be one of the variables relating to any recovery process.

Historically, there has been considerable rheologic study of the inflammatory process, even though fragmented and carried out without formal consideration of fluid dynamics per se. A more systematized or unitarian approach to the rheology of inflammation would produce significant progress in this important aspect of the problem.

References

Chien, S., Luse, S. A., and Bryant, C. A. (1971). *Microvasc. Res.* **3**, 183.
Dintenfass, L. (1964). *J. Lab. Clin. Med.* **64**, 594.
Garvin, J. E. (1961). *J. Exp. Med.* **114**, 51.
Lichtman, M. A. (1970). *N. Engl. J. Med.* **283**, 944.
Murphy, J. R. (1967). *J. Lab. Clin. Med.* **69**, 758.
Mustard, J. F., Murphy, E. A., Rowsell, H. C., and Downie, H. G. (1962). *Amer. J. Med.* **33**, 621.

Rand, R. P. (1964). *Biophys. J.* **4**, 303.

Rand, R. P., and Burton, A. C. (1964). *Biophys. J.* **4**, 115.

Schmid-Schönbein, H., and Wells, R. (1971). *Ergebn. Physiol., Biol. Chem. Exp. Pharmakol.* **63**, 147.

Schmid-Schönbein, H., Wells, R., and Goldstone, J. (1969). *Circ. Res.* **25**, 131.

Siperstein, M. D., Unger, R. H., and Madison, L. L. (1968). *J. Clin. Invest.* **47**, 1973.

Teitel, P. (1967). *Nouv. Rev. Fr. Hematol.* **7**, 321.

Usami, S., Chien, S., and Gregersen, M. I. (1971). *Biorheology* **6**, 277.

Weed, R. I., LaCelle, P. L., and Merrill, E. W. (1969). *J. Clin. Invest.* **48**, 795.

Wells, R. (1965). *In* "Shock and Hypotension" (L. C. Mills and J. H. Moyer, eds.), pp. 80–86. Grune & Stratton, New York.

Wells, R. (1967). *Bibl. Anat.* **9**, 520.

Wells, R., and Merrill, E. W. (1962). *J. Clin. Invest.* **41**, 1591.

Wells, R., and Schmid-Schönbein, H. (1969). *J. Appl. Physiol.* **27**, 213.

Wells, R., Merrill, E. W., Gabelnick, H., Draper, C. S., Gilinson, P. J., and Dauwalter, C. R. (1962). *Trans. Soc. Rheol.* **6**, 19.

Wells, R., Gawronski, T. H., Cox, P. M., and Perera, R. D. (1964). *Amer. J. Physiol.* **207**, 1035.

Wiedeman, M. P. (1963). *Circ. Res.* **12**, 375.

Wiederhielm, C. A. (1968). *J. Gen. Physiol.* **52**, 29.

Chapter 6

THE LYMPHATIC SYSTEM IN INFLAMMATION

J. R. CASLEY-SMITH

I. Introduction

Recently there has been an increasing awareness of the parts played by lymphatics in most disease processes, their major roles in many of them, and their importance for the normal functioning of the body. This system was previously the most neglected in the body. It has recently been reviewed by Courtice (1971), Földi (1969), Mayerson (1963), Rusznyák *et al.* (1967), and Yoffey and Courtice (1970).

The neglect has largely been caused by the difficulties of observing and handling the lymphatics. In particular, it is hard to preserve the form and contents of these very thin-walled fragile vessels with routine histological techniques. There are also great difficulties in collecting the lymph from circumscribed areas. Improvements in fixation and other techniques, the electron microscope, and small bore polyethylene cannulas have immensely facilitated the study of the lymphatics.

II. Structure

The lymphatic system is very similar to the blood vascular system from the venous capillaries onward. There are innumerable, small, thin-walled vessels which merge centrally into progressively larger ones. The peripheral vessels have been termed "lymphatic capillaries," "terminal lymphatics," "small lymphatics," and "peripheral lymphatics." All these terms have deficiencies, and, for reasons given elsewhere (Casley-Smith, 1970a), I prefer the term "initial lymphatics." These, which perform the system's primary function of removing material from the tissues, may be contrasted with the larger, thicker-walled "collecting lymphatics," which perform the system's secondary function of transporting the material. There are great structural differences between these two classes of vessels which correlate with the differences in their functions.

A. Initial Lymphatics in Normal Tissues

1. GENERAL

The initial lymphatics are usually about 100–500 μm long and of very irregular shape. They have "maximal diameters" of $\sim$15–75 μm when completely filled (Casley-Smith, 1972d), but they are usually quite flattened.

Fig. 1. Mouse ear lymphatic (L) injected with thorium dioxide. Its endothelium is slightly thicker, but less electron opaque than that of the blood capillary (C), which is also considerably smaller in diameter. There are a number of closed junctions (J) in the lymphatic endothelium. (8000 $\times$; the line indicates 1 μm in this and the other Figs., unless some other value is stated.) (From Casley-Smith, 1965.)

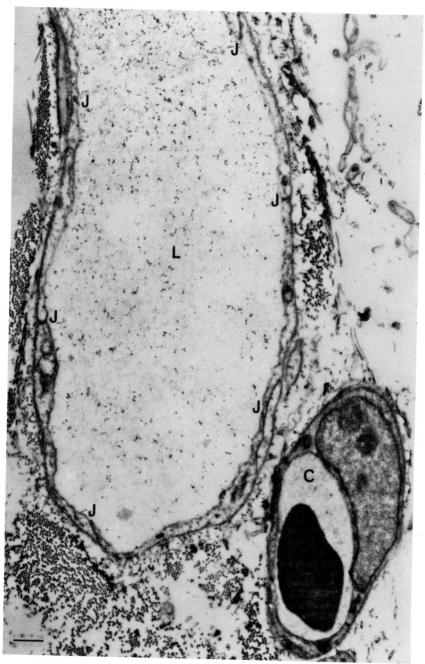

Fig. 1

They are normally arranged in complex, approximately two-dimensional networks, especially in the connective tissue capsules surrounding the lobules, etc., of organs (Rodbard, 1969). Details of the specialized distributions are reviewed by Kampmeier (1969), Rusznyák *et al.* (1967), and Yoffey and Courtice (1970).

The fine structure of the intial lymphatics has been reviewed by Casley-Smith (1967c,d, 1969a,f, 1970a), Collin (1969), Dobbins (1971), Fawcett *et al.* (1969), Lauweryns and Boussauw (1969), Leak (1970), Leak and Burke (1966, 1968), Ohkuma (1970), Ottaviani and Azzali (1965), Viragh *et al.* (1966), and Yoffey and Courtice (1970) (see Figs. 1–11). The endothelium of lymphatics is very similar to that of blood vessels (Chapter 2). It is usually a little thicker in lymphatics, but it appears to be thinner because of their much greater diameters (Fig. 1). It is rather less electron opaque and never contains fenestrae. The basement membrane is much less developed than in blood capillaries, especially in active areas where it is sometimes not visible at all. On the lumenal surface of the cells, in nondistended lymphatics, there are many projections into the lumen (Fig. 4); on the ablumenal surface, there are often processes projecting into the connective tissue (Figs. 3, 10, 12, 14). Many connective tissue filaments attach to these and to other regions of the cell, both generally and at specialized sites which resemble hemidesmosomes (Figs. 10, 14). There are two classes of filaments. Some (~ 5 mμ) are thin, branched, and irregular and may well be coagulated plasma proteins; others (~ 10 mμ) are thicker, straight, long, and probably tubular. These pass into and around the collagen bundles and general ground substance, thus anchoring the cells to these structures.

2. INTERCELLULAR JUNCTIONS

Like the blood capillaries (Chapter 2), the lymphatic endothelium intercellular junctions at their narrowest cross section usually have either tight or close portions (i.e., zonulae occludentes; Figs. 4–6, 10). The intercellular gaps in these are ~ 1 and ~ 4 mμ, respectively (Karnovsky, 1968); but even these probably contain some mucopolysaccharide. There is also, however, a

Fig. 2. Rat foot pad. There are a number of lymphatics (L), which are unusually close together, but whose flattened form is typical of those of normal, relatively quiescent regions. (4000×.) (From Casley-Smith, 1967a.)

Fig. 3. A lymphatic in a lymphedematous tongue. There is much protein in the lumen (L) and in the connective tissue, especially where there are "channels" between the collagen bundles. These might be termed "prelymphatic pathways." There are two long ablumenal projections (P) into the tissue; at higher magnifications these were found to have long, straight (~ 10 mμ) filaments attached to them, which could be clearly distinguished from the smaller, shorter, irregular fibrils (probably protein). (15,000 ×.)

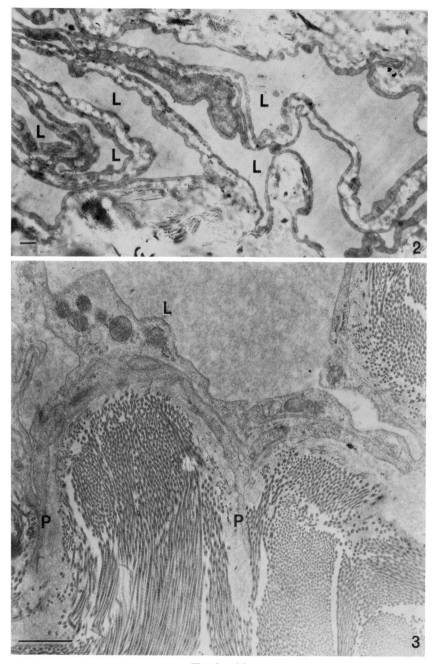

Figs. 2 and 3

varying amount of open junction, as seen only in blood vessels after injuries and in sinusoids (Figs. 1–4). Here the gaps may even be some microns across, although ~100 mμ is usual. In much of the rest of this chapter, the close and tight junctional regions will be classed together as closed junctions, contrasting with the open junctions. This is the essential distinction when considering lymphatic permeability and function.

In quiescent areas, e.g., the pinnas of the mouse ear, only 1–2% of the junctional regions are open; in active areas (e.g., near muscle), they may amount to 20–50%. Similarly large proportions are found in injured areas (Section II,B,2). In the intestinal villi, Dobbins and Rollins (1970) found that of 254 sections of junctions 6 were open, 10 were close, 89 were tight, and 149 could not be visualized clearly enough to be identified. [These workers and Ottaviani and Azzali (1965) consider that this proportion of open junctions is too little for them to be important for permeability; but all other investigators disagree, and it can be shown by calculation that it is likely to be quite sufficient (Elhay and Casley Smith, 1973).] Commonly, the proportion of tight junctions is far less than in blood capillaries. The junctions vary along their lengths, in some places securing the cells firmly and in others allowing them to separate (Majno, 1965). The two-dimensional nature and extreme thinness of the electron microscope sections (~50 mμ) mean that, often, junctions which only appear open over parts of their lengths in the section are actually completely open in some other plane. This has often been shown by serial sectioning. No doubt, the openings also vary greatly with time and tissue movements (Section IV,A). Initial lymphatic junctions have another peculiarity in that there is often considerable cellular interdigitation (Fig. 10). It may be that this, together with the lumenal projections, allows excessive amounts of plasma membrane to be stored when the vessel is almost empty; it may assist in uniting the cells at some points. It also appears that some lymphatic junctions, at least in the dog, have "pockets" external to some closed junctions, formed by ablumenal processes from both cells (G. L. Todd, 1972, personal communication). These contain filaments similar to the anchoring filaments, but here they join one cell to the next rather than the cells to the connective tissues. Presumably, these are additional devices for firmly connecting the cells together over parts of their junctions, while leaving them free to separate over other parts.

Fig. 4. Diaphragmatic lymphatic (L). A junction (J) contains a tight portion (T), with its typical fusion of the outer lamellas of the unit membranes and its intracytoplasmic filaments. There is also a lumenal process (P), which is typically adjacent to the junction. In the endothelial cells there are many vesicles (V). The basement membrane is almost invisible around the lymphatics in this active area. (150,000×.) the line shows 0.1 μm.

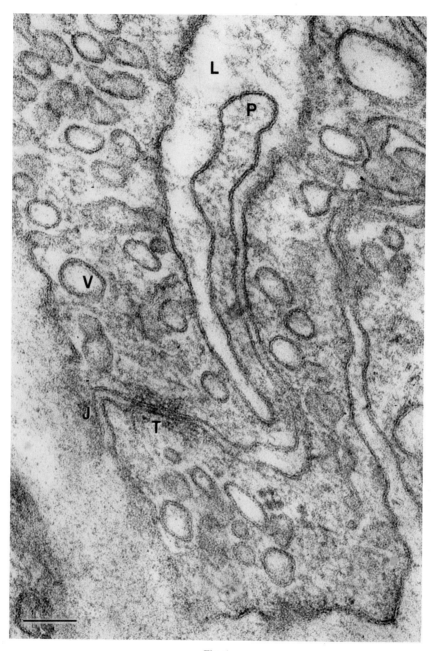

Fig. 4

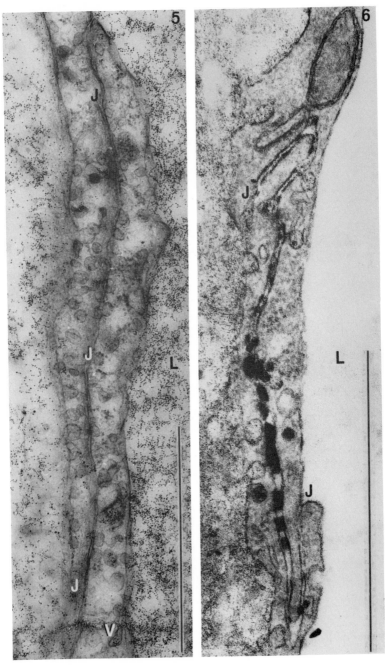

Figs. 5 and 6

Great gentleness is necessary to avoid artifactually opening the junctions. Thus, if the pinnas of the ears are depilated (Leak and Burke, 1966), many more open junctions are found than if this is not done (Casley-Smith, 1965). However, they are certainly not all artifacts, as shown by the frequent findings of tracers and cells lying in them and by the association of the presence of many open junctions with great increases in vessel permeabilities (Section III,A,1).

3. VESICLES

The small (~ 70 mμ) smooth vesicles, which are found in all cells, are also present in lymphatic endothelium (Fig. 4). Here they account for $\sim 35\%$ of the cytoplasmic volume, with about one-half of their volumes being taken up by their limiting membranes (Casley-Smith, 1969a). About 120 are attached to each square micron of endothelial surface by necks ~ 10 mμ in internal diameter and ~ 20 mμ in length. Those free in the cytoplasm number about 300 per square micron of lumenal surface, or about 1000 per cubic micron of cell volume.

The endothelium also contains a few smooth and rough-surfaced endoplasmic reticular elements and a few ropheosomes ("hairy" or "coated" vesicles—~ 200 mμ). Phagocytic vesicles (0.1–5 μm) are found if there are particles, etc., to stimulate their formations, e.g., chylomicrons (Fig. 9). If the small vesicles contain particles which are mutually adherent, many of them with coalesce to form large (0.1–5 μm) vesicles, very similar to those formed by phagocytosis (Casley-Smith, 1964, 1965), but with much more concentrated contents initially (Fig. 15). These have been termed "symphyosomes" (Casley-Smith, 1969f). Cells containing large amounts of material in large vesicles (of either kind) may migrate away from the lymphatic wall after some months and lie in the tissues looking similar to loaded macrophages (Casley-Smith, 1964). These tissues also become quite fibrotic (Section VI,A,4).

Fig. 5. Mouse ear after the injection of ferritin into the lymphatics (L). There is a long, close junction (J), which contains very little tracer. Some particles are visible in small vesicles (V). (60,000×.) (From Casley-Smith, 1965.)

Fig. 6. A close junction (J) in a diaphragmatic lymphatic (L). Ferric chloride and sodium ferrocyanide were administered separately. Ferriferrocyanide has been precipitated in those sites where the ions encountered each other. The large amount of precipitate in the junction shows that this was the preferred pathway. Some is also present in vesicles, but they are likely to be too slow to contribute significantly to its passage. (80,000×.) (From Casley-Smith, 1967b.)

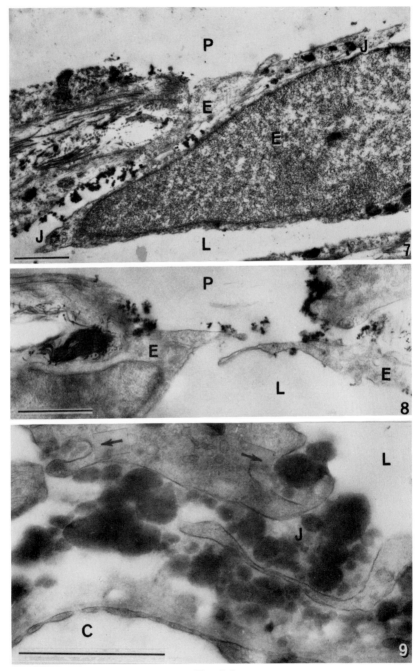

Figs. 7–9

4. Recognizing Lymphatics

With the light microscope, the chief difficulty is to see the lymphatic at all; once seen, it can usually be distinguished from blood vessels, although confusion is possible. Electron microscope verification is therefore desirable (Lauweryns and Boussauw, 1969). Even with the electron microscope, it is not possible to be completely sure that any given vessel is a lymphatic and not a blood vessel, unless the lymphatics have first been microinjected with tracers. However, after considerable experience with tracers, it is possible to be certain without them (most of the time). Lymphatics are usually bigger than blood capillaries, have very irregular walls, and are often rather collapsed. Their endothelium is usually slightly thicker, but appears thinner because of their greater diameters. It is normally paler, and has no fenestrae. The lymphatic basement membranes tend to be more tenuous, and their junctions may be open. They often have lumenal projections, and always have ablumenal ones, often with filaments attached. They normally contain far fewer erythrocytes and less plasma protein than do blood vessels.

None of these criteria are absolute. They are especially fallible in primitive animals, where the blood vessels, particularly the venous capillaries, have most of the characteristics of mammalian lymphatics (Section II,D).

5. Prelymphatic Pathways

In normal tissues, one often sees gaps between the formed elements of the connective tissue, sometimes ending at a lymphatic junction. These are easily visible when tracers or many proteins are present in the tissues (Figs.

Fig. 7. Mouse diaphragm. There is a long, closed junction (J) between two lymphatic endothelial cells (E); the mesothelial cells and the connective tissue are separated at this point. The junction contains some carbon, which was injected into the peritoneal cavity (P). There is obviously a very narrow, slitlike connection between this and the lymphatic lumen (L), but the overlap of the cells implies that the junction is, at present, effectively only permeable to small molecules, and is closed to large ones. This was during diaphragmatic contraction when the junctions are closed, preventing the egress of large molecules from the compressed lymphatics. (15,000×.)

Fig. 8. Mouse diaphragm. Here the diaphragm was more relaxed, and there is a gap between two lymphatic endothelial cells; the lymphatic and the peritoneal cavity communicate directly, and large molecules can pass through. The overlapping nature of the junction implies that it would be readily closed on diaphragmatic contraction. (20,000×.) (From Casley-Smith, 1964.)

Fig. 9. A lacteal (L) in a fat-fed rat's intestinal villus has many chylomicrons entering via an open junction (J) from the connective tissue. Some lipid is also entering or leaving the cell via large vesicles (arrows). [The direction of such passage is better determined in other experiments (Casley-Smith, 1964).] There is a fenestrated blood capillary (C); one can see that chylomicrons cannot fit through fenestrae. (40,000×.) (From Casley-Smith, 1962.)

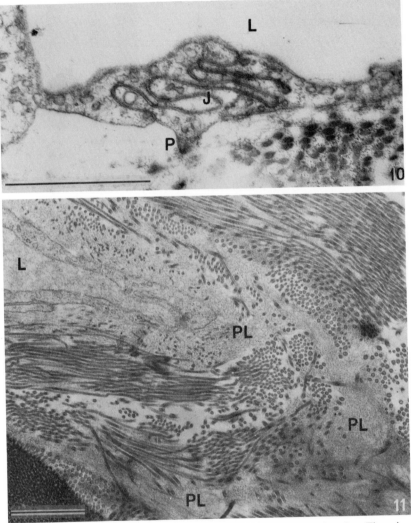

Fig. 10. Mouse ear lymphatic (L), with a very convoluted close junction. There is an ablumenal endothelial projection (P), with some filaments attaching at a hemidesmosome-like area. (40,000×.) (From Casley-Smith and Florey, 1961.)

Fig. 11. A lymphatic in a lymphedematous tongue. There is much protein in the lumen (L) and in prelymphatic pathways (PL) in the connective tissue between some of the collagen bundles. (20,000×.) (From Casley-Smith *et al.*, 1969.)

3, 11). They become particularly prominent in inflamed regions when the edema forces the cells and fiber bundles further apart. It is, of course, evident that some regions of the tissues contain more fluid and fewer formed elements than others: to many workers, this hardly seems to justify designating those which happen to open at a lymphatic junction with the term "prelymphatic" or "paralymphatic." This argument is especially forceful when one considers primitive animals (Section II,D). With these, the peripheral blood vessels, sometimes even without basement membranes, are often directly continuous with the tissue spaces. (True lymphatics are absent in these animals, and the blood vessels perform their functions.)

Some prelymphatics, however, are quite large and follow definite, well-defined courses (Földi et al., 1968a,b; Ottaviani and Azzali, 1965; Várkonyi et al., 1969, 1970; Wallace, 1969). This is particularly evident in the brain and retina, which have no true lymphatics. Inflammation, or lymphedema produced by ligating the cervical lymphatics, cause the marked dilation and filling with protein of what are evidently preformed paths in the adventitia of the larger blood vessels. There is considerable evidence that these non-endothelialised paths perform the functions of lymphatics and empty into them. They therefore certainly deserve some special designation, such as "prelymphatics." This being so, it appears to be only a question of degree if one excludes the smaller, less regular vessels elsewhere in the body. Perhaps this whole system could be termed "prelymphatic pathways," with the more major vessels being "prelymphatics."

B. Initial Lymphatics in Inflamed Tissues

1. GENERAL

The appearances of injured cells are considered in this volume in Chapter 1 and in Volume I, Chapter 3. Injured lymphatic endothelium shows similar changes, ranging from none in very mild injuries to complete derangement in very severe ones (Casley-Smith, 1965, 1967d, 1969f, 1970a; J. C. Chin, unpublished, 1971; Collin, 1969; Leak and Burke, 1965; Leak and Kato, 1970; Virágh et al., 1966) (see Figs. 12, 17, 23). Initially, there is contraction and darkening for a few minutes, followed by profound swelling, the formation of blebs, and the breaking of the plasma membranes (Fig. 14). The swelling of the endoplasmic reticulum gives rise to large (0.1–1 μm), empty vesicles, often studded with ribosomes (Fig. 13). While the small vesicles may become slightly more numerous in mild injuries, they are almost absent in severe ones; perhaps they become incorporated into the tightly stretched plasma membranes (Fig. 14).

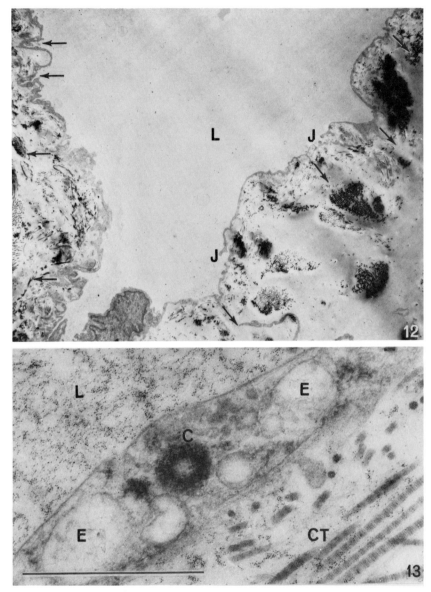

Fig. 12. A rat foot pad which had been inflamed with dextran. A lymphatic (L) is dilated, with open junctions (J). Portions of endothelium have been pulled out by filaments (arrows); the intervening portions bulge inward. (3000×.) (From Casley-Smith, 1967a.)

Fig. 13. Swollen lymphatic endothelium in a mouse ear injured by heat (54°C for 4 minutes). There are dilated portions of endoplasmic reticulum (E). Ferritin was injected into the connective tissue (CT); it has been considerably concentrated in the lumen (L). A centriole (C) is present. (50,000×.) (From Casley-Smith, 1972d.)

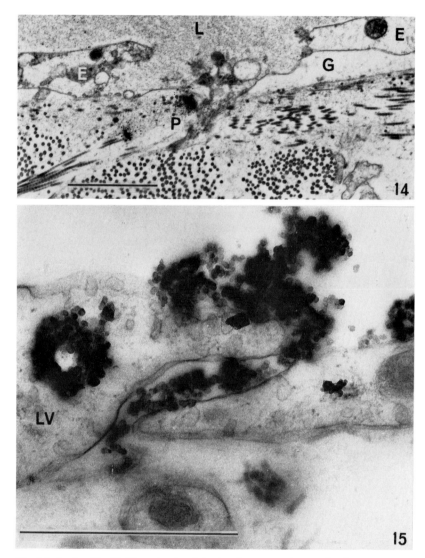

Fig. 14. As for Fig. 13. There is a break in the plasma membrane, allowing much protein to enter the cell. A gap (G) is present between the ablumenal plasma membrane and the basement membrane, but the bulging of the cell toward the lumen is prevented at an ablumenal projection (P), to which filaments are attached. The cytoplasm is very watery with few vesicles. (25,000×.) (From Casley-Smith, 1964.)

Fig. 15. As for Fig. 13. Carbon is passing down an open junction. Other particles are present in a large vesicle (LV), which is probably a symphyosome. (60,000×.) (From Casley-Smith, 1964.)

The vessels are greatly dilated (Fig. 12), sometimes being almost circular in cross section. Their content of protein often has an increased electron opacity, as does that in the tissues. They frequently contain erythrocytes, other cells, and cell debris.

2. JUNCTIONS

A characteristic finding is that even after the mildest injury there are many open junctions (Casley-Smith, 1965, 1967a, 1969f, 1970a; Collin, 1969; Leak and Burke, 1965; Leak and Kato, 1970; Virágh et al., 1966, 1971) (see Figs. 12, 15, 23). This has been seen after very light touch, heat, microinjections of KCN, bacterial and chemical injuries, and after the peritoneal injection of dextran which causes edema of the snout and foot pads of the rat. In quiescent regions, where the open junctions comprise normally only 1–2%, their proportion rises to 20–50%. It is of interest and considerable importance (Section VI,A,1) that lymphatic blockage also causes the initial lymphatics to dilate and to become filled with concentrated proteins (Figs. 3, 11) and the junctions to open (Casley-Smith, 1965; Casley-Smith et al., 1969).

3. EXTRACELLULAR FILAMENTS

These are very important in inflammation. Pullinger and Florey (1935) showed that the fibers "attached" to the lymphatic walls become tight and pull the vessels open when the tissues become edematous, even against the raised solid tissue and hydrostatic pressures (Section IV,A,1). Virágh et al. (1966, 1971) queried this and showed that collagen fibers are often detached from the endothelium in inflammation. Casley-Smith (1967a) and Collin (1969) found, however, that the fine filaments are still attached to the endothelium and continue to allow the swollen tissues to dilate the vessels. There is other evidence supporting this role of the filaments (Casley-Smith, 1967a): those regions of the walls where there are the most filaments are pulled first and furthest out into the tissues (Figs. 12, 23). The intervening regions of wall are often bowed inward by the pressures outside the vessels; indeed, at times the endothelium is pushed inward, separating from the basement membrane for some distance (Figs. 16, 23). Finally, the injection of hyaluronidase weakens the unions of the filaments with the ground substance and allows the lymphatics to collapse (Figs. 16, 17). This last was not confirmed by Virágh et al. (1971), but similar results were obtained by L. V. Leak and J. F. Burke (personal communication, 1968).

Virágh et al. (1971) also found that the filaments remain attached to the cells, but claimed that because they were not continuous between the endothelium and the dense connective tissue of the epimyseum or the cutis they could not exert traction on the lymphatics. This view ignores the fact that

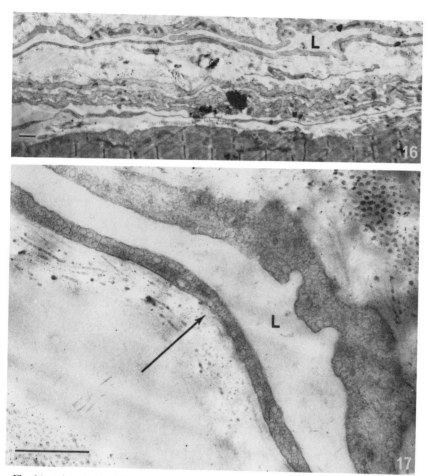

Fig. 16. A lymphatic (L) in the foot pad of a rat, which had been inflamed with dextran, but whose dilated lymphatics had been collapsed by the local administration of hyaluronidase, cf. Fig. 12. This collapse is so complete that this vessel was mistaken for one in a normal foot pad. This error was fortunately pointed out by Virágh *et al.* (1971). (4000×.) (From Casley-Smith, 1967a.)

Fig. 17. A higher magnification of a portion of Fig. 16. Part of the lymphatic wall (arrow) has been forced in toward the lumen by the high external pressure after the connections of the filaments with the ground substance had been destroyed by the hyaluronidase. (20,000×.) (From Casley-Smith, 1967a.)

even edematous connective tissue has considerable viscosity and is capable of adhering to the filaments with tenacity. It seems clear, then, that the original views of Pullinger and Florey were correct: in edema, the swollen tissues pull on the filaments, which thus dilate the initial lymphatics in spite of the raised pressures in the tissues.

C. Collecting Lymphatics

Passing from the initial lymphatics to the great ones, one finds that gradually fewer and fewer of the junctions are open, that there are more and more
close and tight regions, and that the basement membranes become more and
more prominant (Casley-Smith, 1969b; Mislin and Schipp, 1967; Moe, 1963;
Pressman et al., 1967; Yamagishi, 1960). (An exception is the thoracic duct
where the basement membrane vanishes, its place probably being taken by
a well-developed internal elastic lamina, paralleling what happens in the
great arteries and veins.) The walls of these larger lymphatics acquire more
elements. The pericytes, rather than being only occasional, become almost
continuous. They give way to true smooth muscle cells, which eventually
form as continuous and thick a tube as in the great veins. The noncellular
elements increase, notably the collagen and elastic tissue. There are also
unmyelinated nerve fibers (B. Morris, personal communication, 1971),
which correlate with the observations on lymphatic spasm in inflammation
and its release after sympathetic blocking (Section V,A).

The vessels in the lymph nodes are similar to those outside them. There
are a few open junctions in the more peripheral nodes, particularly in the
internal vessels, rather than in the peripheral sinuses. The larger, more
central nodes have only closed junctions.

D. Comparative Morphology of Blood Vessels and Lymphatics

The gross and light microscopical aspects have been reviewed by Drinker
(1942) and Kampmeier (1969), and the fine structure by Casley-Smith
(1971a, 1972a) (see Figs. 18, 19, 21). Briefly, passing from primitive verte-

---

Fig. 18. Amphioxus, the hepatic vein (V) has large openings between its endothelial cells
(E). Only a basement membrane lines an adjacent sinusoid (S), which contains lipoproteins.
(5000×.) (From Casley-Smith, 1971a.)

Fig. 19. A venous capillary in the kidney of an elasmobranch. There is a junction (J) which
is open over part of its length; the endothelial cells have ablumenal projections (P); and the
basement membrane is poorly developed: All of these features resemble those of mammalian
lymphatics. Fenestrae (arrows) are also present; this is the most primitive animal in which they
have so far been found. (12,000×.) (From Casley-Smith and Mart, 1970.)

Fig. 20. Fenestrated venous blood capillary (C) in the renal medulla of the mouse. Ferritin molecules were microinjected into the connective tissues (CT). They approach the fenestrae (arrows), are found in their diaphragms, and presumably pass through them into the blood.
They do not approach fenestrae on the arterial limbs, but ferritin injected into the blood leaves
via these, rather than via those on the venous limbs. Thus, proteins probably leave the vessels
via the arterial fenestrae, and reenter them via the venous ones. (150,000×; the line indicates
0.1 μm.) (From Casley-Smith, 1970b.)

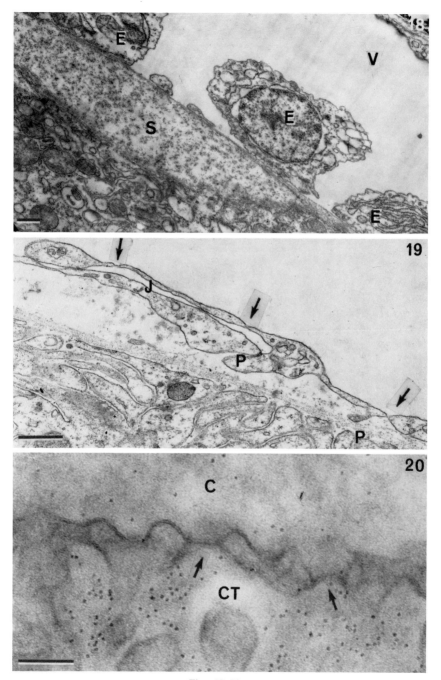

Figs. 18–20

brates or invertebrates toward the higher forms, one finds that the blood vessels, which originally consist of just basement membrane with scattered endothelial cells, become more and more fully lined with endothelial cells and pericytes. This is also the sequence when one passes from the small, peripheral vessels toward the larger, central ones. Eventually, the linings become complete, and relatively impermeable junctions develop. (These are between the endothelial cells in vertebrates and between the pericytes in invertebrates.) These changes are almost certainly correlated with the increasing blood pressures and plasma protein concentration. The pericytes develop contractile fibrils in both vertebrates and invertebrates (except, curiously, in amphioxus where they occur in the endothelium.)

In the elasmobrachs, which lack true lymphatics, the junctions in the small venous vessels in the body wall appear very similar to those of mammalian lymphatics (Casley-Smith and Mart, 1970) (Fig. 19). Presumably, swimming motions can still force fluid, etc., into the vessels against the low blood pressure. After this stage, in the torpedoes and teleosts, true lymphatics developed (i.e., a separate system of vessels which do not normally contain blood). This corresponds to a marked elevation in blood pressure (especially venous pres-

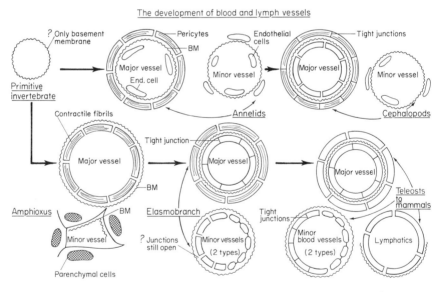

Fig. 21. A diagram showing the similar, yet divergent, development of the vascular systems in the vertebrates and invertebrates. The relationships of open capillary junctions, fenestrae, and lymphatics are indicated. (The hagfish have been found to occupy a position between amphioxus and the elasmobranchs in their vascular systems, as in the rest of their morphology.) (From Casley-Smith, 1971a.)

sure) which presumably either necessitated the junctions in the venous vessels being closed all the time or would not allow material to be forced into the vessels by body movements, or both—hence, the necessity for the lymphatic system to develop separately.

It is of interest, in view of the similarity of some of the roles of lymphatics and fenestrae (Section VI,C) (Fig. 20) that fenestrae antedate lymphatics and are found in the visceral blood capillaries of elasmobranchs (Figs. 19, 21). They are not found in the hagfish or amphioxus, where the many permanently open junctions would render them unnecessary and nonfunctional (Casley-Smith, 1971a, 1972a).

III. Permeable Paths through the Lymphatic Wall

A. Junctions

1. PERMEABILITY

It now appears almost certain that the intercellular junctions of blood vessels correspond to Pappenheimer's (1953) "pores" or, better, to his "slits" (Chapter 2). (This is in continuous capillaries; in fenestrated ones (Clementi and Palade, 1969), the fenestrae almost certainly let much more material through than do the junctions.) It has been shown that ions traverse even the tight junctions of blood vessels and of both initial and collecting lymphatics (Casley-Smith, 1967b, 1969c,d; Cotran and Majno, 1967) (Fig. 6). The close junctions of blood capillaries allow small macromolecules (mw $\sim 40,000$) to pass through them (Karnovsky, 1968), as they also do in the lymphatics (J. R. Casley-Smith, unpublished, 1971). Larger macromolecules (mw $\sim 500,000$) rarely or never penetrate them (Casley-Smith, 1969b; Clementi, 1971) (Fig. 5). It has been suggested that even the penetration of the small macromolecules is an artifact because the tracer used, peroxidase, can open the close junctions to wider than normal (Clementi, 1971). Certainly in both blood vessels (Garlick and Renkin, 1970; Grotte, 1956; Landis and Pappenheimer, 1963; Renkin, 1971) and in lymphatics (Mayerson, 1963; Strawitz *et al.*, 1968; Rusznyák *et al.*, 1967, pp. 456–459), there is a dramatic falling off in the permeability of the junctions for molecules of over a few thousand molecular weight.

The situation changes completely as soon as some of the junctions become open, both in blood capillaries (Chapter 2) and in lymphatics (Casley-Smith, 1962, 1964, 1965, 1970a; Fawcett *et al.*, 1969; Leak and Burke, 1968; Kato, 1966; Yoffey and Courtice, 1970, pp. 18–21, 74–77). All the blood constituents, including cells, pass with ease through the open junctions in the walls of the vessels (Figs. 7, 9, 15). In particular, the greatly increased permeability of injured initial lymphatics (McMaster and Hudack, 1932) can be seen to be associated with all the material pouring through these open junctions (Casley-Smith, 1965; Leak and Burke, 1965; Leak and Kato, 1970). This association, together with the lack of markedly increased passage via other paths, shows that the open junctions cause the increased permeability. Similar great increases in lymphatic permeability caused by the presence of many open junctions can be seen when active regions are compared with quiescent ones. Additional proof of this causation is provided by certain specialized sites, such as the diaphragm (Casley-Smith, 1964). Here, the location of the lymphatics relative to the pleural and peritoneal cavities is almost identical. However, those on the peritoneal aspect have open junctions which communicate with the peritoneal cavity; lymphatics on the other side do not communicate with the pleural cavity. There is a concomitant enormous difference in the permeability to macromolecules on the two sides.

2. SELECTIVITY

The principles of restricted diffusion and steric impedence (Pappenheimer, 1953; Landis and Pappenheimer, 1963) can account for the selectivity which the junctions exhibit against the larger particles. This selectivity can be seen in lymphatics (Casley-Smith, 1969f, 1970a; Rusznyák *et al.*, 1967, pp. 455–461; Yoffey and Courtice, 1970, pp. 73–77) as well as in the blood capillaries (Chapter 2). Naturally, the extent of these impedences will vary according to the particular molecular dimensions, configurations, and surface charges, as compared with those of the junctional walls. (During passage through the tissues, the ground substance and basement membranes will add selectively also by similar mechanisms; see Chapter 4).

3. WHY THE JUNCTIONS OPEN

The primary reasons that the junctions open are the poor support given to the junctions by the tenuous basement membranes and the paucity of close junctions, especially if the bonds of these are weakened during inflammation (Chapter 2). [It may be that lymphatic endothelium contracts in inflammation just as blood vascular endothelium does (Majno *et al.*, 1969), and preliminary results (Casley-Smith, 1972e) suggest that this may also occur in lymphatics.] Movements of the tissues and any pulling apart of the endothelial cells by the attached filaments during edema will assist the junctions to open. It is important to note that the filaments are not attached to any portions of the cells overlapped by and on the lumenal side of another. Since the cells are very flexible, this means that the inner flap will be pushed aside by the inflowing fluid. This process will be assisted by the passage of any large particles or cells, which will act as dilators as they are forced in.

B. Vesicles

1. SMALL VESICLES

There is mounting evidence that these small vesicles account for the slow leakage of macromolecules out of the continuous blood capillaries (Chapter 2; Bruns and Palade, 1968; Casley-Smith, 1969a; Casley-Smith and Chin, 1971; Garlick and Renkin, 1970; Jennings and Florey, 1967; Karnovsky, 1968; Majno, 1965; Renkin, 1971; Palade, 1961; Shea *et al.*, 1969). It is also evident that they transport material across lymphatic endothelium and mesothelium (Casley-Smith, 1964, 1965, 1969a,e; Casley-Smith and Chin, 1971) (Figs. 5, 6). In fact, it is likely that large macromolecules can enter the vesicles more readily in lymphatic endothelium than in blood endothelium because there is likely to be a form of "micro-plasma-skimming" in the swiftly flowing blood. This will keep the macromolecules a short distance away from the mouths of the vesicles opening at the lumenal surface (J. R. Casley-Smith, unpublished, 1971).

It is probable that the vesicles are separated from the plasma membranes, are moved randomly about the cells, and are reunited with the membranes through the action of Brownian motion (Casley-Smith, 1969a,e; Casley-Smith, and Chin, 1971; Green and Casley-Smith, 1972; Jennings and Florey, 1967; Shea *et al.*, 1969). They do not need cellular energy to take up material or to transport it across the cell. It has been calculated that about seven vesicles cross the cells per square micron per second (Casley-Smith, 1969a; Garlick and Renkin, 1970; Shea *et al.*, 1969), that they have median transit times of ~3–5 seconds and median attachment times of ~2–3 seconds (Casley-Smith and Chin, 1971; Green and Casley-Smith, 1972). It is also likely that the vesicles approach the plasma membranes many times before fusing, possibly because of the repulsion of identical charges on the two stuctures: thus, nearly 50% of those which leave one side of the cell eventually reach the other.* The random movements mean that material will be carried in quanta in the direction of (and in amounts proportional to) any concentration gradients existing across the endothelium. (Hence, foreign macromolecules injected into the tissues will be slowly removed by the

---

*J. R. Casley-Smith and H. I. Clark (*J. Microsc.* 1972, in press) reexamined this problem using the vesicular numbers and dimensions found in the hindlegs of dogs, the same species as was used for most of the gross physiological measurements by other workers. They found that approximately 6.2 vesicles crossed the cells (in each direction) per second per 1 μm^2 of lumenal surface area; the median transit times and median free lives of the vesicles were about 1 second, while the median attachment times were about 8 seconds. (These refer to the periods between one attachment and the next. The actual life-spans of the vesicles are likely to be of the order of hours at the least.) They were also able to calculate the cytoplasmic viscosity as about 0.1 poise.

vesicles of the blood vessels, as well as by the lymphatics and by the fenestrae, if fenestrated capillaries are present; see Section VI,C.)

Similar selective factors to those mentioned for junctions no doubt also operate for the vesicles (Casley-Smith, 1970a). This has been demonstrated in the case of ferritin (Casley-Smith and Chin, 1971). It can also be seen that the very small volumes of the vesicles, as well as their relatively long transit times, allow only a very slow transfer of material. Hence, while they can cause the slow passage of proteins out of the continuous blood capillaries, their effect is insignificant compared with that of the junctions for substances which can pass through the latter (Casley-Smith, 1970a; Garlick and Renkin, 1970; Renkin, 1971). [It should be mentioned, however, that a few workers consider that even the slow leakage of proteins is via occasionally opened junctions (Hurley, 1972).]

2. LARGE VESICLES

Material which is contained in those large vesicles formed by coalescence (the "symphyosomes") remains in the cells for months (Casley-Smith, 1964), unlike that in the small vesicles, which soon leaves the cells.

Material also enters the cells via large, phagocytic vesicles. These need cellular energy to form, which occurs only after triggering by a stimulus. The ingested matter also usually stays in the cells for long periods. An apparent exception is the case of chylomicrons, which may traverse the lymphatic endothelium relatively quickly via these large vesicles (Casley-Smith, 1962, 1964, 1969b; Dobbins, 1971, Ottaviani and Azzali, 1965) (Fig. 9).

C. Direct Passage through the Cytoplasm

It has been strongly suggested by Pappenheimer (1970) that water can pass through the endothelial cytoplasm. Presumably, other small molecules which can enter the cytoplasm will also do so. While such considerations are of great importance for the details of permeability and precise functioning of various kinds of junctions and the fenestrae (Casley-Smith, 1972c; Elhay and Casley-Smith, 1973), they can be ignored when dealing with the more general functioning of whole lymphatics.

It was earlier thought that even macromolecules can pass directly through normal cytoplasm (Casley-Smith, 1964, 1965), but this is now known to have been an artifact of fixation. In severely injured cells, however, there is no doubt that large amounts of macromolecules pass through the watery cytoplasm via the large gaps in the plasma membranes (Casley-Smith, 1965) (Fig. 14.).

IV. Functioning of the Lymphatic System

It is generally agreed that the principal functions of the system are to remove particles, macromolecules, and excess fluid from the tissues and to transport them to the blood. In this regard, Mayerson, in 1963, remarked that there were two main unsolved problems: how material entered the system, and how it was retained in it. Recent evidence has largely allowed us to answer these questions. The first concerns the initial lymphatics; the second involves all the vessels.

A. Initial Lymphatics

1. Entry of Material

It is evident that macromolecules and particles diffuse so slowly that they must be carried by any bulk flow of fluid (Pappenheimer, 1953). It is also evident that fluid enters the lymphatics almost entirely via the open junctions. What, however, causes the fluid to flow into the vessels?

a. Hydrostatic Pressure. It has long been held that there is a slight gradient of hydrostatic pressure from the tissues into the lymphatics (McMaster, 1947; Wiederhielm, 1968). However, the techniques used to establish this have been increasingly criticized (Guyton, 1963, 1965, 1969; Landis and Pappenheimer, 1963; Mayerson, 1963; Rusznyák et al., 1967, pp. 384–386, 418–419). While micropipettes can measure the pressures within the lymphatics with reasonable accuracy, they cannot measure the pressures in normal tissues because here free pools of fluid, of comparable size to the pipette tips, do not exist. In inflamed, edematous tissues there is no such problem, and, indeed, quite large hydrostatic pressure gradients into the vessels do occur (Guyton, 1965, 1969; McMaster, 1946a,b, 1947). In one so-called normal tissue, the wing of the bat, pools of fluid have also been found and a slight inward gradient measured (Wiederhielm, 1968); it is, however, doubtful if these results can be extrapolated to the normal, dry tissues of other animals.

Almost certainly, the "tissue resistance," which is what has been measured in the normal tissue by micropipettes really corresponds to the true "tissue hydrostatic pressure" plus the "solid tissue pressure" of Guyton (1969).* This is the force exerted on relatively large objects (such as the lymphatic walls) by the cells, fiber bundles, and the more solid, contin-

*A recent review of the whole problem of interstitial fluid pressure by Guyton et al. (1971) discusses these concepts in considerable detail.

uous portions of the connective tissue. The true hydrostatic pressure of the minute collections of fluid is more likely to be recorded by techniques such as Guyton's capsules (1963, 1965, 1969) or the "wicks" of Scholander *et al.* (1968). Both these quite independent methods indicate that tissue hydrostatic pressure is normally ~ 5–10 cm H_2O less than atmospheric pressure. This may be compared with the slight (~ 1 cm) positive pressure found in the initial lymphatics. (This small positive pressure must be carefully distinguished from the much larger pressures found in the collecting lymphatics, which are caused by pressures on and by the vessel walls.) If the negative tissue and positive lymphatic hydrostatic pressure measurements are correct, the hydrostatic pressure difference is much more likely to remove fluid from the lymphatics, rather than to force it in.

When fluid is entering the tissues (because of raised venous pressure), the hydrostatic pressures rise rapidly until at ~ 0 cm visible edema commences; then the rate of increase becomes much less (Guyton, 1969). It is during this initial rise that lymph flow increases greatly (about twentyfold; A. C. Guyton, personal communication, 1971). It reaches a maximum, and edema commences when the lymphatic capacity is saturated (Section VI,A). Presumably, the same happens during inflammation.

b. OTHER FACTORS.   Other forces causing fluid to enter the lymphatics have been suggested. Active pumping of fluid through the cells (cf. Dobbins and Rollins, 1970; Mayerson, 1963; Virágh *et al.*, 1966) is most unlikely. The cells do not resemble those in which this occurs; cyanide does not prevent lymphatic filling (Casley-Smith, 1965); passage can be in either direction; the vesicles are likely to be able to give rise only to very slow rates of transport; and there is very strong evidence indicating that passage is principally via the junctions (Section III,A,1).

It is conceivable that the first few segments of the collecting vessels could exert a suction force, due to their being pulled open by the tissues via attached filaments, etc., after the vessels had been compressed or had contracted (B. Morris, personal communication, 1971). However, this does not overcome the difficulty of measurements showing that the hydrostatic pressures in the initial lymphatics are probably higher than in the tissues. Also, such attached filaments are not prominent features of the collecting vessels.

c. OSMOTIC PRESSURE (FIG. 22)   One force which has not been considered is osmotic pressure (Casley-Smith, 1972b,d; Elhay and Casley-Smith, 1973). The proteins in the initial lymphatics of two sites have been shown by a number of methods to have mean concentrations of about three times those in the tissue space (Fig. 13). Such a difference could well produce an inwardly directed osmotic pressure difference greater than the outwardly

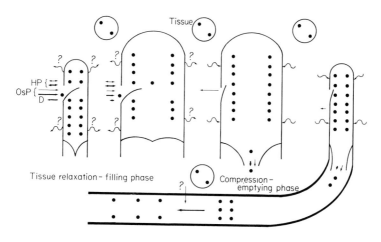

Fig. 22. A diagram of the initially lymphatic cycle. The dilation filling, and compression and telescoping during emptying are shown. The thick arrows indicate protein movement; the thin ones indicate fluid flow. Their lengths show the presumed variations in flow rates during the cycle. The wavy arrows indicate the solid tissue pressure or the pull by the filaments (which may not be important in normal tissue, although they are in inflammation, hence the "?"). Proteins (dots) are represented in their presumed relative concentrations in the tissues (circles), in the initial lymphatics during the cycle, and in the (thick-walled) collecting lymphatic before and after their hypothesized dilution by the inflow of fluid through its wall. During filling, material enters the initial lymphatics via the open junctions. The hydrostatic pressure difference (HP) is shown as either inward or outward, according to circumstances, although it probably is only directed inward during edema (see text). The hypothesized osmotic pressure difference (OsP), due to the differences in protein concentration, causes fluid and proteins to enter the vessels. It varies in force with variations in the concentrations of the intralymphatic proteins. There is also similarly variable outward diffusion (D) of proteins. During compression, the junctions become closed; the net hydrostatic–osmotic pressure difference forces only fluid out of them. This flow presumably decreases as the contents become more concentrated. A relatively small amount of the lymph fluid and protein is passed to the collecting lymphatics, leaving the concentrated remaining protein to provide the osmotic pressure needed to cause the cycle to continue. Thus, the lymph concentration and volume should be inversely proportional to each other.

directed hydrostatic pressure difference suggested by Guyton's measurements. (This is in spite of the relatively large openings of the junctions.) It is suggested that this concentration of the proteins is caused by the escape of much fluid into the tissues via the "closed" junctions (Section IV,A,2) during the intermittent tissue compressions. The compression will relax any stretched filaments dilating the lymphatics, allowing the solid tissue pressure to compress the vessels. Since this is considerably greater than the tissue hydrostatic pressure and since the intralymphatic pressure will become approximately equal to the solid tissue pressure, fluid will be forced out of the closed junctions. (These are too small for the macromolecules to traverse.) The expelled fluid will rapidly diffuse throughout the tissues without significantly altering local protein concentrations.

If only a portion of the protein (8–50%, depending on the conditions) passes with the lymph into the collecting lymphatics, the remainder will be sufficient to cause the initial lymphatics to refill with fluid during the next relaxation (filling) phase. This inflowing fluid will bring with it more protein to replace that lost to the collecting lymphatics, and the whole cycle can continue indefinitely. Such a low efficiency of the lymphatics is perhaps *a priori* unexpected, but it has, in fact, been shown to be very likely (Casley-Smith, 1972b). Normal lymphatic efficiency was found to be ~ 0.1–1% at a number of sites, with that of the intestinal lacteals being about fifty times greater. The probable reason for this increased efficiency on the part of the lacteals is that they are very short and discharge into adjacent, uncompressed collecting lymphatics; those in the rest of the body discharge into collecting vessels which are also compressed during the compression phase. These must often run many centimeters before emptying into uncompressed vessels external to the organ or muscle. Hence, the ratio of the resistances to flow via the orifices into the uncompressed collecting ducts to those via the junctions are much lower in the lacteals than elsewhere. In the lacteals then, more fluid will flow out of the orifices, relative to amount which flows out of the junctions.

A mathematical model (Elhay and Casley-Smith, 1973) shows that these processes are quite likely, biophysically, and there is also some experimental evidence supporting them.* The whole series of processes involving osmotic pressure is only hypothetical at present, however, but it is difficult to see what other force is available to cause fluid to enter the initial lymphatics in normal tissues.

2. The Retention of Material

During tissue compression, when lymph is being expelled into the collecting lymphatics, the open junctions almost certainly close, thus preventing the escape of the large molecules into the tissues (Casley-Smith, 1967c,d, 1969f, 1970a, 1972b,d) (Figs. 7, 22, 24). The changes in the relative pressures have been mentioned in the preceding section; such compression is occasioned by adjacent contracting muscle, respiration, the pulse, etc. This closure was originally suggested by Allen and Vogt (1937) for the diaphragm,

*It has recently been shown (J. R. Casley-Smith and T. Bolton 1973, *Microvasc. Res.*, in press) that quite considerable effective colloidal osmotic pressures do exist across holes even up to some microns wide *in vitro*. An *in vitro* model of the initial lymphatics (J. R. Casley-Smith, unpublished) is giving results in accordance with this concept.

but the morphology of the junctions, coupled with the increased overlapping of the endothelial cells as the vessels' diameters and lengths are reduced, indicate that it is likely to occur everywhere. An exception is during lymphedema when the incompetency of the intralymphatic valves may cause the initial lymphatics to become so dilated that their junctions are also no longer competent: during extreme, high lymph flow edema (including inflammation), the filaments may so dilate the vessels that a similar situation occurs. Breaks in the plasma membranes caused by injury would also vitiate the effect of the junctions closing. Usually, however, the overlapping endothelial cells will act as inlet valves. These, with the intralymphatic valves, mean that the lymphatic system commences as millions of tiny force pumps.

3. Effects of Inflammation

These changes have been mentioned in various sections. In summary (Fig. 23), inflammation opens the lymphatic junctions because edema causes the filaments to dilate the vessels and to drag the cells apart. In extreme cases, these might cause the junctions to become incompetent during the compression phase of the initial lymphatic cycle. Injurious substances may also damage the tight junctions, and apparently may cause endothelial contraction. Any breaks in the plasma membranes will help to destroy the effectiveness of the pumping. The accumulation of fluid in the tissues reduces the outwardly directed hydrostatic pressure difference, until, eventually, edema appears, and the pressure difference becomes directed into the vessels. In moderate burns there, is still about a threefold concentration of proteins inside the lymphatics (Casley-Smith, 1972d), suggesting that, here, osmotic pressure may still be an important force, but this is unlikely to be the case in the presence of the incompetent junctions and broken plasma membranes of very severe injuries.

B. Collecting Lymphatics

1. Retention of Material

Macromolecules are retained in the collecting lymphatics simply because the predominantly closed junctions are too small to let them pass, and the vesicles are too slow (Casley-Smith, 1969a,b,f). There is a slight loss from these causes (Garlick and Renkin, 1970; Mayerson, 1963; Strawitz et al., 1968), but this is relatively insignificant. On the other hand, the closed junctions are quite permeable to small molecules (Casley-Smith, 1969c; Mayerson, 1963; Rusznyák et al., 1967, pp. 456–459; Strawitz et al., 1968; Yoffey and Courtice, 1970, pp. 79–82).

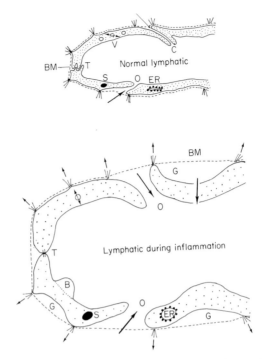

Fig. 23. The effects of inflammation on the initial lymphatics. The vessel is dilated and the cells are pulled apart by the filaments attached to the ablumen surfaces; intervening portions are forced inward, leaving gaps (G) between them and the basement membrane (BM). The close junctions (C) become open (O); the tight ones (T) probably remain closed. However, the convolutions and projections tend to disappear as the very swollen cells stretch and break their plasma membranes. Probably for the same reason, the vesicles (V) decrease in numbers, with their membranes becoming incorporated in the plasma membranes. Blebs (B) are seen on the cells, and the endoplasmic reticulum (ER) dilates. Fluid (thin arrows) and fluid and proteins (thick arrows) pass via the junctions, vesicles, and broken plasma membranes in directions and amounts which depend on the conditions, phase of the cycle, and their relative dimensions. Symphosomes (S) are present under both conditions.

These permeability differences have a number of consequences. First, small molecules removed from one region may readily enter the blood system other than via lymphaticovenous anastamoses (Fig. 24). Second, there must be a hydrostatic–osmotic equilibrium between the lymph in the collecting lymphatics and the tissues through which they pass [and also the vasa vasorum; Yoffey and Courtice (1970) p. 80]. During contractions of the lymphatics, the pressures can rise to ~150 cm H_2O in occluded vessels, though they are usually 5–25 cm (Yoffey and Courtice, 1970, pp. 181–183); these should cause some expulsion of fluid, which will reenter during the

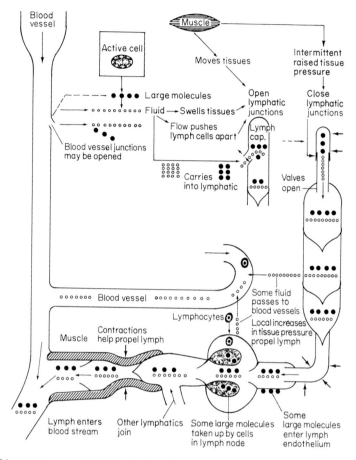

Fig. 24. A summary of the functioning of the whole lymphatic system. (The effects of lymphatic spasm or thrombosis are not shown, nor are some of those factors which appear in Figs. 22 and 23.) (From Casley-Smith, 1967c.)

relaxation phase. If, however, the hypothesis relating to osmotic pressure is correct, the lymph entering the collecting lymphatics will be quite concentrated; this will be diluted again during its passage along the vessels by the entry of more fluid, presumably until the lymph nearly reaches the concentration of the proteins in the tissues through which the vessels are passing (Fig. 22). It is therefore likely that the concentrations of proteins obtained from the more central collecting lymphatics reflect those in the tissues through which they pass as well as of those in the tissues where the lymph originated. Some workers, however, consider that there is little alteration in the lymph during its passage (Yoffey and Courtice, 1970, pp. 80–82).

2. TRANSMISSION OF MATERIAL

Lymph is pumped onward in the collecting vessels by the combined actions of the intralymphatic valves and the periodic contractions of the segments of the vessels ("lymphangions"; Mislin, 1967, Mislin and Schipp, 1967) (Fig. 24). These are brought about either by the actions of the smooth muscle in their walls or by varying external pressures—adjacent muscles, respiration, or the pulse.

The lymph is discharged into lymphaticovenous communications. These are usually in the neck, but appear to exist, at least potentially, at other sites (Threefoot *et al.*, 1967a,b; Rusznyák *et al.*, 1967, pp. 555–564; Yoffey and Courtice, 1970, pp. 27–32). These other communications usually seem to function only when the collecting lymphatics central to them are occluded; it appears, however, that more lymph is produced than can be collected from the thoracic and right lymph ducts, so these other communications may function normally to some extent. One of their more dramatic appearances is as bleeding esophageal varices which seem to occur only when there is an increased hepatic lymph flow coupled with a relative inability of the thoracic duct to handle it (Dumont and Witte, 1969). One wonders if they may also be functional in other states in which much lymph is produced (e.g., in inflammation) if the central lymphatics become unable to carry it all and the pressures in them rise.

V. Effects of Inflammation on the Lymphatic System

These effects have been considered from the point of view of the functioning of the initial lymphatics (Sections II,B; III,A,C;VI,A). They will now be discussed for the lymphatic system as a whole.

A. Composition and Flow of Lymph

Inflammation causes a considerable increase (ten- to twentyfold) in the flow of lymph from a region and also a rise in protein concentration, *viz.*, from 1 to 2 gm per 100 ml to ~5 gm (Drinker, 1942, pp. 88–96; Florey, 1970, pp. 107–117; Yoffey and Courtice, 1970, pp. 339–409, 414–416). There are also often a large number of erythrocytes, other cells, and cellular debris in the lymph. The reasons for these changes are evident when one considers the increases in the permeability and functioning of the initial lymphatics and the great increase in the amounts of protein, cells, and debris in the tissues. In keeping with their general removal of proteins in inflammation, the lymphatics also contain unusual proteins, some of which are enzymes, which probably originate in the injured tissues, rather than in the blood (Section VI,B,3).

The lymph flow naturally varies with time. Roberts and Courtice (1969) found that in acute thermal injury flow rose to a peak during the first hour and then decreased as the turnover from plasma to lymph fell, i.e., it depended on the rate of arrival of the proteins and fluid at the lymphatics. Again, enclosing the region in a pressure bandage or cooling it lessens the rate of lymph formation (Section VII); this is increased when the treatments are reversed (Barnes and Trueta, 1941; Glenn et al., 1943; Courtice and Sabine, 1966).

Menkin (1940) showed that the coagulation of the inflammatory exudate in the tissues tended to prevent its entering the lymphatics, while similar fibrin thrombi in the lymphatics themselves tended to prevent what did arrive from passing along them. Injection of a coagulating tissue extract (Glenn et al., 1942) supported this view by causing a marked reduction in lymph flow, with a concomitant rise in protein concentration (Section VI,A). It is held, however (Rusznyák et al., 1967, pp. 415–417, 507–510), that this concept of fixation is much more complex than suggested by Menkin and that far from being beneficial it is often a disadvantage (Drinker, 1942, pp. 90–96). While it will help prevent the spread of any bacteria, it will also reduce the removal of debris and cause the accumulation of protein, with consequent fibrosis and keloid formation (Section VI,A,2,a).

A further most important factor which interferes with the functioning of the lymphatics in inflammation is the spasm of the collecting vessels proximal to the lesion (Rusznyák et al., 1967, pp. 549–554). This has been demonstrated histologically, radiographically, and by releasing the spasm by blocking the sympathetics. Danese et al. (1963) independently confirmed this lymphatic spasm, which they showed was present in septic thrombophlebitis, but not in that produced aseptically. As with coagulation, this spasm can be both a defense or a disadvantage, depending on the circumstances.

B. Lymphangitis

This is produced by the spread of injurious stimuli (bacterial or chemical) from the inflamed area along the draining lymphatics. This often extends to the regional lymph nodes. These act as filters, and virulent bacteria can proliferate in them (Volume III, Chapter 1), so they can be inflamed even if the intervening lymphatics are not. If the lymphangitis or lymphadenitis leads to fibrosis, cicatrization can produce chronic lymphedema in the distal region (Section VI,A).

C. Lymphatic Regeneration

It is a truism of lymphology that it is extremely difficult to permanently deprive a region of its lymphatic drainage. The initial lymphatics rapidly invade the healing region, although not as rapidly as blood capillaries do (Clark, 1922–1923, Clark and Clark, 1932; Cliff, 1963; McMaster, 1942; Pullinger and Florey, 1937). There is initially a growth of innumerable fine vessels by endothelial sprouting from existing ones. Later, some of these enlarge to form normal-sized initial lymphatics; the others regress. The fine structure of the growing lymphatics is very similar to that of growing blood capillaries (Cliff, 1963). It has been suggested (Yoffey, 1954) that the slower growth of lymphatics compared with capillaries allows much protein to lie in the tissues, especially as the growing capillaries are very permeable. This tends to cause fibrosis, hypertrophy, and keloid formation (Section VI,A,4). Any preexisting fibrosis will slow the lymphatic regrowth even more than that of the capillaries.

The collecting lymphatics can also regenerate, especially in inflammation. In addition, they have many collateral channels which will readily dilate to replace those which are obstructed. This is more important than is regeneration (L. C. Yong, 1972, personal communication), which is much more a feature of the initial lymphatics.

VI. Effects of the Lymphatic System on Inflammation

A. Causes and Effects of Lymphatic Failure

1. CAUSES

It is first necessary to consider the causes of edema. Moderate amounts of excess fluid are essentially removed by the blood system. With large amounts, the lymphatic system will assist in this—its "safety valve" or "spillway" function. Excess macromolecules, however, can only be removed via the lymphatics, since their concentrations are less than in the blood. This is because the concentration gradient is outward from the blood vessels, and the vesicle system acts only in the direction of this gradient; fenestrae only remove lower concentrations than in the tissues because of molecular sieving. Naturally, proteins produced in the tissues, or injected there, will also pass into the capillaries via the vesicles, but plasma proteins (whose plasma concentration excedes their tissue concentrations) will have a net passage outward from the capillaries via the vesicles. In general, then, macromolecules rely on the lymphatics for their removal. While they remain in the tissues, their osmotic pressures tend to cause the accumulation of edema fluid. Edema is therefore an indication that the lymphatics are failing to remove all the proteins and fluid that they should. It is basically a lymphatic failure.

Földi (1969, pp. 12–21) divided edema into two main categories: that caused by mechanical insufficiency of the lymphatic system (low lymph—flow failure) and that caused by its dynamic insufficiency (high lymph—flow failure). In the former, the protein content is high (1–5 gm per 100 ml); in the latter, it is low (0.1–0.5gm). (These differences are caused by the differences in the amounts of molecular sieving at the different flow rates through the two endothelial and the connective tissue barriers.) These two conditions can be distinguished clinically by the rates of flow of dyes along the lymphatics (McMaster, 1942) or by radiological lymphography (Földi, 1969). Földi includes a third class—safety valve insufficiency—in which large amounts of high protein fluid enter the tissues and overwhelm the capacity of the lymphatic system. This is obviously one of the main causes of edema in inflammation.

Mechanical insufficiency edema also occurs in inflammation. It is produced by lymphatic spasm and thrombosis in acute inflammation and by fibrosis in chronic inflammation. It adds the effects of lymphedema to those already being produced by the increased permeability of the blood vessels. The increases in intralymphatic pressures (up to 150 cm H_2O) are transmitted back to the initial lymphatics as the collecting lymphatics dilate and as their valves become incompetent. The initial lymphatics, in turn, dilate; their junctions become incompetent; and the raised pressures are transmitted back to the tissues. Thus, they become swollen and full of stagnant fluid and protein. The effects of the two forms of edema occurring in inflammation summate, and may be so extreme that the skin bursts.

2. EFFECTS

It has been mentioned (Section IV,A,1,a) that as fluid enters the tissues both the lymph flow and the tissue hydrostatic pressure rise until lymph flow reaches a maximum at a pressure of about 0 cm. Further increases in the rate of entry of fluid cause no further increase in lymph flow, showing that the capacity of the lymphatics is being exceeded. Then the tissue hydrostatic pressure becomes positive, and edema commences. These experiments used raised venous pressure, so it was lymphatic dynamic insufficiency which caused the edema. Similar mechanisms should operate in inflammation also, but it appears that the necessary experiments have not been done, not even those showing effects of lymphatic occlusion on the amount of inflammatory reaction and edema after regulated doses of an inflammatory stimulus.* (It is, of course, well known that infection develops readily in lymphedematous limbs, but this could be because the conditions were particularly favorable, and it gives no information relating lymph drainage to the pathogenesis of the inflammatory response itself.) It is, however, almost certain that inflammatory edema is caused by safety valve failure of the lymphatic system, to which are usually added the effects of mechanical insufficiency.

Apart from edema, the effects of lymphatic failure are to allow the accumulation of proteins, debris, and wastes. The resolution of inflammation must be impeded if there is an insufficient through flow of fluid carrying nutrients and antibodies, assisting in the passage of phagocytes and in removing wastes and debris. Even highly diffusible small molecules must be impeded in their passages into and out of edematous regions by the increased intercapillary distances in the swollen tissues. The raised tissue hydrostatic and solid tissue pressures, produced by safety valve lymphatic failure combined with back pressures transmitted by lymphedema, will reduce the flow of fluid out of the capillaries and of macromolecules carried by it; if the pressures rise greatly, blood flow itself may be arrested. These will impede the arrival of material needed for healing.

As mentioned in the next sections, lymphatics do assist in the spread of virulent bacteria and injurious substances. If lymph flow is prevented by mechanical insufficiency, these will be reduced. If lymph flow is high, with only safety valve failure causing the edema, the spread will be high also. As pointed out in Section VI,A, however, such lymphatic blocking is more often detrimental than helpful.

After acute cardiac ischemia, the degrees of necrosis, fibrosis, and calcification are greater if lymphedema is present (Kline *et al.*, 1963; Rusznyák *et al.*, 1967, pp. 623–636). Similar results in many other injured tissues are also described by Földi (1969, pp. 22–28) and by Rusznyák *et al.* (1967, pp. 462–468, 636, 661–669, 676–678, 727, 733–737, 767–783, 811).

a. Elephantiasis.   The accumulation of proteins in the tissues, especially if chronic, promotes excessive fibrosis (Drinker, 1942, pp. 89–95; Rusznyák *et al.*, 1967, pp. 463–468; Yoffey and Courtice, 1970, pp. 368–369, 376–381). This tends to contract and block the lymphatics, causing chronic lymphedema with still more accumulation of proteins. Such a lymphedema, produced by inflammation or in another way, is very prone to infection because

---

*Since this was written, Casley-Smith and Piller (1973) have shown that after a standard mild burn (54°C, 60 seconds) the edema produced in rats' legs is much greater if the lymphatics are occluded. Hence, the lymphatic system must be of considerable importance in limiting the extent of edema for this sort of inflammation.

of the accumulation of proteinaceous fluid and the ease with which the tense, unwieldy limb is injured. It appears that this secondary infection is an important factor in the production of the typical changes of elephantiasis (Földi, 1969, pp. 46–49, 61; Rusznyák *et al.*, 1967, pp. 831–832; Yoffey and Courtice, 1970, pp. 376–383); presumably, it adds even more protein to the pool and promotes fibrosis and contraction in the skin as well as in the deeper tissues. Infection seems to be needed for elephantiatic changes even in filariasis (Marques and Pereira, 1963).

B. Effects of Lymphatic Functioning

1. CLEARING THE TISSUES

The lymphatics remove cells, debris, bacteria, particles, macromolecules, and fluid from the inflamed site. This aids in the resolution of the inflammatory reaction, as is best shown by the results of lymphatic failure (Section VII,A,2). The transport of antigens to the regional lymph nodes is vital for the development of immunity (Volume III, Chapter 8).

2. BACTERIAL SPREAD

Virulent bacteria can be carried along the lymphatics to cause lymphangitis, and can also multiply in the regional lymph nodes to cause lymphadenitis (Section VI,B). From these, the infection can spread to the thoracic duct, the blood, and the body generally (Cole *et al.*, 1968). Even local dissemination via the lymphatics can be very important, e.g., in pulmonary tuberculosis. They also provide pathways toward regional vulnerable sites, e.g., from the middle third of the nasopharynx to the adjacent meninges. The direction and amount of such transmission will be affected by the direction of fluid flow, the sites of the regional lymph nodes, bacterial motility, the extent of tissue compression, etc., e.g., forceful blowing of the nose could reverse the normal flow of lymph, thus forcing it and any bacteria it contained up to the meninges. Similarly, pressure on the nodes greatly lessens their effectiveness as filters (Drinker *et al.*, 1934).

3. TRANSPORT OF INJURIOUS SUBSTANCES

Lymph from injured limbs, particularly in acute thermal injury, carries abnormal enzymes and other proteins together with some normal ones at abnormally high levels (Mayerson, 1963; Yoffey and Courtice, 1970, pp. 414–416). It has been suggested that these may cause injuries elsewhere in the body, particularly in association with the toxemia and the concept of autoimminity in burns (Yoffey and Courtice, p. 416). While much more work is necessary in this area, it is of great interest that Földi-Börcsök (1972), using burn injury, finds that the inflammatory reaction is greatly reduced in rats if the thoracic duct lymph is removed from the animal, rather than being allowed to recirculate in the blood. Similar findings in animals and man have been reported for thoracic duct cannulation in acute pancreatitis (Dumont and Witte, 1969).

C. Fenestrated Blood Capillaries and the Lymphatic System

Fenestrated capillaries are common in certain regions (Casley-Smith, 1971b,c; Karnovsky, 1968; Majno, 1965). These are, notably, where macromolecules are made or ingested, where the excretion of fluid leaves the tissues containing high concentrations of proteins, or where the lymphatics are likely to function poorly; it appears that the fenestrae help remove the macromolecules from the tissues (Casley-Smith, 1970b, 1971b,c, 1927c; Casley-Smith and Mart, 1970). They also almost certainly greatly increase the local turnover of water and small molecules through a region.

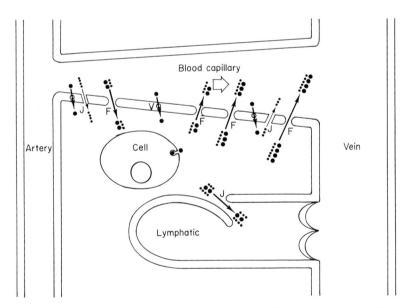

Fig. 25. The normal relationships of fenestrated blood capillaries and lymphatics. The passage of fluid (thin arrows) and fluid and proteins (thick arrows) into and out of the vessels is shown, with the lengths and numbers of the arrows giving some representation of their relative importances. As the hydrostatic pressure decreases along the capillary, the outflow through the junctions (J) and fenestrae (F) decreases, and then becomes an increasing inflow. Some of the material also passes into the lymphatic; the relative amount of this must depend on the conditions, the dimensions of the molecules, junctions and fenestrae, and their numbers.

There is rapidly accumulating evidence—morphological, experimental, and biophysical—which supports this conclusion (Fig. 20). (This uptake is, however, only by the fenestrae on the venous limbs of capillaries; those, relatively much fewer, on the arterial limbs seem to be devices for allowing far more large molecules to reach the tissues than could possibly pass via the vesicular system.) There is likely to be, then, a very considerable local circulation of proteins in these regions, which never passes to the lymphatics at all (Fig. 25).

It is very difficult to define the relative roles of the lymphatics and fenestrae. Fenestrae antedate true lymphatics (Section II,D). They probably evolved in the viscera of the ancestors of the elasmobranchs because these organs were too far from the body wall for swimming motions to cause material to pass through the venous blood vascular junctions. Subsequently, true lymphatics evolved in the body wall and then invaded the viscera. However, the problem of their present relative roles still remains.

In the elasmobranchs (Casley-Smith and Mart, 1970), small lipoprotein molecules ($\sim 10–20$ mμ) enter the blood vessels via the fenestrae. Chylomicrons ($\sim 0.1–1$ μm) can only be formed when lymphatics are available, since fenestrae large enough to pass these would be unlikely to function (Casley-Smith, 1972c) (Fig. 9). In mammals, the long chain fatty acids are absorbed in chylomicrons via the lymphatics; short chain ones can enter the blood stream, and may be carried by albumen, via the fenestrae (Vodovár et al., 1967; Yoffey and Courtice, 1970, pp. 119, 219–221). While small and medium macromolecules may well be removed by the fenestrae, it seems that large ones (e.g., γ-globulin) are too big and must travel via the lymphatics (Yoffey and Courtice, 1970, pp. 277–228).

There is, however, almost no information about the relative roles of the two systems in inflammation. Edema certainly occurs during inflammation of regions with fenestrated capillaries, e.g., in the intestine. It is perhaps not as severe as in other regions where fenestrated capillaries are very rare, e.g., skin and lung, but this is certainly not established. No doubt, both the fenestrae and the lymphatics can become overloaded, causing proteins to accumulate in the tissues and edema to commence. Unfortunately, however, the roles of the two systems in this situation, as in most others, remains to be elucidated. It is particularly unfortunate that inflammation is only rarely studied in regions with fenestrae.

VII. Therapeutic Measures

The purpose of this section is not to discuss the therapy of inflammation as it relates to the lymphatic system in general, but rather to mention some of the factors involved where these are either important in their own right or where they have important implications for the interactions of inflammation and the lymphatic system.

A. General Measures

The most important treatment, naturally, is to remove the cause of the inflammation (e.g., with antiobiotics) or to ameliorate its effects (e.g., with antihistamines). The use of thoracic duct cannulation for removing injurious products has been mentioned (Section VI,B,3). While it is sometimes desirable to confine bacteria, etc., to the inflamed area by restricting lymph flow, normally one prefers to assist the resolution of the inflammation by removing the proteins and edema fluid or by preventing their occurrence.

B. Treating Lymphatic Insufficiency

Since edema is caused by both mechanical and safety valve insufficiency, both need to be treated. The mechanical insufficiency caused by lymphatic spasm has been treated with chemical or surgical sympathectomies with apparent success (Rusznyák et al., 1967, pp. 553–554, 836). Anticoagulants have been suggested to prevent thrombosis in the vessels and tissues (Lowenberg, 1952), but attention would have to be paid to hemostasis. In chronic cases, when fibrosis and elephantiasis are well developed, surgery is indicated (Földi, 1969, pp. 55–57).

Various physical methods, which are of use in edemas generally, are also helpful in inflammatory edema, provided care is taken not to increase the spread of virulent bacteria or to disrupt the healing processes. Some of these are elevating the part; compression by means of plaster, pneumatic, or compression bandages; massage and exercise; heat (once the blood vascular junctions have closed) or cold (before this). Heat will help wash the debris out of the site, but is only of use if the lymphatics can handle the increased flow reaching them. Cold, pressure, and elevation all help to reduce the outflow from the blood vessels, thus aiding the lymphatic safety valve insufficiency. Compression, massage, and exercise all help the mechanical insufficiency and improve the lymph flow. They make the initial lymph pumps more efficient, particularly by raising the tissue hydrostatic and solid tissue pressures. Also they, and elevation, improve flow in the collecting lymphatics. Diuretics, by reducing the blood volume and the water-loading of the tissues, have been found to be effective (Földi, 1969, p. 52; Rusznyak et al., 1967, pp. 836–837).

C. Pharmaceutical Methods

Large doses of pyridoxine (~25 mg per kilogram per day) and pantothenic acid (~125 mg per kilogram per day) are very effective in preventing lymphedema or in removing it in both animals and man (Casley-Smith *et al.*, 1969; Földi, 1969, pp. 51, 106–111; Földi *et al.*, 1970a,b; Jóo *et al.*, 1967). This has been found not only in the more usual lymphedemas of the body generally, but also in the edema of the brain and retina produced by mechanical insufficiency of the cervical lymphatics (Section II,A,4). Recently, coumarin (~25 mg per kilogram per day) and/or rutin (~400 mg per kilogram per day) have been shown to do the same (Casley-Smith *et al.*, 1972; Földi *et al.* 1970a,b; Földi-Börcsök, 1972; Casley-Smith and Piller, 1973). These are also most effective in reducing the inflammatory reaction, including edema, after severe thermal injuries, presumably in the same manner. (This effect is even more marked when it is combined with cannulation of the thoracic duct.)

How these substances work is in doubt. It appears that they affect neither the outflow from the capillaries nor the uptake by the lymphatics per se, but they may cause the cells in the tissues either to remove the edema-producing macromolecules or not to form them. Casley-Smith and Piller (1973) found that far from reducing the outflow of macromolecules from injured blood vessels these substances increased this to some extent. However, after the injection of labeled proteins, there was a most marked increase in the amount of label leaving a region, if coumarin was administered to the animal. This was not just via the lymphatics since in some experiments these were occluded. [Also Földi-Börcsök (1972) has shown that the reduction in the volume of an inflamed limb after this therapy is much more than the total lymph flow from it.] An increase in labeled small polypeptides was found, implying increased proteolysis.

It is considered that this proteolysis occurs in the tissues, particularly in the inflamed or lymphedematous regions where there is an accumulation of proteins. The resulting small polypeptides, with their smaller sizes and greatly increased diffusion velocities, and with their concentration gradients being directed from the tissues to the blood, would easily enter the blood stream through the closed endothelial junctions of the venous capillaries and small venules. (These junctions are too small to permit the passage of the intact protein molecules and their concentration gradients are directed outward from the blood vessels.) Much more work is needed to elucidate their effects, but, meanwhile, they offer safe and substantial improvements in the therapy of many edemas, including those of inflammation.

References

Allen, L., and Vogt, E. (1937). *Amer. J. Physiol.* **119**, 776.

Barnes, J. M., and Trueta, J. (1941). *Lancet* **1**, 623.

Bruns, R. R., and Palade, G. E. (1968). *J. Cell Biol.* **37**, 277.

Casley-Smith, J. R. (1962). *J. Cell Biol.* **15**, 259.

Casley-Smith, J. R. (1964). *Quart. J. Exp. Physiol. Cog. Med. Sci.* **49**, 365.

Casley-Smith, J. R. (1965). *Brit. J. Exp. Pathol.* **46**, 35.

Casley-Smith, J. R. (1967a). *Brit. J. Exp. Pathol.* **48**, 680.

Casley-Smith, J. R. (1967b). *Quart. J. Exp. Physiol. Cog. Med. Sci.* **52**, 105.

Casley-Smith, J. R. (1967c). *In* "New Trends in Basic Lymphology" (J. M. Collette, G. Jantet, and E. Schofeniels, eds.), pp. 19–36 Birkhauser, Basel.

Casley-Smith, J. R. (1967d). *In* "New Trends in Basic lymphology" (J. M. Collette, G. Jantet, and E. Schoffeniels, eds.), pp. 124–137. Birkhaeuser, Basel.

Casley-Smith, J. R. (1969a). *J. Microsc.* **90**, 251.

Casley-Smith, J. R. (1969b). *Lymphology* **1**, 15.

Casley-Smith, J. R. (1969c). *Experientia* **25**, 374.

Casley-Smith, J. R. (1969d). *Experientia* **25**, 845.

Casley-Smith, J. R. (1969e). *J. Microsc.* **90**, 15.

Casley-Smith, J. R; (1969f). *In* "Proceedings of the Sixth International Congress of Angiology" (R. Saleras, ed.), pp. 1–30. Swets & Zietlinger, Amsterdam.

Casley-Smith, J. R. (1970a). *In* "Progress in Lymphology II" (M. Viamonte *et al.*, eds.), pp. 51–54, 122–124, and 255–260. Thieme, Stuttgart.

Casley-Smith, J. R. (1970b). *Experientia* **26**, 852.

Casley-Smith, J. R. (1971a). *Lymphology* **4**, 79.

Casley-Smith, J; R. (1971b). *Microvasc. Res.* **3**, 49.

Casley-Smith, J. R. (1971c). *Electron Microsc. Proc. Int. Cong., 1970* Vol. 3, p. 49.

Casley-Smith, J. R. (1972a). *Rev. Suisse Zool.* (accepted for publication).

Casley-Smith, J. R. (1972b). *Proc. Aust. Physiol. Pharmacol. Soc.* **3**, 32.

Casley-Smith, J. R. (1972c). *Microvasc. Res.* (submitted for publication).

Casley-Smith, J. R. (1972d). *Lymphology* (submitted for publication).

Casley-Smith, J. R. (1972e). *Experientia* (submitted for publication).

Casley-Smith, J. R., and Bolton, T. (1973). *Microvasc. Res.* **5**, (in press).

Casley-Smith, J. R., and Chin, J. C. (1971). *J. Microsc.* **93**, 167.

Casley-Smith, J. R., and Clark, H. I. (1972). *J. Microsc.* **96**, 263.

Casley-Smith, J. R., and Florey, H. W. *Quart. J. Exp. Physiol. Cog. Med. Sci.* **46**, 101.

Casley-Smith, J. R., Földi-Börcsök, E., and Földi, M. (1972). *Brit. J. Exp. Pathol.* (accepted for publication).

Casley-Smith, J. R., and Mart, P. (1970). *Experientia* **26**, 508.

Casley-Smith, J. R., and Piller, N. B. (1973). *In* "Lymphedema, Pathophysiology and Treatment" (L. Clodius, ed.). In preparation.

Casley-Smith, J. R., Földi, M., and Zoltán, Ö.T. (1969). *Lymphology* **2**, 63.

Clark, E. R. (1922–1923). *Anat. Rec.* **24**, 181.

Clark, E. R., and Clark, E. L. (1932). *Amer. J. Anat.* **51**, 49.

Clementi, F. (1971). *Electron Microsco. Proc. Int. Congi., 1970* Vol. 3, p. 45.

Clementi, F., and Palade, G. E. (1969). *J. Cell Biol.* **41**, 33.

Cliff, W. J. (1963). *Proc. Roy. Soc., Ser. B* **246**, 305.

Cole, W. R., Petit, R., Brown, A. B., and Witte, M. H. (1968). *Lymphology* **1**, 52.

Collin, H. B. (1969). *Exp. Eye Res.* **8**, 102.

Cotran, R. S., and Majno, G. (1967). *Protoplasma* **43**, 45.

Courtice, F. C. (1971). *Lymphology* **4**, 9.

Courtice, F. C., and Sabine, M. S. (1966). *Aust. J. Exp. Biol. Med. Sci.* **44**, 23.
Danese, C., Diaz, R., and Howard, J. M. (1963). *Arch. Surg. (Chicago)* **86**, 5.
Dobbins, W. O. (1971). *Amer. J. Clin. Nutr.* **24**, 77.
Dobbins, W. O., and Rollins, E. L. (1970). *J. Ultrastruct. Res.* **33**, 29.
Drinker, C. K. (1942). "Lane Medical Lectures: The Lymphatic System." Stanford Univ. Press, Stanford, California.
Drinker, C. K., Field, M. E., and Ward, H. K. (1934). *J. Exp. Med.* **59**, 393.
Dumont, A. E., and Witte, M. H. (1969). *Advan. Intern. Med.* **15**, 51.
Elhay, S., and Casley-Smith, J. R. (1973). In preparation.
Fawcett, D. W., Heidgen, P. M., and Leak, L. V. (1969). *J. Reprod. Fert.* **19**, 109.
Florey, H. W. (1970). *In* "General Pathology" (H. W. Florey, ed.), 4th ed., pp. 103–121. Lloyd-Luke, London.
Földi, M. (1969). "Diseases of Lymphatics and Lymph Circulation." Thomas, Springfield, Illinois.
Földi, M., Csillik, B., and Zoltán, Ö. T. (1968a). *Experientia* **24**, 1283.
Földi, M., Csillik, B., Várkonyi, T., and Zoltán, Ö. T. (1968b). *Vasc. Surg.* **2**, 214.
Földi, M., Zoltán, Ö. T., and Obál, F. (1970a). *Arzneim. Forsch.* **11a**, 1626.
Földi, M., Zoltán, Ö. T., and Piukovich, I. (1970b). *Arzneim-Forsch.* **11a**, 1629.
Földi-Börcsök, E. (1972). *Brit. J. Pharmacol.* **46**, 254.
Garlick, D. G., and Renkin, E. M. (1970). *Amer. J. Physiol.* **219**, 1595.
Glenn, W. W. L., Peterson, D. K., and Drinker, C. K. (1942). *Surgery* **12**, 685.
Glenn, W. W. L., Gilbert, H. H., and Drinker, C. K. (1943). *J. Clin. Invest.* **22**, 609.
Green, H. S., and Casley-Smith, J. R. (1972). *J. Theor. Biol.* **35**, 103.
Grotte, G. (1956). *Acta Chir. Scand., Suppl.* **211**, 1.
Guyton, A. C. (1963). *Circ. Res.* **12**, 399.
Guyton, A. C. (1965). *Invest. Ophthalmol.* **4**, 1075.
Guyton, A. C. (1969). *Circ. Resp. Mass Transport, Ciba Found. Symp.* pp. 4–20.
Guyton, A. C., Granger, H. J., and Taylor, A. E. (1971). *Physiol. Rev.* **51**, 527.
Hurley, J. V. (1972). In preparation.
Jennings, M. A., and Florey, H. W. (1967). *Proc. Roy. Soc., Ser. B* **167**, 39.
Joó F., Csillik, B., Zoltán, Ö. T., Maurer, M., Sonkodi, S., and Földi, M. (1967). *Angiologica* **4**, 271.
Kampmeier, O. F. (1969). "Evolution and Comparative Morphology of the Lymphatic System." Thomas, Springfield, Illinois.
Karnovsky, M. J. (1968). *J. Gen. Physiol.* **52**, 64s.
Kato, F. (1966). *Nagoya Med. J.* **12**, 221.
Kline, I. K., Miller, A. J., Pick, R., and Katz, L. N. (1963). *Arch. Pathol.* **76**, 424.
Landis, E. M., and Pappenheimer, J. R. (1963). *In* "Handbook of Physiology" (Amer. Physiol. Soc., J. Field, ed.), Sect. 2, Vol. II, pp. 961–1034. Williams & Wilkins, Baltimore, Maryland.
Lauweryns, J. M., and Boussauw, L. (1969). *Lymphology* **2**, 108.
Leak, L. V. (1970). *Microvasc. Res.* **2**, 361.
Leak, L. V., and Burke, J. F. (1965). *Anat. Rec.* **151**, 489.
Leak, L. V., and Burke, J. F. (1966). *Amer. J. Anat.* **118**, 785.
Leak, L. V., and Burke, J. F. (1968). *J. Cell Biol.* **36**, 129.
Leak, L. V., and Kato, F. (1970). *Proc. Int. Cong. Lymphol., III, 1970* p. 149.
Lowenberg, E. L. (1952). *Va. Med. Mon.* **79**, 351.
McMaster, P. D. (1942). *Harvey Lect.* **37**, 227.
McMaster, P. D. (1946a). *J. Exp. Med.* **84**, 473.
McMaster, P. D. (1946b). *Ann. N. Y. Acad. Sci.* **46**, 743.
McMaster, P. D. (1947). *J. Exp. Med.* **86**, 293.
McMaster, P. D., and Hudack, S. S. (1932). *J. Exp. Med.* **58**, 239.

Majno, G. (1965). *In* "Handbook of Physiology" (Amer. Physiol. Soc., J. Field, ed.), Sect. 2, Vol. III, pp. 2293–2375. Williams & Wilkins, Baltimore, Maryland.

Majno, G., Shea, S. M., and Leventhal, M. (1969). *J. Cell Biol.* **42**, 647.

Marques, R., and Pereira, L. (1963). *Lancet* **2**, 778.

Mayerson, H. S. (1963). *In* "Handbook of Physiology" (Amer. Physiol. Soc., J. Field, ed.), Sect. 2, Vol. II, pp. 1035–1073. Williams & Wilkins, Baltimore, Maryland.

Menkin, V. (1940). "Dynamics of Inflammation." Macmillan, New York.

Mislin, H. (1967). *In* "New Trends in Basic Lymphology" (J. M. Collette, G. Jantet, and E. Schoffeniels, eds.), pp. 87–96. Birkhauser, Basel.

Mislin, H., and Schipp, R. (1967). *In* "Progress in Lymphology" (A. Rüttimann, ed.), pp. 360–364. Thieme, Stuttgart.

Moe, R. E. (1963). *Amer. J. Anat.* **112**, 311.

Ohkuma, M. (1970). *Bull. Tokyo Med. Dent. Univ.* **17**, 103.

Ottaviani, G., and Azzali, G. (1965). *In* "Morphologie Histochimie Paroi Vasculaire, Fribourg," Vol. 2, p. 325.

Palade, G. E. (1961). *Circulation* **24**, 368.

Pappenheimer, J. R. (1953). *Physiol. Rev.* **33**, 387.

Pappenheimer, J. R. (1970). *In* "'Capillary Permeability" (C. Crone and N. A. Lassen, eds.), pp. 278–290. Academic Press, New York.

Pressman, J. J., Dunn, R. F., and Burtz, M. (1967). *Surg., Gynecol. Obstet.* **124**, 963.

Pullinger, B. D., and Florey, H. W. (1935). *Brit. J. Exp. Pathol.* **16**, 49.

Pullinger, B. D., and Florey, H. W. (1937). *J. Pathol. Bacteriol.* **45**, 157.

Renkin, E. M. (1971). *Proc. Int. Congr. Physiol Soc. 25th.*, 1971, pp. 263–264.

Roberts, J. C., and Courtice, F. C. (1969). *Aust. J. Exp. Biol. Med. Sci.* **47**, 421.

Rodbard, S. (1969). *Curr. Mod. Biol.* **3**, 27.

Rusznyák, I., Földi, M., and Szabó G. (1967). "Lymphatics and Lymph Circulation," 2nd ed. Pergamon, Oxford.

Scholander, P. F., Hargens, A. R., and Miller, S. L. (1968). *Science* **161**, 321.

Shea, S. M., Karnovsky, M. J., and Bossert, W. H. (1969). *J. Theor. Biol.* **24**, 30.

Strawitz, J. G., Eto, K., Mitsuoka, H., Olney, C., Pairent, F. W., and Howard, J. M. (1968). *Microvasc. Res.* **1**, 58.

Threefoot, S. A., Kossover, M. F., Kent, W. T., Hatchett, B. F., Pearson, J. E., Cabrera-Gil, C., and Aiken, D. W. (1967a). *In* "New Trends in Basic Lymphology" (J. M. Collette, G. Jantet, and E. Schoffeniels, eds.), pp. 102–119. Birkhäeuser, Basel.

Threefoot, S. A., Pearson, J. E., Cabrera-Gil, C., and Bradburn, D. M. (1967b). *In* "New Trends in Basic Lymphology" (J. M. Collette, G. Jantet, and E. Schoffeniels, eds.), pp. 173–191. Birkhäeuser, Basel.

Várkonyi, T., Csillik, B., Zoltán, Ö. T., and Földi, M. (1969). *Beitr. Pathol. Anat. Allg. Pathol.* **139**, 344.

Várkonyi, T., Polgár, J. Zoltán, Ö. T., Csillik, B., and Földi, M. (1970). *Experientia* **26**, 67.

Virágh, Sz., Papp, M., Törö, I., and Rusznyák, I. (1966). *Brit. J. Exp. Pathol.* **47**, 563.

Virágh, Sz., Papp, M., and Rusznyák, I. (1971). *Acta Morphol. Acad. Sci. Hung.* **19**, 203.

Vodovár, N., Flanzy, J., and François, A. C. (1967). *Ann. Biol. Anim., Biochim., Biophys.* **7**, 423.

Wallace, S. (1969). *In* "Procedings of the Sixth International Congress of Angiology" (R. Saleras, ed.), pp. 62–66. Swets & Zeitlinger, Amsterdam.

Wiederhielm, C. A. (1968). *J. Gen. Physiol.* **52**, 29s.

Yamagishi, T. (1960). *Nagoya Med. J.* **6**, 634.

Yoffey, J. M. (1954). *Proc. Int. Surg. Congr., 15th* p. 131.

Yoffey, J. M., and Courtice, F. C., eds. (1970). "Lymphatics, Lymph, and the Lymphomyeloid Complex." Academic Press, New York.

Chapter 7

THE STICKING AND EMIGRATION OF WHITE BLOOD CELLS IN INFLAMMATION

LESTER GRANT

I. Introduction

An important, and little understood, phenomenon characterizing many inflammatory reactions is the sticking of white cells to endothelium and their emigration across membrane of small vascular beds. The adherence of such cells to endothelial interfaces may be virtually the sole manifestation of the inflamatory process, or it may occur in concert with, or in sequence with, changes in both the caliber and the permeability of the vessels. Extravascular cells, such as macrophages, may also be mobilized at various stages of the process, and luminal precipitates, such as fibrin, may take their appearance in the course of the reaction (Wood *et al.*, 1951). Proteolytic breakdown products and the release of subcellular hydrolases (see Volume I, Chapters 4 by Hirschhorn, 7 by Hirsch, 8 by Steinman and Cohn, and Thomas, 1965), are believed to enter the reaction at as yet undetermined intervals. In this extremely complex situation, the sticking and emigration of white cells is the dominant microscopic event, barring those circumstances where severe, direct injury causes hemorrhage. In this event, the early extravasation of red cells and stasis occur in relatively rapid succession (see von Haller, 1757; Thoma, 1896).

The sticking of white cells seems to be not necessarily dependent on other well-known hallmarks of inflammation (Allison *et al.*, 1955), but until recently it has been a difficult process to study as an isolated event, with an experimental guarantee that only sticking has occurred accompanied by no other pathological changes. Grant *et al.* (1962) suggested that, if one limited the intensity of an ultraviolet burn of connective tissue, one could limit the gross reaction of the tissue to white cell sticking. Under these conditions, with little or no emigration of neutrophils and with white cell sticking predictably of a transient nature, the sticking itself could be blocked with high doses of hydrocortisone, but was unaffected by heparin. The procedure yielded no evidence for gross edema formation, for red cell sticking, or for platelet participation in the reaction. The white blood cells themselves could not have been injured by the UV stimulus because there was a latent period before the reaction occurred. Those white cells in the path of the UV light almost certainly were not the same white cells that later returned to the site of the reaction to affix to the vessel wall. This experiment suggests that the critical alteration in the tissue caused by the UV stimulus—possibly the only alteration in the tissue—is some change in the membrane of the endothelial cell which converts this cell from a nonadhesive to an adhesive state. This embeds an important mechanism of the inflammatory reaction in the vessel wall itself not in the formed elements of the blood, or, for that matter, not even in changes in plasma proteins or other plasma constituents.

Cohnheim placed the reaction in the vessel wall almost 100 years ago (see Cohnheim, 1882). In a century that has often tended to ignore Cohnheim's assertion that "molecular" changes in the endothelial wall are the critical events in the inflammatory process, it is of interest that experimental pathology may now be turning up direct evidence to support his view. For example, Grant and his colleagues (Grant, 1965; Grant and Becker, 1965, 1966; Grant and Epstein, 1973) have used a laser beam to select discrete areas in small vascular beds upon which to inflict microburns. If one aims a laser beam at transparent extravascular tissue, there is no effect whatever on the tissue because there is no color in the tissue to absorb laser energy (laser injury is caused when the absorbed energy is converted to heat and imparted to nearby structures). But, if one aims the beam at a blood vessel, the absorption of laser energy by red blood cells permits the infliction of discrete microburns on the vessel wall, yielding thrombi of varying severity, starting, in the usual case, with a lesion 5–15 μm in diameter. The intraluminal diffusion of a heat stimulus can affect any one or all of the five possible components of an inflammatory reaction: any of the three formed elements (white cells, platelets, and red calls), the plasma, or the vessel wall. If, however, one perfuses the capillary bed with saline and dye solutions or other appropriate media, it is possible to wash out four of the five potential reactants: the three formed elements and the plasma. Admittedly, plasma residues may stick to the vessel during perfusion—the point has not been settled—but it is quite clear that there are no formed elements present during the perfusion and that the bulk of the fluid in the vessel is a dye-saline solution. Because the dye has color, it can absorb laser energy. Therefore, in this circumstance, an injury to the vessel wall can be only an endothelial injury in the absence of the formed elements of the blood. After the injury has been inflicted, normal blood flow is permitted to return to the vessel. Under circumstances where the genesis of the reaction can be ascribed only to an alteration of the blood vascular endothelium, this yields white cell and platelet sticking at the injury site, but not red cell sticking. With minimal stimuli, the reaction is dominated by white cell sticking. With severe stimuli, such as those creating breaches in the wall, the reaction is dominated by platelet sticking, suggesting that the platelets function to plug holes in porous and leaking dikes: a point on which there has been general agreement for many years. (For a fuller discussion of the role of platelets in inflammatory reactions, see Volume I, Chapter 9 by Dr. Zucker.)

Thus, the endothelial cell has a certain primacy in inflammatory states, as Cohnheim indicated, but we are as far today from understanding the nature of the membrane changes that must occur in the transition from nonadhesive to adhesive conditions intraluminally as we were at the turn of the century. Actually, a question can even be raised as to the validity of considering sticking a wholly pathological phenomenon. Investigators who have worked with thin, transparent vascular beds in living animals—mesenteries, cheek pouches, and ear chambers—are impressed with the tendency of white cells to be attracted to the endothelial wall in what would seem to be natural physiological states. The flow properties of blood and physical forces that tend to propel the white cells into the plasma sleeve under certain circumstances probably contribute to this phenomenon. Often, as the cells carom off the endothelial wall and off each other, they hesitate in their journey downstream, as though attracted here and there to certain sites, occasionally stopping momentarily and seeming to stretch out before breaking loose and moving on. Under certain circumstances, injury to a small vascular bed seems heralded by the "hesitation" of white cells before they "stick" to the endothelium. It is as though a mounting reaction, in its dimly discernible beginnings, brings into play at the outset a set of attractive forces which when most intense, cause an adherence that cannot be altered, even in vigorous blood flow or, for that matter, if one irrigates the vessels with fluid (Arnold, 1875). It is conceivable that all experimental preparations developed to study this phenomenon are equipped with a built-in artifact that permits the investigator to state that under "normal" circumstances there is a certain amount of white cell hesitation and sticking, a point emphasized in the nineteenth century (Lister, 1858) but sometimes lost sight of in the twentieth century. In an investigative area where the interfaces between physiology and pathology are ultrathin, it is difficult to say where a pathological process departs from a physiological one.

Although the process of white cell sticking can be described at the levels of light and electron microscopy, the mechanisms responsible for this phenomenon are not known. Whether it is of a physical or chemical nature, or both; whether key changes involve alterations in the blood stream, in the formed elements, in the vascular barriers, or even in the connective tissue in certain circumstances, or in all four parameters—these are points that have been debated for many years. The factors related to flow and the

Fig. 1. (a) Pholomicrograph of two thrombotic lesions in the small vasculature of rabbit connective tissue. Photograph depicts three vessels, two venules (V) taking the form of a hairpin and flanking an arteriole (A), which crosses a segment of the venule at upper right. The arteriolar thrombus (AT) has occluded the vessel at a point where construction has occurred (center of photograph). The venular thrombus (VT), larger in size, has created a partial occlusion of the vessel. Both lesions were inflicted by a laser beam, which was absorbed by the red blood cells and released as heat to create an endothelial microburn. Initially, the dominant adhesive reaction took the form of white cell adherence to the vessel wall. In the venule this reaction, some minutes after the injury, is still obvious. The construction and total occlusion of the arteriole has shut off flow distal to the thrombus. (b) Same field as in (a), 30 minutes later, showing presence of two thrombi, one in an arteriole (AT), the other in a venule (VT). Flow has resumed in the arteriole (A), where the thrombus has changed shape and flattened somewhat. The arteriole construction is obvious. Flow is sluggish in the venule (V) with some evidence of rouleaux formation, but blood, though transiently static in the photograph, is actually moving intermittently without vessel occlusion. (c) Same field as (a) and (b) 1 hour after injury, showing clearing of arteriolar lesion with some construction still present, and marked diminution of venular lesion (VT) with the thrombus jutting out into the lumen and without evidence of occlusion. See text for further discussion. All photographs, × 660, rabbit ear chamber tissue; long arrows indicate direction of blood flow.

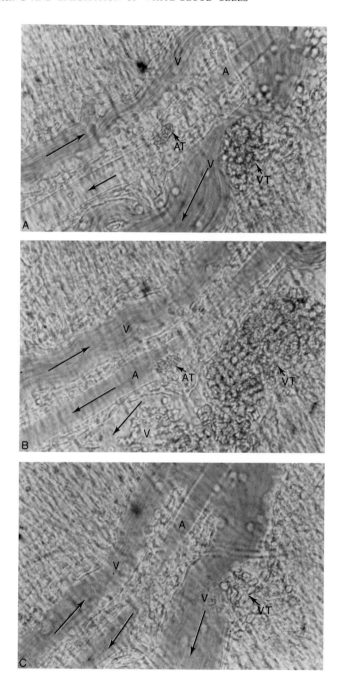

relationship between structure and function in capillary beds also have been the subject of considerable investigation and speculation (see Chapter 1 by Zweifach). At an experimental level, white cell sticking seems to be mainly a venular phenomenon (Illig, 1961), but Allison and his colleagues reported both capillary and arteriolar sticking under heat stimulus (Allison *et al.*, 1955), noting that arteriolar sticking was infrequent, compared with venular sticking, and occurred only where the velocity of flow was reduced drastically by the injury. Ebert and Wissler (1951), in a study of immune rabbits challenged with horse serum, observed arteriolar sticking and emigration, as did Tannenberg (quoted by Illig, 1961) in severe circulatory derangements in the rabbit mesentery. Janoff and Zweifach (1964a,b) were impressed with both venular and capillary sticking in mesenteric vessels subjected to injury by cationic proteins extracted from leukocyte granules.

There is no question that white blood cells can stick to arteriolar walls, in slow or rapid flow, if the stimulus is strong enough. Fig. 1 illustrates the reaction of two vessels, a venule and an arteriole, in close proximity to each other, both subjected to a laser microburn. In both cases, thrombi, composed mainly of white blood cells, ensued, the severity of the thrombus in the arteriole being greater because of the constriction induced by the reaction of the muscular wall of the vessel.

The fact that the use of agents which seem to block white cell sticking has not defined the mechanism of sticking more precisely has been a disappointment to the investigator. But it would be more surprising if the reverse were true; since the mechanism of sticking is unknown and the mechanisms of the action of so-called antiphlogistic agents are unknown, one is in the awkward position of juggling one equation with two unknowns. On logical grounds, if on no other, such a biological equation would seem to be at least as formidable as its mathematical counterpart. Thus, the literature is replete with vivid descriptions of white cells sticking, some of them quite beautiful, but the study of the phenomenon has, since its discovery 140 years ago, hardly gone beyond the descriptive stage, even though it can be analyzed in living preparations and then carried to ultrathin sections, can be elicited in a repeatable and predictable way, can be interrupted and examined at any stage with the white cell attached to the endothelium on the luminal side of the vessel wall or caught in the endothelium between cells or having emigrated into the extravascular space, beyond the basement membrane. The possibilities for manipulation of experimental systems are virtually unlimited in all species from amphibians to mammals, with the investigator able to exercise a very rigorous control over the material, although the segregation of sticking from other phenomena is not easily demonstrated.

Direct injury to the endothelial cell certainly seems to cause white cell sticking (Clark and Clark, 1935; Clark *et al.*, 1936; Zweifach, 1953, 1954,

Grant *et al.*, 1962; Grant and Becker, 1965, 1966; Grant and Epstein, 1973). White cells can be seen, under certain circumstances, to stick to each other in the blood stream. One gets the impression from watching *in vivo* preparations, however, that under most circumstances of injury the white cells stick to localized areas in the endothelial wall which have an affinity for them (Allison *et al.*, 1955; Florey, 1962), and under certain conditions injury can cause them to stick to endothelium when it appears quite clear that the white cells themselves have not been altered by the injury-causing stimulus (Grant *et al.*, 1962; Grant and Epstein, 1973).

Yet injury to the endothelial cell may not be the only basis for the mechanism of stickiness, although the literature on this point is far from clear, being a mixture of speculation, guesswork based on isolated scraps of morphological detail, and probably a good deal of experimental artifact. Whether the sticky material that causes the adherence of white cell and platelet to the endothelial wall is a product of an alteration in white cell or platelet or endothelial cell, or all three, is not known. Whether it involves the production of new material that is sticky or simply the removal of physiological material which normally prevents sticking is not known. It is an interesting fact that if one creates a microinjury in the endothelial wall with a laser beam (Fig. 1a, b) platelets and white cells accumulate at the site of injury forming a thrombus. These cells intermittently break off from the original thrombus and stick downstream at new sites. In most experimental preparations, a question invariably is raised concerning the extent of the original injury, and one often wonders if widespread sticking is simply a reflection of a widespread stimulus. The introduction of laser microinjury by Baez and Kochen (1964, 1965) and Grant and his colleagues (Grant, 1965; Grant and Epstein, 1973) seems to have clarified this point. With a laser beam focused on subcutaneous tissue, it is possible to confine an injury to an area of a blood vessel 5–15 μm in diameter without apparent concomitant extravascular injury. The laser heat stimulus yields a thrombus. The thrombus alternately grows and diminishes in size as white blood cells and platelets adhere to it and then break off, singly and in clumps, to be carried downstream. Often, these embolic fragments adhere to new sites distal to the original injury site where no injury had been inflicted on the endothelial wall. These multiple downstream emboli, which become thrombi at new sites, represent a secondary effect related to the fact that when white blood cells and platelets stick at one site in the vessel wall, they carry the capacity for sticking to other sites and to other white blood cells and platelets.

In the circumstances just described, one can imagine that the laser injury caused an alteration in the property of endothelium that made it sticky, and that this property was imparted to the white cell or platelet. But it could be true that the microburn caused by the laser beam welded platelets and white cells to the endothelial wall, altering a property of the platelets and white cells. In the first instance, newly arrived white cells sweeping past the injury site might pick up stickiness from the altered endothelium, or perhaps, as Zweifach (1940) suggested, there is a release into the blood stream of some substance from the irritated region. In the second instance, such cells would pike up this new property from stuck platelets and white cells. Attempts to stain the sticking sites intravitally have not yet yielded specificity. Alcian blue, an acid mucopolysaccharide stain, colors the injury site, possibly suggesting that the alteration that yields stickiness in white cells, platelets, or endothelium involves an alteration in the mucopolysaccharides of cell surfaces (see Chapter 2 by Luft; see also, Yamaguchi, 1964). But carbon also colors the injury site, as do Evans' blue and other dyes, and, for that matter, even tantalum, which is inert and normally has no affinity whatever for endothelial surfaces (Grant et al., 1973). Thus, it is possible to state that white blood cell, platelet, and endothelium are altered by injury, but it is not clear where the priorities lie or whether one can postulate a single key event as invariable setting off a series of characteristic, stepwise events that lead, always, to the same result.

As noted, one aspect of the problem does seem to have been clarified in recent years, however: the fact that if endothelium is altered, without change in any other parameter of the reaction (white blood cell, platelet, red blood cell, or plasma), inflammatory reactions occur (Grant and Epstein, 1973). This was long suspected by many investigators of the inflammatory process (see Cohnheim, 1882), but the point is an awkward one to study *in vivo*, the only circumstance thus far where the properties of endothelium have been studied with any success, limited though it has been. By perfusing the blood vessels of connective tissue so that all of the formed elements (and possibly even all plasma) are taken from the system, leaving only the endothelial vessel in the path of a laser beam, Grant and Epstein were able to inflict microburns on what amounts to an isolated vessel wall *in vivo*. When the formed elements were permitted to return to the vessel, white blood cells and platelets, but not red blood cells, adhered to the injury site. This evidence tends to argue for the primacy of blood vascular endothelium in the genesis of intravascular injury, including thrombotic states. It also suggests that the adherence of red blood cells is fortuitous, which is not a new idea in any event (see Cohnheim, 1882; Thoma, 1896). But it is also true that altered white cells and platelets, sticking at one site and embolizing downstream, can stick at new sites without evidence that the endothelial cell itself has been altered prior to this adherence. Thus, wheras there is no question about the importance of the endothelial cell in the genesis of inflammatory states intravascularly, there is also no doubt that the white cell and platelet can contribute their own special pathology to this process.

Leaving the question of cell stickiness aside, we can ask how such an alteration could bear on the emigration of the cells from the blood vessel into the extravascular space. As Florey (1962) pointed out, it is well to distinguish between the factors that determine the emigration of cells through endothelium and the factors that control their movement in the tissues outside the perivascular space. It is quite possible that the two phenomena occur under different influences or are controlled by separate, though possibly related, factors. In one case—the adherence of the cells as the first step in their emigration—influence may be completely nonspecific; that is, any noxious stimulus that alters the character of the endothelial membrane may cause it to become sticky. The second circumstance—the emigration of the cell and its extravascular movement—may involve chemotactic influences of a far more specific nature (see discussion of this point in Volume I, Chapter 5 by Ramsey and Grant).

In this chapter, an attempt will be made to cover those aspects of the history of the problem which have influenced current thinking. This will be followed by a discussion of factors that may be related to the sticking phenomenon with some emphasis on experimental studies that make it clear that intravascular and extravascular injury carry their own ground rules. Important aspects of the problem, in other contexts, are discussed by Luft, Chapter 2; Zweifach, Chapter 1; and Macfarlane, Chapter 10; in Volume I, Hirschhorn, Chapter 4; Zucker, Chapter 9; Hirsch, Chapter 7; and Steinman and Cohn, Chapter 8.

II. History of the Problem

A. The Observations of Dutrochet; Sticking and Cement Substance; The Endocapillary Layer; The Junctional Pathway

The first investigator to describe the sticking and emigration of white cells (called "vesicular globules") appears to have been Dutrochet (1824).*

---

*The author is indebted to the National Library of Medicine, Bethesda, Maryland, for making this rare and occasionally cited references available to New York University. Dr. Ian Buckley has called the author's attention to the observations of von Haller (1757) who, in a study of hemorrhagic reactions in the mesenteries of various species of animals, was struck with the appearance of "globules" coating the veins "like a chaplet of beads" and the extravascular appearance of spherical and yellow cells. Although these observations could be interpreted as giving von Haller a priority on the point relating to white cell sticking, it is possible that the yellow globules he described were more often than not, if not in all cases, red cells, not white cells.

He stated:

> What we have just seen concerning the similarity of the organic composition of solids
> and fluids in the living body would indicate that the vesicular globules contained in the
> blood are added to the tissues of the organs and become fixed there to augment and
> repair them so that nutrition consists of a veritable intercalation of fully formed
> and extremely tiny cells. This opinion, though it may seem strange, is however well
> founded, since observation favors this view. Many times I have seen blood cells leaving
> the blood stream, being arrested and becoming fixed to the organic tissue. I have seen
> this phenomenon, which I was far from suspecting, when I observed the movement of the
> blood in the transparent tail of young tadpoles under the microscope. . . . Observing
> the movement of the blood, I have seen many times a single cell escape laterally
> from the blood vessel and move in the transparent tissue . . . with a slowness which
> contrasted strongly with the rapidity of the circulation from which the cell had
> escaped. Soon afterwards, the cell stopped moving and remained fixed in the transparent
> tissue. A comparison with the granulations which this tissue contained showed that
> they were in no way different. There is no doubt that these semi-transparent granu-
> lations were also blood cells which had previously become fixed.

Drutrochet then asked: "In what manner do these cells leave the blood
stream? this is not easy to determine. Perhaps the vessels have lateral openings through which the blood can discharge its elements into the tissues
of the organs." Emperiments on tongue, mesentery, and urinary bladder of
frogs led Arnold (1875) to believe that both white and red cells emigrated
through the "intercellular cement" between endothelial cells. He attributed
an earlier similar observation to Purves (1874). Zweifach (1954) also reached
the conclusion that emigration occurred through the intercellular junctions,
penetrating a cement substance, but Florey et al. (1959) modified the concept
of "cement," producing evidence that cement, as understood by earlier
workers, does not exist; they showed that there appeared to be only a thin
space between endothelial cells which contained some unidentified substance. Recently, Luft (see Chapter 2) has modified the concept of cement
once again, with evidence that a postulated endocapillary layer can be
stained selectively with ruthenium red, and electron-dense material. Leaving
aside the possible relationship between intercellular cement, or some other
such substance, and white cell emigration, electron microscope studies from
Florey's group at Oxford (Marchesi and Florey, 1960; Marchesi, 1961;
Florey and Grant, 1961) confirmed earlier observations demonstrating that
emigration took place through the cell junctions, except in the case of
lymphocytes which may be able to penetrate the endothelial cytoplasm
directly, at least in the postvenular capillaries of the rat lymph node
(Marchesi and Gowans, 1964). This has been disputed recently by Schoefl
(1970, 1972) in a careful analysis by electron microscopy reported by calculations derived from binomial sampling theory.

B. *Addison and Waller; The Problem is Placed on an Experimental Basis*

Dutrochet's observations were either overlooked or did not attract attention at the time. The early English investigators who saw the significance of this phenomenon (Addison, 1843; Waller, 1846; Wharton-Jones, 1851) built upon the work of Rudolph Wagner who stated that lymph granules frequently are arrested and then move (in the blood stream) in irregular propulsive movements (Wagner, 1833) and who emphasized the peripheral position in the blood stream of the white cells (Wagner, 1839). Addison, however, reported two methods to *cause* white cells to adhere to endothelium and thereby seems to have been the first investigator to put the problem firmly on an experimental basis (Addison, 1843). He applied a crystal of salt to the web of a frog's foot, noted that in half an hour the number of lymph globules had increased considerably, and stated that on the next morning the whole interior of the inflamed vessels appeared to be lined with cells, many of them appearing to lie external to the boundary of the vessels. He then heated a frog's foot to 94° F for 30 seconds, again noting the increase in cells. During some of his experiments, the islets of tissue between the capillaries became distinctly cellular, and appeared as if overspread with irregular-shaped cells. Addison's observations impressed Augustus Waller, who thought it curious that a white cell could remain in the same place notwithstanding the rush of red cells past it in the vessel. From the globular form of the white cells, he would have expected, *a priori*, that the contrary would have been the case. He compared the adherence of white cells to vessel walls to that of "so many pebbles or marbles over which a stream runs without disturbing them." In an addendum to his early observations, Waller explained the origin of pus on the basis of the escape of white cells, noting that in some areas the cells are seen protruding half out of the vessel, with the escape route of the vessel wall closing after the emigration of the cell. He stated as established the passage of the white cells *"de toute piece"* throught the capillaries and the "restorative power of the blood," which immediately closed the aperture thus formed. Waller said that these phenomena seemed so improbable to many persons that a theory was expounded that the white cells are not derived from the blood but "like semen or milk, are formed on the secreting surface, in virtue of some plastic power of the fluids which are effused upon it." His observations did not pass without criticism, but he stood his ground, repeating experiments many times and demonstrating them to others who confirmed what he saw. He made many interesting observations, among them that white cells escape more frequently at a bend or angle, where there is a subdivision of the vessel, and that sticking is more prominent at such a site. He had difficulty, as have his successors, in explaining the mechanism of white cell emigration, surmising either that the white cell, after contact with the vessel, exudes a substance with solvent action on the vessel or "that the solution of the vessel takes place in virtue of some of those molecular actions which arise from the contact of two bodies; actions which are now known as exerting such extensive influence in digestion, as are referred to what is termed the catalytic power." But then, by way of refuting his own suggestion, Waller added quickly that white cells are seen adherent to the inner sides of a vessel for long periods without altering their appearance in the least.

C. Cohnheim, Adami, and Metchnikoff; The Central Role of Endothelium; The Ameboid Nature of White Cell Emigration and Evidence That It Is an Active, Not a Passive, Process

When Cohnheim addressed himself to the problem of inflammation in the last half of the nineteenth century (Cohnheim, 1882), he focused attention on the central role of the endothelial cell, formulating a viewpoint that has influenced the thinking of many investigators, although it has not survived without criticism. His argument that molecular changes in the endothelial wall are responsible for the events seen in inflammatory reactions was summarized in the 1899 translation of his "Lectures on General Pathology" (1882). He looked to four systems as potential mediators of inflammation: the blood, the central nervous system, the extravascular connective tissue, and the endothelial wall. He dismissed the first three possibilities succinctly: blood is only momentarily exposed to the local reaction; reflex activities would exhibit themselves more quickly than is characteristic of many inflammatory reactions, and in any event classic inflammatory processes proceed in the absence of a nerve supply; extravascular events would seem unlikely candidates to cause reactions inside the vessels, and he could not imagine the type of diffusion necessary, particularly of solid constituents, to cause an intravascular reaction. This left the endothelial cells as the only remaining focal point of critical alterations in the inflammatory area. For Cohnheim, the exit of the leukocytes from the blood stream did not depend on spontaneous movements of the cells. He asserted that if one interrupted the blood flow in any way (e.g., by compressing the central artery) all further extravasation ceased instantaneously and completely, although previous emigration had been observed in the vessel. The implication is that without pressure there is no emigration. He pointed out, however, that it is not the rise of pressure that forces the cells through the vessel wall; indeed, there is a fall in pressure in the inflamed vessel, and this was further evidence for him that changes in the vessel wall constitute the important fact of adherence and emigration. Cohnheim's conclusion, but not necessarily the reasoning that went into it, remains attractive, and questions he posed still stimulate controversy. In recent years, evidence has accumulated relating diminution of flow and pressure blood in the capillaries to an inhibition of emigration (Delauney et al., 1947; Evans et al., 1948; Miles and Niven, 1950). Miles and Niven demonstrated an association between enhancement of skin infection and shock sufficient to lower the pressure in smaller arteries of the skin below a certain value; the degree of enhancement was directly related to the suppression of leukocytosis in the infected tissues. It was suggested that the absence of tissue leukocytosis may have been due, not to a complete suppression of emigration, but to a diminution in the number of leukocytes passing through the endothelium. If tissue leukocytosis is at any moment dynamic, in the sense that leukocytes are rapidly destroyed or removed and rapidly replaced from the blood, even a partial failure in replacement such as in shock states might soon lead to a virtual absence of leukocytes. Miles and Niven stated that such an explanation would leave inviolate the view that phagocytes traverse capillary endothelium under their own power, but they added a skeptical note:

The view [that phagocytes penetrate endothelium under their own power] is generally held, but we know of no observation proving it. We do not know whether the intracellular forces behind the amoeboid movements of the polynuclear cells in relatively free conditions are sufficient to move a phagocyte through narrow holes in the capillary blood pressure required to help the leucocytes go through the endothelium, either by a direct path, or by stretching the capillary wall so as to produce holes large enough for the passage of leucocytes under their own power; and that in shock the pressure remains for some time below the critical level.

Many investigators have been struck by the active ameboid movement of leukocytes in their progression through vascular wall structures (Thoma, 1896; Metchnikoff, 1893; Adami, 1909; Clark and Clark, 1935; Clark et al., 1936; Ebert and Florey, 1939; Zweifach, 1954; Allison et al., 1955; Florey, 1962). It is interesting that Cohnheim refused to concede the active nature of leukocyte emigration. It was not a revolutionary or even an original thought in his time, and there was reasonable evidence for it (Lavdowsky, 1884; Thoma, 1896). Lavdowsky, indeed, noted that in the inflammed mesenteries of rabbits, guinea pigs, cats, dogs, and rats the leukocytes in the outer zone of the blood stream did not simply adhere passively to the vessel wall, but moved around it, crossing the stream against the current, before attaching themselves and emigrating, as though seeking for a point of less resistance. Admitting that the phenomenon can be characterized only at a descriptive level, one would be hard pressed to define it except by the use of the word ameboid, or its equivalent. Cohnheim, moreover, conceded the ameboid nature of the leukocytes and saw that, once outside the vessel, they moved actively. Adami (1909) stated that Cohnheim's preoccupation with the vessel wall hypothesis "arrested his advance toward a fuller comprehension of the subject." Adami agreed that there is much that would seem to support the doctrine of passivity of leukocytes. No one, he stated, is prepared to attribute active movements to the red corpuscles; nevertheless, in inflammation a few of these escape through the vessel wall. In the inflammation affecting some organs, notably the lung, the number of escaped cells is considerable. If, then, the red cells emerge passively, why should not the emergence of the white cells be passive also? Add to this the observation by Cohnheim that where the circulation is arrested by compression of the artery, there emigration ceases. This, if invariably true, would seem to indicate that when once, by changes in the vessel, the leukocytes adhere to the wall, the further passage through that wall is due to the *vis a tergo* of the blood pressure, a point disputed by Allison *et al.* (1955) and Zweifach (1954). Adami also thought this not a safe deduction to draw. When the artery in an inflamed area is compressed, the stoppage of the blood stream not only reduce the pressure, but also affects the quality of the blood and the conditions of the vessel walls; moreover, it must profoundly affect the vitality or at least the activity of the contained leukocytes, he believed. Again, the outward passage of red corpuscles does not occur in the earliest stages of a reaction to irritation; it does not precede the emigration of the leukocytes (save where there is gross injury), but follows it: a point noted also by Arnold (1875) and by Purves (1874). A capillary or small vein in the frog's web, for example, may be seen completely filled with corpuscles, the peripheral plasma zone being quite annihilated and numerous red corpuscles lying in immediate contact with the walls; nevertheless, at first only leukocytes emigrate. This difference must be due to some special property of these cells. The leukocytes are not necessarily passive globular agents, Adami reasoned, but are capable of independent movement. Finally, Adami noted that if, both within and without the vessels, the leukocytes can be actively ameboid, it is strange that they should be passive in the process of emigration, which to the eye has so characteristically an ameboid movement. Cohnheim's point about compression of the artery led Adami to suggest that this phenomenon may be due to the altered environment of the leukocytes. He asserted that if an embryonic form is used, in which the tissues would seem to possess "greater inherent vitality" coupled with "less sensibility," the arrest of emigration does not occur, thus fortifying an argument advances by Metchnikoff (1893). Metchnikoff and his followers added new evidence that white cells are active, not passive, agents in inflammation and made observations to support the concept of chemotaxis, a term first used by Leber (1888). Metchnikoff diposed of the argument that leukocytes must be forced out of the blood vessel by the pressure of the blood with the observation that the emigration of cells can be seen after stopping the heart of tadpoles with curare.

The upshot of this was that, in the state of knowledge at the turn of the century, the investigator chose to regard the emigration of leukocytes as an active process, with blood pressure, the disposition of the blood stream, and the altered condition of dilated vessels as adjuvants in the process. The slowing of the blood stream and the diminished pressure in the inflamed capillaries would make it easier for the leukocytes to accumulate close to the vessel wall; the dilation of the vessels and subsequent "thinning" of the walls, with the opening, perhaps, of spaces between the cells, made it easier to accomplish the passage, but the movement from within the capillaries to the tissue spaces outside had to be considered an active process due to ameboid movements of the leukocytes themselves. The continuity of the vessel wall once destroyed, other cells—red corpuscles—may be pressed passively through the walls. In this connection, two observations of Allison and his colleagues (1955) are interesting: after thermal injury in the ear chamber, red cells emigrated in small numbers during early inflammation, particularly when they became trapped in endothelial defects left by emigrating leukocytes; additionally, leukocytes adhered in large numbers to the walls of blood vessels which at no time during the experiment exhibited an increase in caliber—indeed, sticking was not uncommonly seen in vessels that were constricted rather than dilated.

D. The Clarks; The Time Sequence of Emigration

At the level of light microscopy, the most extensive studies of white cell sticking and emigration in this century are those of the Clarks (Clark and Clark, 1935; Clark et al., 1936) using the Sandison rabbit ear chamber technique (Sandison, 1924). In a study of emigration in amphibians, Clark and Clark (1935) made the following observations: "A minute protoplasmic knob first appeared on the exterior of the vessel and its size increased rapidly while at the same time the size of the leucocyte in the interior diminished. The process consumed from 2 to 8 minutes between the time of the first appearance of the small knob outside and the emergence of the whole cell on the outside. During the process an actual performed hole was never seen, even under × 700 magnification." The Clarks stated that all types of leukocytes penetrated the endothelium, but the polymorphonuclear leukocyte appeared to make its way through with more ease. It was also noted that sometimes the leukocytes were caught in the endothelial wall, the "outer" portion connected by a fine "thread" to the portion in the lumen, which was distorted by brisk red cell flow, finally being broken off and swept along with the stream. The outer portion remained in the tissue and occasionally showed ameboid movement, although in most cases it assumed a rounded form and was eventually phagocytized by a macrophage. Studying mammalian blood vessels in the rabbit ear chamber, the Clarks found little that contradicted their findings in amphibians. The time occupied in the emigration of a leukocyte, in experiments where the tissue was mechanically traumatized, was 3–9 minutes. They stated that, at times when the endothelium has undergone a change in consistency in which there is marked sticking of cells, there is at the same time an accumulation of free fluid in the outside tissue, indicating a greater permeability of the vessel wall in these situations. They noted, however, that although marked changes in endothelial consistency are accompanied by increase passage of fluid through the endothelial wall increased permeability may also occur in the absence of some of these endothelial changes.

The Clarks took issue with Metchnikoff's view that in chemotaxis lay the explanation of white cell sticking and emigration, and argued, as Cohnheim had, that a change in the endothelium itself is an essential preliminary to the sticking of leukocytes. They formulated, diagrammatically, the series of changes in consistency of the vascular endothelium necessary to achieve various degrees of white cell sticking and emigration (see Fig. 2).

E. Reverse Emigration

Thoma (1896) stated that he had never observed movement of white cells back into the blood stream but said that sometimes a "wandering" cell approaches a capillary, only to pass by it at a higher or lower level. Clark and Clark (1930a) observed intravascular phagocytosis of erythrocytes by macrophages, which were seen to migrate from the tissue into the vessel lumen. It was stated that when "abnormal" erythrocytes in the circulating blood came in contact with the pigmented macrophages, they showed a decided stickiness for them, but "normal" blood cells slipped by without the slightest tendency to adhere. It was concluded that the susceptibility to both intra- and extravascular phagocytosis is associated with a change in the surface of the erythrocyte which makes it sticky toward a macrophage. In studies of aortic lesions in cholesterol-fed rabbits, Poole and Florey (1958) observed monocytes adherent to the endothelium of the aorta overlying the lesions and also reported migration of monocytes through the endothelium. It was not clear whether the monocytes were emigrating from the luminal to the subendothelial side, or vice versa, but, on the basis of the Clarks' observations reported above, either could have been the case, and it is possible that this represents an emigration of monocytes in a reverse direction. Clark *et al.*

(1936) also reported that in tadpoles occasionally a polymorphonuclear leucocyte was seen to make its way back into the lumen of a blood vessel, a very rare observation indeed, or into a lymphatic capillary, which the author has also noted (Grant, 1960).

F. White Cell Sticking and Emigration as Revealed by Ultrastructure Studies

Ultrastructure studies of inflamed small vascular beds have added some interesting morphological details to the description of the reaction, much of the evidence confirmatory of earlier work, but have yielded no clues to the mechanism of the phenomenon. Williamson and Grisham (1960, 1961). Marchesi and Florey (1960), Florey and Grant (1961), Marchesi (1961, 1962), Peterson and Good (1962), Marchesi and Gowans (1964), and Schoefl (1970, 1972) all studied under a variety of circumstances the passage of white cells through small vascular beds.

Williamson and Grisham (1960, 1961) ligated pancreatic lobules and removed tissue adjacent to the ligatures from the side with intact circulation, noting the development of intraluminal cytoplasmic processes and large intracytoplasmic vesicles. The vesicles were described as much larger (1 μm in diameter) than those seen in normal capillaries, but they appeared to arise in an analogous manner and appeared to be formed of infolded plasma membranes. In most instances, the cytoplasmic projections were thought to represent fingerlike processes since many of them were round or oval in cross section. They were quite long (up to 8 μm) and thin (not more than 1 μm), were often irregular in configuration and thickness, and formed hooks or loops. They contained many small vacuoles but few cytoplasmic organelles. In some areas, the endothelial processes were so numerous and extensive as to form a network in the vessel lumen. Leukocytes appeared to become enmeshed in these processes and were then gradually enveloped and surrounded by endothelial cytoplasm. As leukocytes emerged from the extraluminal margin of endothelial cells and began to separate from them, a new basement membrane formed between the two. The outermost layer of basement membrane then disappeared, permitting release of the leukocytes into the extravascular space. In this experimental system, almost all the cells emigrating were polymorphonuclear leukocytes, but occasional lymphocytes and red blood cells were seen. In studies of acute inflammation in rat skin, the authors stated that they did not observe endothelial changes, and, in other acutely inflamed tissues in the dog, endothelial alterations did not appear with the frequency observed in the pancreas, suggesting perhaps that in the endothelium in the pancreas and under the special conditions of the experiment may reside a property not widely shared by other similar vascular membranes.

Marchesi and Florey (1960) and Florey and Grant (1961) studied acute changes in small vascular beds, the former in the rat mesentery inflamed with mild trauma, the latter in the rabbit ear chamber subjected to mild ultraviolet burning. Marchesi and Florey noted that the leukocyte starts its passage through the endothelium by protruding clear hyaloplasm. Having passed the endothelial cell, the pseudopod can continue straight on through the basement membrane, or it may strip the basement membrane from the endothelium and come to lie in the space between the endothelium and the basement membrane. A further bar to the leukocyte passage is formed by the periendothelial cells and the fibers associated with them. It is common to find a vessel lined by a layer of leukocytes external to the endothelium and basement membrane but inside the periendothelial sheat. The leukocyte may turn after passing through the endothelium, but finally a gap is found, apparently between the periendothelial cells and fibers, and the leukocytes streams out into the surrounding connective tissue, clear hyaloplasm again going first. It appeared that once the leukocyte passes through the endothelium, the hole closes up again, for no gaps unoccupied by portions of a leukocyte were seen. Eosinophils and monocytes apparently followed the same pattern, and red cell extrusion from the lumen was noted. No lymphocytes were seen migrating through the vessel wall. The evidence suggested, but did not prove, that emigration occurred through cell junctions, even through occasionally portions of platelets and leukocytes were seen completely surrounded by cytoplasm. Marchesi (1961) carried his observation on sticking a step further, performing series sections in areas of inflammatory reactions. He found that he could trace the relationship between white cell and endothelial cell to the point where it became evident that the white cell was breaching an intercellular junction, although early cuts from the block often had left the point in doubt. Whether this is the only mode of emigration of the polymorphonuclear leukocytes, and other granulocytes, remains to be seen, but the two reported exceptions in the white cell series do not discount the importance of these observations. One of these exceptions is Williamson's observation that in the inflamed dog pancreas endothelium can phagocytize white cells. The other is the observation of Marchesi and Gowans (1963) that small lymphocytes emigrate, under physiological conditions, through the endothelial cytoplasm in the postcapillary venules of the lymph node. This would place the emigration of lymphocytes in a special category and could have some implications for the mechanism of immigration in immune reactions. On the other hand, Schoefl (1970, 1972) restudied this problem in venous vessels of Peyer's patches in the intestine of rats and mice. She found that lymphocytes in the process of emigration lay between endothelial cells, the usual circumstance. Where the white cells were found completely surrounded by endothelial cytoplasm—fewer than 20%—this was of the order of magnitude expected statistically in random sections if one assumed passage exclusively between cells. In some instances, further sectioning showed the "intracellular" lymphocyte to extend into the intercellular space. It was not possible to unequivocally demonstrate in serial sections a lymphocyte within an endothelial cell.

Florey and Grant (1961) found evidence of polymorphonuclear leukocyte and eosinophil emigration, but no evidence of lymphocyte emigration. They noted that the granules of white cells remained intact during passage through the endothelial wall and suggested, as had Marchesi and Florey, that the route might be via the cell junctions. Neither group found evidence for "cement" substance (Arnold, 1875; Chambers and Zweifach, 1940; 1947; Florey et al., 1959) or an electron-dense material that could be considered fibrin, nor was there any evidence for the gelatinous material described by Zweifach (1953). But Florey and Grant (1961) occasionally noted a dense area near the endothelium, sometimes found in the angle formed by endothelium and leukocyte, which could be considered to represent "cement." Since the material was seen so rarely, it seemed unlikely that it had anything to do with sticking. The search for the "glue" that causes white cells to adhere to endothelium has not been a productive one at the level of electron microscopy. It is conceivable that the fixing and dehydrating procedures used in preparing ultra-thin sections may wash out or alter luminal material, thus placing the point beyond the reach of the electron microscope at this time. The idea that there may be a "glue," such as to cause white cells to stick to endothelium as flies stick to flypaper, may be naive. The attractive force may be an electrochemical one, far out of range of a direct morphological approach. It should be noted, however, that Luft (Chapter 2) describes evidence for an endocapillary layer, probably mucoprotein or mucopolysaccharide, which seems to be attached to, or to be part of, the external layer of the unit membrane of the luminal surface of the endothelial cell.

The strong evidence that polymorphonuclear leukocyte emigration occurs through intercellular junctions, and not through the endothelial cytoplasm, raises questions as to whether all molecules, large and small, as well as white cells, may leave small vascular lumina by the same route. Benacerraf et al. (1959) produced data supporting the view that blood vascular endothelium has phagocytic properties, citing evidence reported previously by von Jancsó (1955; see also von Jancsó, 1947; Biozzi et al., 1948). Marchesi (1962), however, injected colloidal carbon intravenously, noting that it accumulated in the walls of the venules in the inflamed mesentery of the rat. Electron micrographs showed that the carbon passed through open intercellular junctions of the endothelial wall. It was found to be contained within the walls of venules by the basement membrane of the endothelium and also by the periendothelial sheath of cells and their basement membrane. Little carbon was found within the cytoplasm of inflamed endothelial cells, although small amounts were found there, apparently in vacuoles similar to the phagocytosis vacuoles described by Karrer (1960) in macrophages in the lung. Marchesi reached the conclusion that inflamed endothelium is not as actively phagocytic as Jancsó and Benacerraf had suggested. Along parallel lines, Majno and Palade (1961) disputed Alksne's (1959) conclusions that there is a vesicular transport of macromolecules in dermal capillaries (for a further discussion of endothelial phagocytosis, see Altschul, 1954; Majno, 1964, 1965). Once past the endothelium, masses of carbon were held up by the basement membrane of the endothelial cells, Marchesi noted. Policard *et al.* (1957) and Palade (1959) argued for a central role of the basement membrane as a protein filtration mechanism, but Marchesi noted that his experiments left this point in a state of uncertainty. In Marchesi's experiments, the periendothelial sheath seemed to act as a further barrier to the passage of the carbon into the extravascular spaces, as it had acted as a barrier to the white cells (Marchesi and Florey, 1960; Florey and Grant, 1961).

Peterson and Good (1962) studied the morphology of vascular permeability in passive cutaneous anaphylaxis, noting the escape of thorium dioxide particles exclusively through the intercellular spaces. A study by Cotran (1965) confirmed the ability of endothelial cells outside the reticuloendothelial system to phagocytize carbon particles under certain circumstances. [For a discussion of the problems relating to the use of tracer particles in electron microscopy, see Majno's review (1965).] Even accepting the fact, however, that the normal route of white cells through the endothelial wall in inflamed tissues is via the intercellular junctions and that vascular leaks occur at these sites (Majno and Palade, 1961), the mechanism of sticking and emigration remains obscure, for the relationship between sticking and permeability is by no means clear. This will be referred to later.

G. Red Cell Sticking

Factors that influence the sticking of red cells to endothelium and the diapedesis of the red cells through the endothelial wall are largely unknown, but it is possible that the *vis a tergo* of blood flow is more important in red cell diapedesis than in white cell emigration. Even this point, however, is in doubt. Although flow and pressure factors may be important, the state of the endothelial wall is also of some consequence. Clark and Clark (1935) described a situation in the rabbit ear chamber where, after compression of the chamber cover slip for some time such as to cause opposing endothelial surfaces to remain in contact with each other, delicate threads of endothelium extending across the wall from lumen to lumen made their appearance with the resumption of flow. Erythrocytes were often suspended in these threads, and at the same time there was extensive leukocyte sticking. Temporary compression caused no such adherence of endothelial cells, so the Clarks concluded that the traumatic stimulus had altered a property of endothelium. The strands of endothelium conceivably could have some relationship to the intravascular gelatinous material appearing on endothelial interfaces as reported by Zweifach (1953) under inflammatory conditions.

Florey (1962) called attention to visible roughening of endothelium in the form of "spikes," around which red cells can be seen to be bent double by the force of the blood stream, but whether the spikes represent a special example of erythrocyte sticking is not clear. Thoma (1896) and others (Pfaff and Herold, 1937; Humble, 1949; Spaet, 1952a; Arendt et al., 1953) pointed out that, whereas leukocyte emigration is a relatively slow process, erythrocyte diapedesis is explosively fast and punctate. Arendt et al. (1953), for example, observed that erythrocytes "popped out," one by one, through a single hole (occasionally multiple), in spurts related to blood pressure, and no permanent opening was left. Extravasation ceased without the formation of platelet plugs. Thoma stated that those places in the vessel wall which have allowed the passage of a considerable number of leukocytes later permit the red cells to pass through also: a point also made by Ricker and Regendanz (1921) and Allison et al. (1955). Ricker and Regendanz (1921) thought that diapedesis occurred at the same site as white cell emigration, that is, through what was once considered to be intercellular cement, or intercellular junctions. Marchesi and Florey (1960) showed an electron micrograph of a red cell passing through endothelium, but they pointed out that it was not obviously treading, so to speak, on the heels of a leukocyte. Portions of red cells were found occasionally surrounded by endothelial cytoplasm, but the authors cautioned that this is not unequivocal evidence for the passage through the endothelial cell. Red cells cross the endothelium in capillaries and venules where there is a preference for junction points (Arendt et al., 1953; Spaet, 1952a). Lee and Lee (1947) studied the peripheral vascular system and its characteristics in scurvy in guinea pig mesentery and reported that up to 85% of the petechiae associated with the experimental disease were to be found in collecting venules. Spaet (1952b), however, found bleeding in the smallest arteries as frequently as in the smallest veins in thrombocytopenic mesenteries subjected to positive pressure. Illig (1961) quotes Witte (1958) as stating—and Illig agreed with him—that there exists another less conspicuous and slower form of erythrocyte diapedesis in which the red cells form a thin layer immediately outside the vessels, fringing them like a cuff. In contrast to punctate bleeding, the cells evidently do not pass through the vascular wall at specific sites but rather on a plane. Illig speculates that this form of bleeding may be associated specifically with coagulation defects, but he states that it can also be observed after trauma. This is a confusing point that needs to be examined in more detail.

As in the case of white cell sticking and emigration, damage to endothelium appears to be a prerequisite for red cell diapedesis. Neither vasomotor stimuli, according to Illig (1961), nor anticoagulants alone (Dietrich and Nordmann, 1930, cited by Illig, 1961) were able to produce diapedesis regularly. Apparently, as in the case of white cell emigration, erythrocyte diapedesis does not depend solely on the velocity of blood flow. Arendt *et al.* (1953) and Illig (1961) observed bleeding with a slowdown of blood flow and Illig quotes Witte as stating that bleeding can occur also under normal circulatory circumstances and, for that matter, can be observed from stagnant vessels, for example, during venous congestion or stasis, but apparently only when stagnant blood is under high pressure (Illig, 1961). Illig assumed that under these conditions only those red cells pass through the endothelium which are still affected by the increased pressure, for example, at the beginning of the stasis column, but he conceded that this is an unsolved problem.

Whether fluid passes with red cell diapedesis (i.e., the relationship between capillary permeability and capillary fragility) is not clear. The openings through which the red cells traverse the endothelial wall seem to close immediately after the cells have passed through, but the opening itself can be very small, according to Illig (1961), for the erythrocytes are literally hurled out. It is possible that the right combination of endothelial defect, local pressure, and red cell accumulation could account for all of this, but there are no facts which define the phenomenon precisely.

As for the fate of the red cells in the extravascular tissue, they are phagocytized by tissue macrophages, according to Clark and Clark (1930a), as noted earlier. They suggested that this abnormality was reflected in a change in the surface of the erythrocyte which made it sticky for the macrophage. Whether the stickiness associated with the phagocytosis of foreign bodies by macrophages—if such an idea has merit in the first place—bears any relationship to the stickiness of endothelium is not known.

H. Platelet Sticking

Platelet aggregation is reviewed by Zucker (Volume I, Chapter 9) and Macfarlane (Chapter 10), and the circulatory aspects of the problem are considered by Zweifach (Chapter 1). It is mentioned here only for continuity in the context of white cell sticking which often involves the clumping of platelets in a mass known as a white thrombus. The thrombus may grow so large that it blocks the lumen of the vessel, thereby shutting off flow and leading to stasis and necrosis. Sometimes it seems that the pressure of the blood flow proximal to the thrombus may be strong enough to dislodge it, in which event it moves downstream as an embolic mass. The factors that regulate the sticking of platelets to endothelium and to each other are not known, but recent evidence suggests that exposure of microfibris of basement membrane to platelets may account for the genesis of some thrombi (Ross and Bornstein, 1969; Stemerman et al., 1971). It is of interest that subsequent to Cohnheim's dictum that molecular events in the vessel wall are responsible for the accumulation of formed elements of the blood at injury sites (Cohnheim, 1882), a period followed when the focus of many investigators was trained on such extravascular factors as thromboplastin and foreign surfaces and the role of these factors in initiating intravascular fibrin deposition (Macfarlane, 1965; French and Macfarlane, 1970). When the importance of platelets in hemostasis was appreciated, it was first assumed that platelets were bound together passively by fibrin, but then it was realized that platelet aggregation preceded fibrin formation (French and Macfarlane, 1970).

Hellem (1960) and Ollgaard (1961) described a factor from red blood cells that caused platelet aggregation; this later was characterized as adenosine diphosphate (ADP), a point that has been confirmed by many investigators (Gaarder et al., 1961; Zucker and Borrelli, 1962; Born and Cross, 1963; Clayton et al., 1963; Hovig, 1963; Haslam, 1964). The importance of some vessel wall constituent in initiating platelet aggregation resulting from vessel injury was emphasized by Bounameaux (1959), Hugues (1962), and Roskam (1964), the first two demonstrating that platelets adhere to fibers in the mesentery near injured vessels and to fragments of aorta. Kjaerheim and Hovig (1962) observed that the mesenteric fibers to which platelets adhered were collagenous in character, and then Hovig examined tendon extracts and discovered that they caused a release of ADP from platelets (Hovig, 1963). This type of evidence kept the initiating mechanism in the extravascular compartment, where coagulation studies had placed it originally (Spaet and Zucker, 1964; Spaet and Erichson, 1966), but on a quite different basis and having little relationship to thromboplastin. Recently this postulated mechanism has been shifted toward a subendothelial area, possibly on the basis of microfibril exposure (Stemerman et al., 1971). This viewpoint might gain support from recent evidence suggesting that basement membrane, contrary to an older concept that it is mucopolysaccharide in character, does in fact have a collagenous component (Dische, 1964; Lazarow and Speidel, 1964; Misra and Berman, 1966; Kefalides, 1966, 1967; Ross and Grant, 1968). Even so, such evidence may bear on the issue only tangentially.

Grant and Epstein (1973) found, for example, that under minimal stimuli it is difficult to demonstrate platelet sticking, inflammatory reactions being dominated by the adherence of white cells to injured endothelial cells. But under severe stimuli, severe enough to create breaches in the vessel wall, there is an immediate and massive accumulation of platelets at the injury site. These observations were made *in vivo* and correlated with those of Stehbens (1965) *in vitro*. Since there is some platelet sticking even in minimal injuries where there is no evidence of breaches in the vessel wall, there may well be intravascular factors at work to create these, not a surprising possibility in view of the fact that platelets can adhere to endothelium (Marchesi, 1964; Shirasawa, 1966; Ashford and Freiman, 1968; Johnson *et al.*, 1969; Grant and Epstein, 1973). Platelets can also adhere to fibrin (McCallum, 1916; Chandler, 1969; French, 1969; Mustard, 1969; Warren and de Bono, 1970), and platelet agglutination can be initiated by thrombin (Hovig, 1969) and also by fibrinolysis split products (Barnhart *et al.*, 1967; Barnhart and Riddle, 1967; Barnhart *et al.*, 1972). Even in physiological states, where the presence of collagen and microfibril attachment can be excluded, platelet thrombi can form, as shown in the provocative study of placental thrombotic mechanisms by Moe and Jorgenson (1967, 1968). The findings of Majno and his colleagues also could be relevant to this discussion. They have noted that the contraction of endothelial cells causes the cells to bulge into the vessel lumen, creating intercellular gaps. They achieved these changes with such agents as histamine and bradykinin (Majno *et al.*, 1969), and it is possible that such alterations in the shape of the endothelial cell could expose provocative substrate for platelet sticking, a concept similar to one offered by Tranzer and Baumgartner (1967). This suggests a mechanism for the platelet to get access to structures beyond the endothelial luminal membrane.

On balance, the evidence indicates that the mechanisms of white blood cell and platelet sticking differ in a fundamental way, one broad distinction based on the fact that with breaches in the vessel wall intravascular thrombosis is dominated, in its early stages, by platelet accumulation. It would appear, then, that one role for the platelet is to plug a hole in the dike, and the availability of collagenous substrates may accelerate this. But there are probably other reasons for platelet sticking—some of them perhaps shared with white blood cells some not—and these may not require subendothelial or extravascular triggers. It may be of interest to note that mild injury to a small vascular bed yields white cell sticking, and, if the experiment is calibrated carefully, such as to cause white cell sticking but little or no emigration, the reaction can be blocked with high doses of hydrocortisone (Grant *et al.*, 1962). The case for a steroid influence on platelets is much less clear; Mowbray (1967) suggests that cortisone has an antiaggregation effect on platelets, but Caen argues that there is no such effect (Caen *et al.*, 1967), and Gatspar (1970) indicates that cortisone may, in fact, contribute to an adhesive effect on thrombocytes. It would be useful to segregate the differences between white cell and platelet adhesive mechanisms for the light that one might shed on the other. At the moment, apparently the best one can say is that frank breaches in the vessel wall are dominated by platelet aggregation, that less severe injuries are often dominated by white cell aggregation, and that there seems to be an overlapping of adhesiveness of both formed elements in a large gray area of intravascular occlusion where one suspects that membrane changes provide a common basis for pathology. Compounding the riddle is that in some circumstances the white blood cell not only sticks to the vessel wall, but it actively emigrates through it, a phenomenon that defies rationality except on the basis of chemotactic influences.

III. Fate of Emigrated Cells in the Extravascular Tissues

Aside from reactions associated with certain immune states, possibly, for example, delayed hypersensitivity of the tuberculin type, the early inflammatory response yields an extravascular cellular reaction dominated by polymorphonuclear leukocytes. Dienes and Mallory (1932) asserted that the tuberculin reaction was characterized from the beginning by a predominance of mononuclear cells, but Follis (1940) questioned this, contending that the cellular response in the early stages is predominantly a polymorphonuclear one. This is a subject of recurrent dispute through the literature, an important and difficult point to define precisely because in any experimental system where the experiment itself may start with injury to endothelium, the ubiquitous neutrophils will stick to the endothelial wall and, under many circumstances, will emigrate into the tissues. The injunction by Landis (1934) is worth remembering. The most delicate injuries (for example, piercing skin or capillary membranes with a micropipette, 4–8 μm in diameter) yield changes in blood flow and capillary pressure, a reflection of the extraordinary sensitivity of the peripheral vessel. Gentle compression of a single capillary in the frog's mesentery results in increases in permeability with the accumulation of carbon particles in dense masses at the site of injury, an indication of the stickiness of the endothelial wall. Thus, at the outset the artifact of the experiment often tends to swamp the experimental goal, which is to determine whether monocytes or perhaps lymphocytes stick initially in certain immune states. Evidence from studies of contact dermatitis, assuming this to be an adequate model of delayed hypersensitivity, shade the argument in favor of Dienes (see Baer et al., 1957; Baer, 1964), but in Braude's study of brucellosis (1951), where guinea pigs and mice were subjected to infection by intracardiac or intraabdominal puncture, the evidence, gleaned from examination of the liver at varying intervals, suggests that there is a transient predominance of polymorphonuclear leukocytes in the early stages of the reaction, at least under the special circumstances of this experiment. In an electron microscope study of homograft rejection, Wiener *et al.* (1964) were impressed with the invasion of mononuclear cells as being of prime importance in the graft rejection, polymorphonuclear cells being associated with surgical trauma and wound repair as nonspecific concomitants of the reaction. Whether this favors the view that the initial cellular response in graft rejection is a truly mononuclear one, rather than a polymorphonuclear one, is not clear, but it could be construed as evidence supporting Waksman's (1960) emphasis on the importance of infiltrating mononuclear cells in mediating various types of delayed hypersensitivity if one assumes that there is a role for this mechanism in homograft rejection. Bauer (1958) also was impressed with the prominence of mononuclear infiltration in first- and second-set reactions and stated that at no time during a first-set graft destruction was a preponderantly polymorphonuclear invasion observed (for a further discussion of these points, see Volume III, Chapters by Dvorak, and McGregor and Mackaness, and Lawrence, 1956, 1957).

Whether under certain conditions the initial reaction is a polymorphonuclear leukocytic one or a monocytic one, so to speak, the evidence for the hematogeneous origin of mononuclear cells is a strong one (Clark and Clark, 1930b; Kolouch, 1939; Ebert and Florey, 1939; Rebuck and Crowley, 1955; McCluskey *et al.*, 1963; see also discussion by Harris, 1960). A question that remains unsettled, however, is whether mononuclear cells, and possibly lymphocytes, emigrate at the same time as polymorphonuclear leukocytes or emigrate separately, the mononuclear cells following the neutrophilic emigration. In the first instance, the same stimulus could be responsible for sticking and emigration; in the second, the inference could be drawn that the neutrophils in some way help to set the stage for the emigration of mononuclear cells. It is conceivable that the change in the cellular character of the exudate could be associated in some way with the fact that the polymorphonuclear leukocyte is an end cell with a relatively short life history (see Volume I, Chapter 7 by Hirsch), whereas other cells may give rise to other types of cells) (Ebert and Florey, 1939). On this basis, new cell types in the exudate would represent a drying off of the granulocytic series with the continuing emergence of so-called round cell types and their descendants. Page and Good (1958), in studies of a patient with cyclic neutropenia and of rabbits with experimentally induced neutropenia, interpreted their evidence as demonstrating that the sequence and time relationships of events in acute inflammation are a function, in part at least, of the circulating neutrophils. Humphrey (1955a) stated, however, that in rabbits subjected to reversed passive Arthus reactions suppression of polymorphonuclear leukocyte emigration did not prevent the succeeding phase of the reaction from following its usual course. He concluded that the phase of mononuclear cell proliferation and invasion must therefore be directly related to the antigen–antibody reaction, and is not secondary to the polymorphonuclear leukocyte phase. In studies growing out of the observation that 6-mercaptopurine will inhibit the lymphocyte response in inflammation without preventing the early neutrophil exudation, Page and his colleagues (1962) produced evidence supporting the hypothesis that substances released from inflammatory sites induce new protein synthesis in the circulating lymphocyte that is essential for its migration (summarized by Page, 1964).

Paz and Spector (1962; discussion by Spector and Willoughby, 1963) provoked an inflammatory exudate by the injection of macromolecules of various substances into the skin and abdomen of rats and at various times performed differential counts in areas of involved vessels and on smears from peritoneal exudates. Their observations showed that the polymorphonuclear leukocytes and mononuclear cells left the blood vessels concurrently and that there was no detectable selective migration of any cell type. But the polymorphonuclear leukocytes left the vessels faster than did the mononuclear cells so that a dominance of polymorphonuclear cells was soon established in the tissues. Once emigration ceased, however, the polymorphonuclear leukocytes disappeared, but the mononuclear cells remained near the vessels and were transformed into macrophages and then to special cell types whose nature depended on the stimulus. After injection of lipids, for example, they became altered to epithelioid cells. Paz and Spector (1962) concluded with Harris (1960) that where polymorphonuclear dominance persists, as in pyogenic infections, it is due to sustained active emigration because of the intensity of the stimulus but also because of immobilization of the cells at the site of injury. Conversely, responses where mononuclear cells predominate from the early stages were thought to be due to a weak stimulus for emigration, coupled with immobilization of the mononuclear cells, the polymorphonuclear cells escaping unimpaired or suffering destruction. It was suggested that long-lasting mononuclear exudates, for example as in tuberculosis, were due to such a process, augmented by repeated fresh waves of emigration and local proliferation of exuded or tissue cells.

IV. The Influence of pH on the Emigration of White Cells

Menkin (1934) claimed that the cytological character of an exudate elicited by intrapleural injection of turpentine could be correlated with the pH of the exudate. He stated that in an alkaline pH the polymorphonuclear leukocytes predominated and that with the mounting acidosis at the inflammatory site there was a shift from polymorphonuclear leukocytes to mononuclear cells. Steinberg and Dietz (1938) and Lurie (1939) found no such correlation. Menkin (1950) viewed the changes in hydrogen ion concentration at the site of an acute inflammatory reaction as merely an expression of the survival of a given type of leukocyte, the pH apparently having nothing to do with the mobilization of these cells around the lesion. Such changes may not constitute cellular determinants in the chain of events leading to small vascular damage, but they may influence the course of reactions in other ways. Thomas and Stetson (1949), Stetson and Good (1951), and Stetson (1951) produced evidence from the Shwartzman and Arthus reactions that skin sites prepared for these reactions showed a pronounced increase in aerobic glycolysis, a metabolic abnormality reflected, *in vivo*, by a measurable increase in the concentration of lactic acid in the prepared skin. Some increase in anaerobic glycolysis also occurred, this of less degree than the increase in aerobic glycolysis. The change in glycolysis was attributed largely to the influx of polymorphonuclear leukocytes. Crabtree (1928) indicated that such "exudate leukocytes" exhibited a high degree of aerobic glycolysis. These observations were supported by Miles (1958–1959, 1961) who pointed to the evidence of Barron and Harrop (1929) which permitted the conclusion that 10^9 polymorphonuclear leukocytes under optimum conditions of anerobic glycolysis can in 1 hour produce about 10 μg of lactic acid. Given little buffering and not too much removal of the lactic acid formed, a pericapillary mass of leukocytes might well raise enough free lactic acid for a local and sustained increase of permeability, it was argued. Miles (1961) stated that 60 μg of lactic acid will cause marked vasodilation in 1 gm of guinea pig skin. Thomas and Stetson (1949) showed that normal skin produced up to 0.5 mg of lactic acid per hour per gram (net weight) of skin. Skin prepared for the Shwartzman reaction was found to contain up to 2 mg of lactic acid per gram of skin. Stetson (1961) suggested that this point might be extended to cover reactions of delayed hypersensitivity of the tuberculin type, reporting that the permeability change induced by the injection of lactic acid is slow in onset and prolonged in duration and occurs at those concentrations of lactic acid actually found in the inflamed lesions. While considering the point worth investigating, Miles (1958–1959) cast doubt on the significance of lactic acid accumulation in inflammatory lesions, and Thomas and Stetson (1949) in their original paper offered evidence that tends to minimize the generality of this phenomenon: other substances that produced a visible inflammatory reaction did not elicit the marked aerobic glycolysis characteristic of samples prepared with meningococcal or *Serratia marcescens* toxin.

V. Relationship between White Cell Sticking and Vascular Permeability

Most studies of "capillary permeability" or small vessel permeability, as Majno (1964) prefers to refer to the phenomenon, deal with the transport of macromolecules across the endothelial barrier, in most cases dye–protein complexes. Landis (1946) noted that the rate of escape of dye into the tissues does not depend solely on capillary permeability, and cautioned that alleged changes in permeability, based simply on dye passage, are surrounded with doubts unless elaborate control observations are supplied to prove that special factors or artifacts have been eliminated completely. Landis (1934) also stated that whatever may be the mechanism by which leukocytes pass through the capillary wall, it appears to have no direct relation to the normal filtration of fluid and dissolved substances. Burke and Miles (1958) observed that permeability to indicator dye is not necessarily associated with permeability to edema fluid or white blood cells.

Thoma (1896) stated that the emigration of leukocytes gives rise to increased permeability of the vessel wall. This might be too insignificant to be demonstrated with mild stimuli, but with stronger stimuli the increase in permeability would be more considerable. Such an increase in permeability would then, in turn, increase the retardation of the blood stream. Thus, a vicious cycle would be set up, the emigration of the white cells injuring the vessel wall and increasing its permeability and, vice versa, a considerable increase in permeability giving rise to emigration. The fact that a great increase in the permeability of the vessel wall causes emigration of leukocytes can be seen under circumstances where caustic alkalis or acids (or other strong reagents or pyogenic bacteria) injure tissue, leading, Thoma stated, to the following chain of events: the vessels first dilate and the stream becomes accelerated; arteries then contract slightly, the stream in the veins is slowed, and the marginal arrangement and emigration of leukocytes result; this marginal arrangement persists for some time, probably due to increase in the permeability of the vessel wall (a somewhat dubious assumption said to be supported by the fact that the fluid which, under these circumstances, passes through the vessel wall is of abnormal composition and manifests the general characteristics of an exudation); the increase in permeability of the vessel wall causes slowing of the blood stream in the capillaries and veins because under such circumstances the greater part of the blood plasma passes over to the tissues and, additionally, because the white cells which have passed into the marginal stream are apposed to the permeable wall in great numbers and thus diminish the lumen; later, the emigration becomes more extensive because of the greater permeability of the vessel wall, leading ultimately to diapedesis of red blood cells when permeability is greatly increased. If permeability exceeds certain limits, stasis may ensue, with much of the blood plasma passing into the tissues. In Thoma's view, then, injury leads to sticking and emigration, which increases permeability, which increases sticking—a cycle broken by stasis.

Carscadden (1927) incised the liver aseptically and charted the inflammatory reaction by histological sections of the organ. He found that within 3 minutes there was an exudation of plasma, within 30 minutes a margination of white cells and stasis in dilated vessels, and within 1–3 hours emigration of white cells into the extravascular space. On the basis of a study of inflammatory reactions in the subcutaneous tissues of rats challenged with turpentine, Ernst (1926) noted a mounting edema production within 15 minutes, with a migration of leukocytes starting within 1 hour. Allison et al. (1955) injured connective tissue in rabbit ear chambers with heat, noting the onset of white cell sticking within 10–15 minutes, with marked sticking at 30 minutes, and with a subsidence within 6–9 hours. Red cell agglutination and rouleaux formation were obvious within 10 minutes, and stasis mounted until active circulation ceased within 4–6 hours. A second study (Allison and Lancaster, 1959), using the same stimulus and combining this with an injection of Evans' blue dye at appropriate intervals before and after the stimulus, attempted to define permeability changes in relation to other phenomena. Under these circumstances, extravascular dye was most often seen in injured tissue as early as 3 minutes after administration, in some cases not until 30 minutes. One to three hours after injury, endothelial permeability was greatly enhanced, but apparently there was no abrupt increase at this time, for changes were gradual and varied slightly with different animals. After 3 hours there was a fall in tissue staining, possibly due to obstruction of flow by stasis. Dye loading apparently did not influence the course of the reactions, as noted in Allison's first set of experiments (Allison et al., 1955), for sticking was apparent in the dye experiments within 15–30 minutes, was fully developed within 1–2 hours, and had diminished in intensity between 6–9 hours. From this data, one can conclude that permeability increases occur early, before sticking, that intensive sticking follows within a few minutes, mounts for a few hours to subside within 6 hours, and that before 3 hours there is a secondary increase in permeability which occurs gradually, not abruptly.

Burke and Miles (1958), using guinea pigs injected intracutaneously with a variety of bacteria, drew a more precise relationship between permeability and sticking, noting two permeability phases: a transient one during the first half hour and a second, larger and more intense one at 3–4 hours. These alternations more or less paralleled endothelial stickiness in most cases. Burke and Miles noted a decreased exudation of dye (pontamine blue) during the fifth hour at the periphery of the lesion, where the pathogen was in a subnecrotizing concentration. Both macroscopically evident edema and microscopically detectable leucocytosis increased as the permeability curve rose. But tissue leukocytosis tended to increase, as did induration, after the fifth hour, facts which were difficult to reconcile with a recovery of low capillary permeability at this time. In two infections (*Corynebacterium diphtheriae* and *Listeria monocytogenes*), moreover, tissue leukocytosis and edema increased, and a substantial inflammatory induration developed in the absence of any second phase. As noted earlier, they concluded that permeability to indicator dye is not necessarily associated with permeability to edema fluid or white blood cells.

Clark and Clark (1935) set up morphological criteria for analyzing white cell sticking *in vivo*, noting six changes of consistency in endothelial change from the normal state to necrosis, the first three associated with white cell sticking, the fourth with emigration (see Fig. 2). They described changes in permeability in some inflammatory reactions in ear chambers, but associated these changes only with phases 3 and 4 (prolonged sticking and emigration).

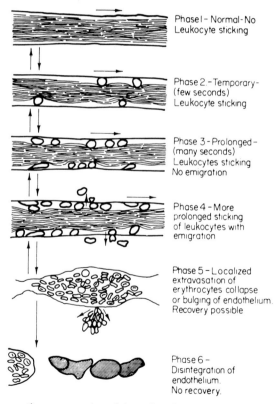

Fig. 2. Diagrammatic representation of the series of changes in consistency which vascular endothelium may undergo in response to external or internal stimuli of varying intensity. Pairs of arrows indicate reversibility of endothelial change in phases 2–5. (From Clark and Clark, 1935.)

The point was left on a doubtful note, however, for they stated that no "appreciable" accumulation of extravascular fluid was observed in cases in which only slight stickiness of the endothelium occurred (phase 2). Clark *et al.* (1934) described a situation where, after an intravenous injection of methylene blue, vessels of the ear chamber became distended and fluid appeared extravascularly, a condition which persisted for several days with loss of tonicity of the vessels and some hemorrhage, but presumably neither stasis nor interruption of flow. During this period there was "practically" no sticking of leukocytes or emigration of white cells from the vessels. They interpreted this to mean that, although marked changes in endothelial consistency (to phases 3 and 4) are accompanied by an increased passage of fluid through the wall, increased permeability may also occur in the absence of some of these endothelial changes. No speculations were offered relating the lack of sticking to possible hydrostatic pressure changes intravascularly, but it should be noted again that both Zweifach (1954) and Allison *et al.* (1955) reported white cell emigration in vessels in which blood flow apparently had stopped altogether.

Humphrey (1955a) studied the reversed passive Arthus reaction in rabbits and related edema formation with polymorphonuclear emigration, but not with mononuclear emigration. In a similar study in guinea pigs, Humphrey (1955b) reported that an early increase in vascular permeability was uninfluenced by polymorphonuclear leukocyte depletion. Miles (1961) reported, however, that in the guinea pig, at least, neither whole granulocytes nor material liberated by freeze-thaw or sonic disruption have any permeability effect. If anything, they are antagonistic to permeability effects, partly neutralizing the action of histamine and histamine liberators and inhibiting the glass activation of globulin factors in plasma. (It is of interest that several investigators have attributed antihistaminic functions to eosinophils; see discussion in Volume I, Chapter 7 by Hirsch and Chapter 8 by Wilhelm.) This issue has been reopened on two fronts—by Janoff and Zweifach (1964) and by Thomas (1964a). Janoff and Zweifach report that a cationic protein fraction isolated from the granules of rabbit polymorphonuclear leukocytes does, in fact, cause white cell sticking and emigration in rat and rabbit mesenteries in concentrations and under circumstances where the postgranule supernatant of lysed leukocytes (cell sap fraction) elicits no such response. A fraction containing lysozyme and ribonuclease, which are also cationic proteins, failed to cause the sticking reaction. The fraction that causes sticking is free from the acid hydrolases, such as cathepsin, acid phosphatase, and β-glucuronidase, which have been implicated in lysosomal studies in other ways. Two other groups have worked with similar materials: Frimmer and Hegner (1963) extracted nuclear histones from the thymus to achieve similar reactions in the mesentery, and Golub and Spitznagel (1964) recorded inflammatory reactions in skin with cationic proteins. Thomas (1964a) found that the granules of polymorphonuclear leukocytes of rabbits augmented the lesion when injected intradermally at the site of reversed passive Arthus reactions and under circumstances where a local Shwartzman reaction is evoked. In the experiments involving the Arthus phenomenon, however, it was possible to elicit the reaction in leukopenic animals, an unexpected finding and one open to a number of interpretations, including the possibility that the granules of polymorphonuclear leukocytes injure endothelium directly, leading, where white cells are absent from the blood, to hemorrhage. Halpern (1963) extended this point, reproducing Thomas' experiments with granules and then blocking the reaction with a protease inhibitor isolated from beef parotid gland, a polypeptide of 11,500 molecular weight which inhibits several proteolytic enzymes including trypsin, chymotrypsin, and plasmin. The data were interpreted to support the view that the release of cathepsins may be the basis for the observed tissue damage. Thus the lysosome, or, in the case of the preparation used by Janoff and Zweifach (1964a), a protein fraction of the white cell, have become the latest candidates for the role of inflammatory agents, a hypothesis growing out of the observations of de Duve (1959, 1964) that the acid hydrolytic enzymes contained a subcellular organelles may be of importance in the production of damage to cells and tissues if released into the cell sap or extracellular space. Cohn and Hirsch (1960) showed that the granules of leukocytes possess the properties and enzymic composition of lysosomes (for a fuller discussion of these points, see Volume I, Chapters by Hirschhorn, Steinman and Cohn, and Hirsch). How direct the link is to the inflammatory process remains an open question, but lysosomes join a long and celebrated list of agents that have been alleged to influence inflammatory reactions in one way or another. These range from such improbable experimental candidates as spirits of wine (Thomson, 1913) to leukotaxine (Menkin, 1950) and including peptides with an average chain length of 8–14 amino acid residues (Spector, 1951), uterine extracts (Spector and Storey, 1958), polysaccharide or lipopolysaccharide components of microorganisms (Meier and Schar, 1957), and the products of lipoprotein dissociation (Buckley, 1963b), as well as histamine (Wolf, 1923), a point denied by Bloom (1922), Grant and Wood (1928), and Morgan (1934), and qualified by Hurley (1963), bradykinin (Lewis, 1961) and, for that matter, normal saline, that paragon of innocuous agents (Bloom, 1922; Harris, 1960; Hurley and Spector, 1961b; McGovern and Bloomfield, 1963). [Harris' review (1954) covers some of these points and many others relating to alleged chemotactic properties of a variety of substances; see also the review by Spector and Willoughby (1963).]

Hurley (Hurley and Spector, 1961a,b; Hurley, 1963) summarized his evidence in a communication to the New York Academy of Sciences (1964). Using intradermal injections into rats of various substances as a test system and with careful attention to the time course of the reactions, he demonstrated two distinct types of leukocyte emigration, dissociating them from permeability effects. The first type involved a relatively nonspecific escape of white cells, the majority of them being polymorphonuclear leukocytes, occurring several hours after the injection of a variety of solutions, notable among them being histamine, physiological saline, and homologous serum (Fig. 3). The second type yielded an emigration starting immediately after injection and reaching massive proportions in 30–40 minutes; these injected agents included (1) extracts of burned skin, (2) saline extracts of polymorphonuclear leukocytes, and (3) serum after incubation *in vitro* with certain tissues, including liver and spleen. It is suggested that all three sources in the early reaction represent a specific endogenous system for inducing leukocyte emigration after injury. In the first instance, where the nonspecific (late) reaction occurred, the reaction was unrelated in extent and time to any increase in vascular permeability caused by the material injected. This was also true in the second instance where no correlation existed between the presence of edema in the burned area of skin and the ability of extracts from such an area to induce leukocyte emigration. Logan

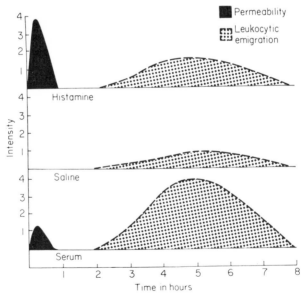

Fig. 3. Diagrammatic representation of time course and degree of leukocytic emigration and of increased vascular permeability following a single intradermal injection of normal saline, histamine, and serum, respectively. (From Hurley, 1963.)

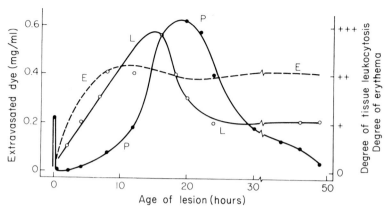

Fig. 4. Maturation of erythema (E), the diphasic increase of vascular permeability (P), and tissue leukocytosis (L) in the inflammatory reaction evoked by ultraviolet injury in guinea pig skin. (From Logan and Wilhelm, 1963.)

and Wilhelm (1963; see also Chapter 8 by Wilhelm), in a study of ultraviolet injury of guinea pig skin, demonstrated early and late permeability increases and showed a parallelism between the late phase of permeability increase and tissue leukocytosis. This led them to wonder if the emigration of white cells was relevant to late permeability events. They induced neutropenia with nitrogen mustard and found that both early and late permeability changes were unaltered. Thus, in bacterial infection, tissue leukocytosis follows the second phase of increased permeability, but in ultraviolet injury, it precedes it (Fig. 4).

The generalization that seems to come from all this is that it is possible to show that increased vascular permeability and white cell sticking and emigration are (a) related temporally and (b) not related temporally, depending on the particular experimental method and conditions. Even conceding that they may be related temporally, there is no evidence that the mechanism of each is the same; in other words, substances that are said to elicit white cell sticking and emigration, whatever this mechanism is, do not seem to betray a consistent relationship to small vascular permeability to noncellular materials, whatever this mechanism is.

VI. Chemotaxis

Chemotaxis is discussed in some detail in Volume I, Chapter 5 and will not be reviewed here in depth. Although chemotaxis is an extremely difficult phenomenon to prove under direct observation *in vivo*, the circumstantial evidence for it is overwhelming. In one way or another, but in all cases through the use of transparent connective tissue preparations, the Clarks (Clark and Clark, 1920, 1922), Allison (Allison *et al.*, 1955), Buckley (1963a), and Grant (1973) have demonstrated chemotaxis *in vivo*, but not with total, rigorous, unquestionable scientific certitude. If one imagines an inflammatory continuum, starting with the adherence of the white blood cell to the vessel wall and ending with the engulfment by the white cell of some noxious material far from the site where the cell emigrated from the vessel, then it is easy to imagine that an intermediate link between the two events is represented by the phenomenon of chemotaxis. And, in fact, one can demonstrate, with some precision, both ends of the reaction. Minimal stimuli cause white blood cells to stick; they do not emigrate. Severe extravascular reactions, such as Arthus reactions incited outside of the blood vessels (Grant *et al.*, 1967), cause white blood cells to stick, emigrate, and phagocytize immune complexes. To explain such remarkable events by any postulate other than a chemically directed chemotactic gradient is virtually to defy common sense, almost to suggest that the white blood cell either has a central nervous system or psychic endowment. Having settled for this explanation, as virtually all biologists have, the question arises as to what chemical signal is necessary to induce a white blood cell to move from one site to another. It has been accepted for years that bacteria and starch granules have chemotactic character, and in recent years immune complexes and other agents, including complement, have been added to a growing list. But chemotaxis can also proceed in the absence of such factors as complement. One can question how complement can be involved in extravascular events, but Alper and Rosen (1967) suggest that there is an extravascular complement pool, approximately 30% of the total vascular pool, lending plausibility to complement mediation inside or outside of blood vessels. With the present state of knowledge, it is not possible to pinpoint a single chemotactic factor. The chances are that in the next decade, however, investigators will follow the leads provided by the microbiologists who have accumulated some evidence for receptor systems in microbes. It is not difficult to imagine that the white cell, too, has a receptor system delicately balanced to pick up chemical chemotactic signals.

VII. Electrochemical Factors

The hypothesis that a changing electrical potential could account for white cell sticking and emigration stimulated McGovern (1957) to postulate that the natural defense against sticking might be found in the tissue stores of heparin and, conversely, heparin itself could have anti-white cell sticking properties. His reasoning was that heparin, a negatively charged molecule, maintained tissue negatively under physiological conditions, thereby providing an electrostatic barrier between the tissues and the negatively charged white cells in the blood stream. With injury, the depletion of heparin caused white cells to be attracted to relatively positively charged tissue. McGovern then subjected rats to chemical injury (ethanolamine) and cold, demonstrating a typical inflammatory reaction by histological tissue section. Under the protection of heparin, there was reduced tissue leukocytosis. In a subsequent communication, McGovern and Bloomfield (1963) were unable to alter traumatically induced white cell sticking with heparin and, indeed, found that heparin could initiate the events leading to leukocyte emigration, a fact noted by other investigators, many of them working with hamster cheek pouches (Copley, 1948; Fleck, 1949; Lutz *et al.*, 1951; Fulton *et al.*, 1953; Sullivan and Masterson, 1953; Berman *et al.*, 1955). Allison *et al.* (1955), however, found that heparin interfered with white cell sticking, but in subsequent communications took the position that this was not the case (Allison and Lancaster, 1960, 1961). Zweifach (1954) also found that heparin modified white cell sticking caused by direct trauma to the endothelial cell in the rat mesentery, but Grant *et al.* (1962) found no effect of heparin in modifying white cell sticking in rabbit ear chambers subjected to mild ultraviolet burning. Miller and Page (1963) found that heparin and a variety of other sulfated mucopolysaccharides inhibited the lymphocyte response to inflammation without inhibiting neutrophil exudation. They speculated that the effect may be due to the binding and inactivation of positively charged substances that are responsible for inducing lymphocyte emigration. Wood and his colleagues (1956, 1957) presented evidence that heparin treatment of mice with subcutaneous tumor implants retarded the tumor growth rate and reduced the number of metastases. Wood noted, however, that the endothelial adherence by tumor cells appeared to be independent of white cell sticking, vasomotor activity, or capillary flow rate, on the basis of ear chamber studies. Von Jancsó (1961) found that heparin did not interfere with "angiotaxis," or what he preferred to consider endothelial phagocytosis, but that other anticoagulants did, notably those compounds containing rare earth metals; they also inhibited vascular permeability. Whatever merit there may be to the concept that alterations in an electrostatic barrier may account for white cell sticking and emigration, an experimental extension of this view to the use of heparin, a negatively charged molecule, as an anti-inflammatory agent has produced results at wide variance with each other.

On the other hand, the possible relationship between a current of injury and white blood cell sticking has been a repeating theme in literature since Abrahamson's studies of 50 years ago (Abrahamson, 1924) and has found expression in many experiments by Sawyer, Pate, and their colleagues in the intervening period (Sawyer and Pate, 1953a,b; Sawyer *et al.*, 1953, 1965; Ogoniak and Sawyer, 1965). As Spector and Willoughby (1963) pointed out, it does not seem unreasonable that the phenomenon of leukocyte adhesion is explicable in terms of electrochemical forces opeative at cell surfaces. Evidence along these lines has come from some quite stimulating work by Bangham and his colleagues (summarized by Bangham, 1964). These investigators have demonstrated that, whereas the adhesive properties of leukocytes cannot be ascribed to surface-carrying charge of opposite sign, the adherence of white cells to other surfaces possibly can be explained on the basis of calcium bridging between cells, this property being based on the anionic species present on the white cell. The data, derived from micro-electrophoresis studies, show that both erythrocytes and leukocytes have only anions on their surfaces and that the surface charge density of the two types of cells is very similar at physiological pH. As Bangham noted, this evidence epitomizes the physical paradox of these two types of quite different cells, both presumably composed of similar chemical compounds and therefore subject to similar van der Waals constants, and both having similar forces of repulsion. In biological systems, however, where both cells are suspended in a common protein pool, at a common bulk pH, and in the presence of a common concentration of uni- and divalent cations, the behavior of these cells is quite different. White cells are phagocytic and adhesive, whereas red cells remain dispersed under circumstances where white cells become sticky, and do not normally adhere to glass. Bangham *et al.* (1958) opened an experimental approach to this problem with the suggestion that the differential adhesive properties of blood cells might be attributed to the presence on their surfaces of different ionic species. Thus, although two types of cell might have the same charge density, e.g., erythrocytes and leukocytes at pH 7.2, the anions contributing to the charge might be different and therefore form different solubility products with a common divalent cation, e.g., calcium. Evidence showed that the anions on the erythrocyte and leukocyte do have different pK' values. Then Seaman and Heard (1960) showed that the acid groups of human erythrocytes are derived from sialic acid, and Wilkins *et al.* (1962a,b) suggested that the anions on sheep leukocytes may be those of a typical carboxyl. Bangham *et al.* (1958) had suggested that if two leukocytes could be brought within a calcium ion radius of each other, bridging between the calcium and the carboxyl groups might occur and binding ensue. Even if this were so, however, a problem would arise in overcoming an energy barrier to enable the two charged surfaces to approach within a necessary postulated 5-Å barrier of each other. Bangham and Pethica (1960) suggested, therefore, that if local areas of a cell were to form villi or small pseudopodia the local charge density in the vicinity of the tip might be proportionately reduced. The process might be likened to the flexing of a brush to which bristles are uniformly attached. A calculation confirmed that if a microvillus had a radius of curvature of about 0.1 μm, two such tips could approach to within the necessary distance with the necessary interaction energy. Lesseps (1963) found structures that fit these calculations in aggregating embryonal tissue cells and suggested that this may be a fundamental mechanism for initial contact.

Bangham summarizes his hypothesis as follows: the differential adhesive properties between cells having the same overall energies of both attraction and repulsion may be refined down to a mechanism whereby local protuberances, having a small radius of curvature, enable close approach at ordinary thermal energies. Such a close approach might then result in successful bonding by calcium bridging, provided that the anion sites of the two cells were of the right type, e.g., carboxyl. The point of contact would then spread to other areas of the cell surface.

As noted by Spector and Willoughby (1963), it is possible that injury leads to a great increase in the number of reaction groups at the endothelial cell surface, perhaps owing to a reorientation with the molecules composing the membrane. It is of interest that Garvin (1961) reported that the adhesion of polymorphonuclear leukocytes (but not lymphocytes) to glass columns is dependent upon the presence of divalent cations, magnesium being at least as important as calcium.

VIII. Summary

In reviewing the problem of white cell sticking and emigration, two prominent hallmarks of inflammation, it becomes clear that, whereas there is agreement on a few basic facts, there is disagreement on most of the critical issues.

Perhaps the most important single fact about white cell sticking is the unassailable one that when blood vascular endothelium is injured, it becomes "sticky." In the wake of this event, formed elements of the blood adhere to the endothelial wall. Other materials, less obvious to the morphological eye, also may adhere, but whether they do or not, some alteration takes place in injured endothelium that causes it to lose its "nonwettable" character for white cells, platelets, and red cells. Since "sticky" and "nonwettable" are literary, not scientific, terms, they provide no insight into the mechanism of the phenomenon.

Scores of agents, some physiological, some not, have been implicated as accomplices in eliciting white cell sticking, and these include normal saline.

Probably sterile needles should be added to the list, and the combination of needle and the injection of fluids under high pressure to rip apart tissue interfaces may be responsible for the initiation of many of the reactions. All noxious stimuli, including heat, direct trauma, and infection, cause sticking, and this adherence appears to be nonspecific, the intensity varying only with intensity of stimulus and the breadth and depth of the injury. It seems reasonable, if not compelling, to assume, therefore, that a significant denominator, if not the common denominator, of the reaction is the alteration in the character of the endothelial wall. This does not minimize the importance of the pneumococcus in causing pneumonia, or a hot stove in causing a burn, or a fall down a stairway in causing a bruise. But at the capillary level it suggests that the altered state of endothelium is a critical event on the final common pathway of the inflammatory process. If the problem is formulated in this light, it seems not irrational to recognize that in many cases, if not in all cases, white cell sticking to blood vascular endothelium is secondary to endothelial damage. One problem for the investigator, then, is to determine what factors are involved in alterations in the character of the endothelial cell. This is a rather difficult point to pin down, and the precise entry into this problem, at this time, is not obvious.

Acknowledgments

This work was supported in part by Public Health Research grant AM 07501-09.

References

Abrahamson, H. A. (1924). *Amer. J. Med. Sci.* **167**, 702.
Adami, J. G. (1909). "Inflammation, An Introduction to the Study of Pathology." Macmillan, New York.
Addison, W. (1843). *Trans. Prov. Med. Surg. Assoc.* **11**, 233.
Alksne, J. F. (1959). *Quart. J. Exp. Physiol. Cog. Med. Sci.* **44**, 51.
Allison, F., Jr., and Lancaster, M. G. (1959). *Brit. J. Exp. Pathol.* **40**, 324.
Allison, F., Jr., and Lancaster, M. G. (1960). *J. Exp. Med.* **111**, 45.
Allison, F., Jr., and Lancaster, M. G. (1961). *J. Exp. Med.* **114**, 535.
Allison, F., Jr., Smith, M. R., and Wood, W. B., Jr. (1955). *J. Exp. Med.* **102**, 655.
Alper, C. A., and Rosen, F. S. (1967). *J. Clin. Invest.* **46**, 20201.
Altschul, R. (1954). "Endothelium: Its Development, Morphology, Function, and Pathology." Macmillan, New York.
Arendt, K. A., Shulman, M. H., Fulton, G. P., and Lutz, B. R. (1953). *Anat. Rec.* **117**, 595.
Arnold, J. (1875). *Arch. Pathol. Anat. Physiol. Klin. Med.* **62**, 87.
Ashford, T. P., and Freiman, D. G. (1968). *Amer. J. Pathol.* **53**, 599.
Baer, R. L. (1964). Presidential Address before Society for Investigative Dermatology, San Francisco, California, June, 1964.

Baer, R. L., Rosenthal, S. A., and Sims, C. F. (1957). *AMA Arch. Dermatol.* **76**, 549.

Baez, S., and Kochen, J. (1964). *Fed. Proc. Fed. Amer. Soc. Exp. Biol.* **23**, 22.

Baez, S., and Kochen, J. (1965). *Ann. N.Y. Acad. Sci.* **122**, 738.

Bangham, A. D. (1964). *Ann. N.Y. Acad. Sci.* **116**, Art. 3, 945.

Bangham, A. D., and Pethica, B. A. (1960). *Proc. Roy. Phys. Soc. Edinburgh* **28**, 73.

Bangham, A. D., Pethica, B. A., and Seaman, G. V. F. (1958). *Biochem. J.* **201**, 12.

Barnhart, M. I., Walsh, R. T., and Robinson, J. A. (1972). *In* "Platelets and their Role in Hemostasis." N.Y. Acad. Sci., New York in press.

Barnhart, M. I., and Riddle, J. M. (1967). *In* "Platelets: Their Role in Hemostasis and Thrombosis," p. 87. Schattauer, Stuttgart.

Barnhart, M. I., Cress, D. C., Henry, R. L., and Riddle, J. M. (1967). *Thromb. Diath. Haemorrh.* **17**, 78.

Barron, E. S. G., and Harrop, G. A., Jr. (1929). *J. Biol. Chem.* **84**, 89.

Bauer, J. A. (1958). *Ann. N.Y. Acad. Sci.* **73**, Art. 3, 663.

Benacerraf, B., McCluskey, R. T., and Patras, D. (1959). *Amer. J. Pathol.* **35**, 75.

Berman, H. J., Fulton, G. P., Lutz, B. R., and Pierce, D. L. (1955). *Blood* **10**, 831.

Biozzi, G., Mene, G., and Ovary, Z. (1948). *Rev. Immunol.* **12**, 320.

Bloom, W. (1922). *Bull. Johns Hopkins Hosp.* **33**, 185.

Born, G. V. R., and Cross, M. J. (1963). *J. Physiol. (London)* **168**, 178.

Bounameaux, Y. (1959). *C. R. Soc. Biol.* **153**, 685.

Braude, A. I. (1951). *J. Infect. Dis.* **89**, 87.

Buckley, I. K. (1963a). *Exp. Mol. Pathol.* **2**, 402.

Buckley, I. K. (1963b). *Int. Rev. Exp. Pathol.* **2**, 241.

Burke, J. F., and Miles, A. A. (1958). *J. Pathol. Bacteriol.* **76**, 1.

Caen, J., Cousin, C., Vainer, H., Gautier, A., and Michel, H. (1967). *In* "Biochemistry of Blood Platelets" (F. Kowalski and S. Niewiarowski, eds.), p. 117. Academic Press, New York.

Cameron, G. R. (1952). "Pathology of the Cell." Oliver & Boyd, Edinburgh and London.

Carscadden, W. G. (1927). *Arch. Pathol.* **4**, 329.

Chambers, R., and Zweifach, B. W. (1940). *J. Cell. Comp. Physiol.* **15**, 255.

Chambers, R., and Zweifach, B. W. (1947). *Physiol. Rev.* **27**, 436.

Chandler, A. B. (1969). *In* "Thrombosis," p. 279. Nat. Acad. Sci., Washington, D.C.

Clark, E. R., and Clark, E. L. (1920). *Amer. J. Anat.* **27**, 221.

Clark, E. R., and Clark, E. L. (1922). *Anat. Rec.* **24**, 137.

Clark, E. R., and Clark, E. L. (1930a). *Amer. J. Anat.* **46**, 91.

Clark, E. R., and Clark, E. L. (1930b). *Amer. J. Anat.* **46**, 149.

Clark, E. R., and Clark, E. L. (1935). *Amer. J. Anat.* **57**, 385.

Clark, E. R., Clark, E. L., and Williams, R. G. (1934). *Amer. J. Anat.* **55**, 47.

Clark, E. R., Clark, E. L., and Rex, R. D. (1936). *Amer. J. Anat.* **59**, 123.

Clayton, S., Born, G. V. R., and Cross, M. J. (1963). *Nature (London)* **200**, 138.

Cohn, Z. A., and Hirsch, J. G. (1960). *J. Exp. Med.* **112**, 983.

Cohnheim, J. (1882). "Lectures on General Pathology," Vol. 1. New Sydenham Soc., London (translated into English, 1889.)

Copley, A. L. (1948). *Fed. Proc. Fed. Amer. Soc. Exp. Biol.* **7**, 22.

Cotran, R. S. (1965). *Exp. Mol. Pathol.* **4**, 1217.

Crabtree, H. G. (1928). *Biochem. J.* **22**, 1289.

de Duve, C. (1959). *In* "Subcellular Particles" (T. Hayashi, ed.), p. 128, Ronald Press, New York.

de Duve, C. (1964). *In* "Injury, Inflammation and Immunity" (L. Thomas, J. W. Uhr, and L. Grant, eds.), p. 283. Williams & Wilkins, Baltimore, Maryland.

Delaunay, A., Lebrun, J., and Cotereau, H. (1947). *Ann. Inst. Pasteur*, **73**, 565.

Dienes, L., and Mallory, T. B. (1932). *Amer. J. Pathol.* **8**, 689.

Dietrich, A., and Nordmann, M. (1930). *Verh. Deut Pathol. Ges.* **25**, 46 (cited by Illig, 1961.)

Dische, Z. (1964). *In* "Small Blood Vessel Involvement in Diabetes Mellitus" (M. D. Siperstein, A. R. Colwell, Sr., and K. Meyer, eds.), p. 201. Amer. Inst. Biol. Sci., Washington, D.C.

Dutrochet, M. H. (1824). "Recherches, anatomiques et Physiologiques sur la structure intime des animaux et des végétaux, et sur Leur Motilité." Baillière et Fils, Paris.

Ebert, R. H., and Florey, H. W. (1939). *Brit. J. Exp. Pathol.* **20**, 342.

Ebert, R. H., and Wissler, R. W. (1951). *J. Lab. Clin. Med.* **38**, 511.

Ernst. T. (1926). *Beitr. Pathol. Anat. Allg. Pathol.* **75**, 229.

Evans, D. G., Miles, A. A., and Niven, J. S. F. (1948). *Brit. J. Exp. Pathol.* **29**, 20.

Fleck, L. (1949). *J. Amer. Med. Assoc.* **139**, 542.

Florey, H. W. (1962). "General Pathology," 3rd ed., Chapters 2 and 3. Saunders, Philadelphia, Pennsylvania.

Florey, H. W., and Grant, L. H. (1961). *J. Pathol. Bacteriol.* **82**, 13.

Florey, H. W., Poole, J. C. F., and Meek, G. A. (1959). *J. Pathol. Bacteriol.* **77**, 625.

French, J. E. (1969). *In* "Thrombosis," p. 300. Nat. Acad. Sci., Washington, D. C.

French, J. E., and Macfarlane, R. G. (1970). *In* "General Pathology" (H. W. Florey, ed.), 4th ed., p. 244. Saunders, Philadelphia, Pennsylvania.

Frimmer, M., and Hegner, D. (1963). *Naunyn-Sckmiedebergs Arch. Exp. Pathol. Pharmakol.* **245**, 355.

Follis, R. H., Jr. (1940). *Bull. Johns Hopkins Hosp.* **66**, 245.

Fulton, G. P., Akers, R. P., and Lutz, B. R. (1953). *Blood* **8**, 140.

Gaarder, A., Jonsen, J., Laland, S., Hellem, A., and Owren, P. A. (1961). *Nature (London)* **192**, 531.

Garvin, J. E. (1961). *J. Exp. Med.* **114**, 51.

Gatspar, H. (1970). *In* "Platelet Adhesion and Aggregation in Thrombosis: Countermeasures" (E. M. Mammen, G. F. Anderson, and M. I. Barnhart, eds.), p. 291. Schattauer, Stuttgart.

Golub, E. S., and Spitznagel, J. K. (1964). *Fed. Proc. Fed. Amer Soc. Exp. Biol.* **23**, (Part I), 509.

Grant, L. H. (1960). D.Phil. Thesis, Lincoln College, Oxford.

Grant, L. (1965). *In* "The Inflammatory Process" (B. W. Zweifach, C. Grant, and R. T. McCluskey, eds.), 1st ed., p. 197. Academic Press, New York.

Grant, L. (1973). *Microvasc. Res.* (in press).

Grant, L., and Becker, F. F. (1965). *Proc. Soc. Exp. Biol. Med.* **119**, 1123.

Grant, L., and Becker, F. R. (1966). *Arch. Pathol.* **81**, 36.

Grant, L., and Epstein, F. (1973). *Microvasc. Res.* (in press).

Grant, L., Palmer, P., and Sanders, A. G. (1962). *J. Pathol. Bacteriol.* **83**, 127.

Grant, L., Ross, M. H., Moses, J., Prose, P., Zweifach, B. W., and Ebert, R. H. (1967). *Z. Zellforsch. Mikvosk. Anal:* **77**, 554.

Grant, L., Martelli, A., and Dumont, A. (1973). *Microvasc. Res.* (in press).

Grant, R. T., and Wood, J. E. (1928). *J. Pathol. Bacteriol.* **31**, 1.

Halpern, B. N. (1963). *Proc. Soc. Exp. Biol. Med.* **115**, 273.

Harris, H. (1954). *Physiol. Rev.* **34**, 529.

Harris, H. (1960). *Bacteriol. Rev.* **24**, 3.

Haslam, R. J. (1964). *Nature (London)* **202**, 765.

Hellem, A. J. (1960). *Scand. J. Clin, Lab. Invest.* **12**, Suppl., 1.

Henry, L., Marshall, D. C., Friedman, E. A., Dammin, G. J., and Merril, J. P. (1962). *J. Clin. Invest.* **41**, 420.

Hovig, T. (1963). *Thromb. Diath. Haemorrh.* **9**, 264.

Hovig, T. (1969). *In* "Thrombosis," p. 374. Nat. Acad. Sci., Washington, D. C.

Hugues, J. (1962). *Thromb. Diath. Haemorrh.* **8**, 241.

Humble, J. G. (1949). *Blood* **4**, 69.

Humphrey, J. H. (1955a). *Brit. J. Exp. Pathol.* **36**, 268.

Humphrey, J. H. (1955b). *Brit. J. Exp. Pathol.* **36**, 283.

Hurley, J. V. (1963). *Aust. J. Exp. Biol. Med. Sci.* **41**, 171.

Hurley, J. V., and Spector, W. G. (1961a). *J. Pathol. Bacteriol.* **82**, 403.

Hurley, J. V., and Spector, W. G. (1961b). *J. Pathol. Bacteriol.* **82**, 421.

Illig, L. (1961). "Die terminale Strombahn." Springer-Verlag, Berlin and New York.

Janoff, A., and Zweifach, B. W. (1964a). *Science* **144**, 1456.

Janoff, A., and Zweifach, B. W. (1964b). *J. Exp. Med.* **120**, 747.

Johnson, S. A., Wojcik, J. D., Webber, A. J., and Yun, J. (1969). *In* "Dynamics of Thrombus Formation and Dissolution" (S. A. Johnson and M. M. Guest, eds.), p. 172. Lippincott, Philadelphia, Pennsylvania.

Karrer, H. E. (1960). *J. Biophys. Biochem. Cytol.* **7**, 357.

Kefalides, M. A. (1966). *Biochem. Biophys. Res. Commun.* **22**, 26,

Kefalides, M. A. (1967). *Fed. Proc., Fed. Amer. Soc. Exp. Biol.* **26**, 822.

Kjaerheim, A., and Hovig, T. (1962). *Thromb. Diath. Haemorrh.* **7**, 1.

Kolouch, F., Jr. (1939). *Amer. J. Pathol.* **15**, 413.

Landis, E. M. (1934). *Physiol. Rev.* **14**, 404.

Landis, E. M. (1946). *Ann. N.Y. Acad. Sci.* **46**, Art. 8, 713.

Lavdowsky, M. (1884). *Arch. Pathol. Anat. Physiol. Klin. Med.* **97**, 177.

Lawrence, H. S. (1956). *Amer. J. Med.* **20**, 428.

Lawrence, H. S. (1957). *Ann. N. Y. Acad. Sci.* **64**, 826.

Lazarow, A., and Speidel, E. (1964). *In* "Small Blood Vessel Involvement in Diabetes Mellitus" (M. D. Siperstein, A. R. Colwell, Sr., and K. Meyer, eds.), p. 127. Amer. Inst. Biol. Sci. Washington, D.C.

Leber, T. (1888). *Fortschr. Med.* **6**, 460.

Lee, R. E., and Lee, N. Z. (1947). *J. Physiol. (London)* **149**, 465.

Lesseps, R. J. (1963). *J. Exp. Zool.* **153**, 171.

Lewis, G. P. (1961). *Nature (London)* **192**, 596.

Lister, J. (1858). *Phil. Trans. Roy. Soc. London* **148**, 645.

Logan, G., and Wilhelm, D. L. (1963). *Nature (London)* **198**, 968.

Lurie, M. B. (1939). *J. Exp. Med.* **69**, 579.

Lutz, B. R., Fulton, G. P., and Akers, R. P. (1951). *Circulation* **3**, 339.

McCallum, W. G. (1916). *In* "A Text-Book of Pathology," p. 7. Saunders, Philadelphia, Pennsylvania.

McCluskey, R. T., Benacerraf, B., and McCluskey, J. W. (1963). *J. Immunol.* **90**, 466.

Macfarlane, R. G. (1965). *In* "The Inflammatory Process" (B. W. Zweifach, L. Grant, and R. T. McCluskey, eds.), 1st ed., p. 465. Academic Press, New York.

McGovern, V. J. (1957). *J. Pathol. Bacteriol.* **73**, 99.

McGovern, V. J., and Bloomfield, D. (1963). *Aust. J. Exp. Biol. Med. Sci.* **41**, 141.

Majno, G. (1964). *In* "Injury, Inflammation and Immunity" (L. Thomas, J. W. Uhr, and L. Grant, eds.), p. 58. Williams & Wilkins, Baltimore, Maryland.

Majno, G. (1965). *In* "Handbook of Physiology," (Amer. Physiol. Soc., J. Field, ed.), Sect. 3. Vol. II, p. 000. Williams & Wilkins, Baltimore, Maryland.

Majno, G., and Palade, G. E. (1961). *J. Biophys. Biochem. Cytol.* **11**, 571.

Majno, G., Shea, S. M., and Leventhal, M. (1969). *J. Cell Biol.* **42**, 647.

Marchesi, V. T. (1961). *Quart. J. Exp. Physiol Cog. Med. Sci.* **46**, 115.

Marchesi, V. T. (1962). *Proc. Roy. Soc. Ser. B* **156**, 550.

Marchesi, V. T. (1964). *Ann. N.Y. Acad. Sci.* **116**, 774.

Marchesi, V. T., and Florey, H. W. (1960). *Quart. J. Exp. Physiol. Cog. Med. Sci.* **45**, 343.

Marchesi, V. T., and Gowans, J. L. (1964). *Proc. Roy. Soc. Ser. B* **159**, 283.

Meier, R., and Schar, B. (1957). *Hoppe-Seyler's Z. Physiol. Chem.* **307**, 103.

Menkin, V. (1934). *Amer. J. Pathol.* **10**, 193.

Menkin, V. (1950), "Newer Concepts of Inflammation." Thomas, Springfield, Illinois.

Metchnikoff, E. (1893). "Lectures on the Comparative Pathology of Inflammation." Kegan Paul, Trench, Trubner, London.

Miles, A. A. (1958–1959). "Lectures on the Scientific Basis of Medicine," Vol. VIII. Oxford Univ. Press (Athlone), London and New York.

Miles, A. A. (1961). *Fed. Proc. Fed. Amer. Soc. Exp. Biol.* **20**, Part II, Suppl. 9, 141.

Miles, A. A., and Niven, J. S. F. (1950). *Brit. J. Exp. Pathol.* **31**, 73.

Miller, T. E., and Page, A. R. (1963). *Fed. Proc. Fed. Amer. Soc. Exp. Biol.* **22**, 255.

Misra, R. P., and Berman, L. B. (1966). *Proc. Soc. Exp. Biol. Med.* **122**, 705.

Moe, N., and Jorgensen, L. (1967). *Acta Path. Microbiol. Scand., Suppl.* **187**, 70.

Moe, N., and Jorgensen, L. (1968). *Acta Pathol. Microbiol. Scand.* **72**, 519.

Morgan, J. R. E. (1934). *Arch. Pathol.* **18**, 516.

Mowbray, J. F. (1967). *Integration Intern. Med., Proc. Int. Congr., 9th, 1966.* Excerpta Med. Int. Congr. Ser. No. 137, p. 106.

Mustard, J. F. (1969). *In* "Thrombosis," p. 496. Nat. Acad. Sci., Washington, D.C.

Ogoniak, J. C., and Sawyer, P. N. (1965). *Proc. Nat. Acad. Sci. U.S.* **53**, 572.

Ollgaard, E. (1961). *Thromb. Diath. Haemorrh.* **6**, 86.

Page, A. R. (1964). *Ann. N. Y. Acad. Sci.* **116**, Art. 3, 950.

Page, A. R., and Good, R. A. (1958). *Amer. J. Pathol.* **34**, 645.

Page, A. R., Condie, R. M., and Good, R. A. (1962). *Amer. J. Pathol.* **40**, 519.

Palade, G. E. (1959). Blood Capillaries. Structure and Function. A lecture delivered at the University of Oxford.

Paz, R. A., and Spector, W. G. (1962). *J. Pathol. Bacteriol.* **84**, 85.

Peterson, R. D. A., and Good, R. A. (1962). *Lab. Invest.* **11**, 507.

Pfaff, W., and Herold, W. (1937). "Grundlagen einer neuen Therapieforschung der Tuberkulose." Thieme, Stuttgart.

Policard, A., Collet, A., and Pregermain, S. (1957). *Acta Anat.* **30**, 624.

Poole, J. C. F., and Florey, H. W. (1958). *J. Pathol. Bacteriol.* **75**, 245.

Purves, L. (1874). *Zentralbl. Med. Wiss.* **41** (as quoted by Arnold, 1875).

Rebuck, J. W., and Crowley, J. H. (1955). *Ann. N. Y. Acad. Sci.* **59**, 757.

Ricker, G., and Regendanz, P. (1921). *Virchows Arch. Pathol. Anat. Physiol.* **231**, 1.

Roskam, J. (1964). *Thromb. Diath. Haemorrh.* **12**, 338.

Ross, M. H., and Grant, L. (1968). *Exp. Cell Res.* **50**, 277.

Ross, R., and Bornstein, P. (1969). *J. Cell Biol.* **40**, 366.

Sandison, J. C. (1924). *Anat. Rec.* **28**, 281.

Sandison, J. C. (1931). *Anat. Rec.* **50**, 355.

Sawyer, P. N., and Pate, J. W. (1953a). *Amer. J. Physiol.* **175**, 103.

Sawyer, P. N., and Pate, J. W. (1953b). *Amer. J. Physiol.* **175**, 113.

Sawyer, P. N., Pate, J. W., and Weldon, C. S. (1953). *Amer. J. Physiol.* **175**, 108.

Sawyer, P. N., Reardon, J. H., and Ogoniak, J. C. (1965). *Proc. Nat. Acad. Sci. U.S.* **53**, 200.

Schoefl, G. I. (1970). "Société française de Micro. Electron.," Vol. 3, p. 589. Paris.

Schoefl, G. I. (1972). *J. Exp. Med.* **136**, 568.

Seaman, G. V. F., and Heard, D. H. (1960). *J. Gen. Physiol.* **44**, 251.

Shirasawa, K. (1966). *Acta Pathol. Jap.* **16**, 1.

Spaet, T. (1952a). *Amer. J. Physiol.* **170**, 333.

Spaet, T. (1952b). *Blood* **7**, 641.

Spaet, T., and Erichson, R. B. (1966). *Thromb. Diath. Haemorrh., Suppl.* **21**, 67.

Spaet, T., and Zucker, M. B. (1964). *Amer. J. Physiol.* **206**, 1267.

Spector, W. G. (1951). *J. Pathol. Bacteriol.* **63**, 93.

Spector, W. G., and Storey, E. (1958). *J. Pathol. Bacteriol.* **75**, 387.

Spector, W. G., and Willoughby, D. A. (1963). *Bacteriol. Rev.* **27**, 117.

Stehbens, W. E. (1965). *Lab. Invest.* **14**, 449.

Steinberg, B., and Dietz, A. (1938). *Arch. Pathol.* **25**, 777.

Stemerman, M. B., Baumgartner, H. R., and Spaet, T. H. (1971). *Lab. Invest.* **24**, 179.

Stetson, C. A. (1951). *J. Expt. Med.* **94**, 347.

Stetson, C. A. (1961). *Fed. Proc. Fed. Amer. Soc. Exp. Biol.* **20**, Part II, Suppl. 9, 150 (discussion of paper by Miles, 1900).

Stetson, C. A., and Good, R, A. (1951). *J. Exp. Med.* **93**, 49.

Sullivan, B. J., and Masterson, W. K. (1953). *Amer. J. Physiol.* **175**, 56.

Thoma, R. (1896). "Textbook of General Pathology, and Pathological Anatomy." Adam & Charles Black, London.

Thomas, L. (1964a). *Proc. Soc. Expt. Biol. Med.* **115**, 236.

Thomas, L. (1964b). *In* "Injury, Inflammation and Immunity" (L. Thomas, J. W. Uhr, and L. Grant, eds.), p. 312. Williams & Wilkins, Baltimore, Maryland.

Thomas, L., and Stetson, C. A. (1949). *J. Exp. Med.* **89**, 461.

Thomson, J. (1913). "Lectures on Inflammation." Edinburgh (as noted by Cameron, 1952).

Tranzer, J. P., and Baumgartner, H. R. (1967). *Nature (London)* **216**, 1126.

von Haller, A. (1757). "A Dissertation on the Motion of the Blood and on the Effects of Bleeding," Whiston & White, London.

von Jancsó, N. (1947). *Nature (London)* **160**, 227.

von Jancsó, N. (1955). "Speicherting; Stoffanreicherung im Retikuloendothel und in der Niere." Akadémai, Kiado, Budapest.

von Jancsó, N. (1961). *J. Pharm. Pharmacol.* **13**, 577.

Wagner, R. (1833). "Zur vergleichenden Physiologie des Blutes," Voss, Leipzig.

Wagner, R. (1839). "Erläuterungstafeln zur Physiologie und Entwicklungsgeschichte," Voss, Leipzig.

Waksman, B. H. (1960). *Cell. Aspects Immunity, Ciba Found. Symp., 1959* p. 280.

Waller, A. (1846). *Phil. Mag.* [3] **29**, 271.

Warren, B. A., and de Bono, A. H. B. (1970). *Brit. J. Exp. Pathol.* **51**, 415.

Wharton Jones, T. (1851). *Guy's Hosp. Rep.* **7**, 1.

Wiener, J., Spiro, D., and Russell, P. (1964). *Amer. J. Pathol.* **44**, 319.

Wilkins, D. J., Ottewill, R. H., and Bangham, A. D. (1962a). *J. Theor. Biol.* **2**, 165.

Wilkins, D. J., Ottewill, R. H., and Bangham, A. D. (1962b). *J. Theor. Biol.* **2**, 176.

Williamson, J. R., and Grisham, J. W. (1960). *Nature (London)* **188**, 1203.

Williamson, J. R., and Grisham, J. W. (1961). *Amer. J. Pathol.* **39**, 239.

Witte, S. (1958). *Thromb. Diath. Haemorrh.* **2**, 146, (cited by Illig, 1961).

Wolf, E. P. (1923). *J. Exp. Med.* **37**, 511.

Wood, J. S., Jr., Holyoke, E. D., and Hardley, J. H. (1956). *Proc. Amer. Ass. Cancer Res.* **2**, 157.

Wood, J. S., Jr., Hardley, J. H., and Holyoke, E. D. (1957). *Proc. Amer. Ass. Cancer Res.* **2**, 260.

Wood, W. B., Jr., Smith, M. R., Perry, W. D., and Berry, J. W. (1951). *J. Exp. Med.* **94**, 521.

Yamaguchi, H. (1964). *Keijo J. Med.* **13**, 46.

Zucker, M. B., and Borrelli, J. (1962). *Proc. Soc. Exp. Biol. Med.* **109**, 779.

Zweifach, B. W. (1940). *Anat. Rec.* **76**, 97.

Zweifach, B. W. (1953). *In* "The Mechanisms of Inflammation" (G. Jasmin and A. Robert, eds.), p. 77. Acta, Inc., Montreal.

Zweifach, B. W. (1954). *Trans. 5th Josiah Macy, Jr., Conf. Connect. Tissue* p. 37.

Chapter 8
CHEMICAL MEDIATORS

D. L. WILHELM

I. Introduction

For more than a century, the vascular phenomena that characterize the early stages of the inflammatory process have been studied by numerous workers including Thompson (1813), Waller (1846), Wharton Jones (1851), Samuel (1890), Cohnheim (1882), and, more recently, Lewis (1927), Clark and Clark (1935, 1936), Chambers and Zweifach (1940, 1947), Florey (1970), and Majno (1965) and their colleagues. Despite all this work, however, our knowledge of inflammation remains largely descriptive, and we still have little precise information concerning the chemical mediation of the characteristic vascular reactions.

In the early stages of inflammation, the main vascular events include vasodilation and augmented blood flow, increased vascular permeability, and the emigration of leukocytes. These events are evoked relatively quickly, even by moderate injury. Furthermore, the pattern of response is remarkably similar in various types of injury, and these two features of the vascular reactions, *viz.*, rapidity of onset and similarity of features, in turn, have prompted the notion that all the principal vascular phenomena in inflammation might be mediated by a common substance, even in different species.

The inflammatory process, however, is a complex reaction in which even the individual vascular events themselves may be complicated. Thus, the permeability response, e.g., in moderate thermal injury, includes both immediate and delayed responses, each of which is probably evoked by a different substance. The permeability changes also vary in both pattern and time course with different kinds of injury, and it is likely that vasodilation and tissue leukocytosis are similarly variable. The notion, then, that a single mediator elicits the whole complex process in early inflammation seems unrealistic.

The study of the chemical mediation of inflammation has been particularly directed at the characteristic increase of vascular permeability. Not only is increased permeability a key response in the inflammatory process (Cohnheim, 1882), but its ready experimental demonstration has made it a popular indicator reaction in the search for mediators of the whole inflammatory process.

The endogenous permeability factors put forward as natural mediators include various groups of substances isolable from normal or inflamed tissue. But, in discussing the chemical mediation of inflammation, I propose to discard the popular approach of first listing the endogenous substances that have been identified and then trying to establish cases for their possible roles as natural mediators. Instead, it seems preferable to review briefly the time course and interrelationships of the three main vascular events and then to discuss which of the known mediators, in fact, might evoke the natural phenomena.

II. Early Vascular Events in Inflammation

A. *Principles of Investigating Chemical Mediators*

The experimental work on the early vascular phenomena of inflammation includes a wide range of injuries induced by factors ranging from mild physical or chemical stimuli to acute burning or advanced infection (see Zweifach, Chapter 1). In severe injury, however, particularly with necrosis of the injured tissue, the pharmacological picture must inevitably be complicated by tissue by-products, with consequent difficulty in the identification of the specific mediators (Miles and Wilhelm, 1960a; Wilhelm and Mason, 1960). It follows that the severity of experimental injury should be minimal. This approach, in turn, offers a further advantage, in that the rate of development of the inflammatory process is roughly proportional to the severity of injury—hence, in mild injury, the component vascular events mature relatively slowly, permitting the whole process to be "dissected" into its component reactions.

One further point seems relevant to the investigation of chemical mediators. Although the increase of vascular permeability in inflammation usually begins within minutes, it often persists for hours or even days, whereas most endogenous permeability factors have short-term effects lasting only about 15 minutes. These short-term effects of isolated factors may raise doubts concerning their natural role in injury, but they also emphasize that the investigation of their natural roles requires a knowledge of the precise time course of the events in inflammation. And however the mediators are identified—whether by isolating the factors or by demonstrating suppression of the vascular reactions in animals depleted of the factors, treated with specific inhibitors or analogues—this argument seems equally valid (for a further discussion of this point, see Zweifach, Chapter 1).

B. Methods of Evaluating the Vascular Reactions in Inflammation

To avoid depression of the vascular reactions (see Miles and Miles, 1952), the inflammatory process is best studied in unanesthetized animals. On the other hand, this technique limits the evaluation of vasodilation and increased blood flow in skin to an assessment of superficial erythema or temperature changes at the injured site. Vasodilation can be measured directly in microcirculatory preparations, but assessment of the actual rate of blood flow requires that the animals be anesthetized (Hilton and Lewis, 1956).

Leukocytic sticking and emigration can be observed directly in similar preparations, e.g., rabbit ear chambers (Clark and Clark, 1935, 1936; Marchesi and Florey, 1960; Florey and Grant, 1961), or tissue leukocytosis can be gauged in histological sections of the injured tissue.

Increased vascular permeability manifests itself by the formation of a fluid exudate containing 1–6 gm of plasma protein per 100 ml. The amount of resulting exudate may be assessed by various methods, including gravimetric or volumetric analysis of plasma proteins labeled with aniline dyes or radioactive isotopes (see Spector, 1958; Spector and Willoughby, 1963).

Permeability changes are commonly evaluated in the skin of laboratory animals by the exudation of a circulating vital dye such as Evans' blue (T-1824), pontamine sky blue 6BX, or trypan blue, each of which becomes bound to the plasma proteins, particularly the albumins (Rawson, 1943), and therefore indicates a movement of the proteins across the wall of the peripheral vascular bed. This technique was developed as a qualitative test by Ramsdell (1928), but lends itself to reasonably precise assays of the potency of permeability factors (PF's) when log dose PF injected intracutaneously is plotted against mean diameter of the area of exuded dye (Miles and Miles, 1952; see, also, Wilhelm et al., 1958; Logan and Wilhelm, 1966a). Later workers have estimated the amount of exuded dye extracted by an ether–ethanol–pyridine technique from skin previously disintegrated by freezing and percussion (Judah and Willoughby, 1962), extracted with Somogyi reagents from skin disintegrated with a simple homogenizer (Carr and Wilhelm, 1964), or extracted with formamide from minced skin (Mustard et al., 1965). A variant of the dye technique involves the use of intravenous albumin labeled with ^{131}I or ^{125}I and determination of radioactivity in lymph (Wasserman et al., 1955) or inflammatory exudate (Spector, 1956; Faulk et al., 1971).

A method for the continuous recording of permeability responses in skin has recently been developed by Baumgarten and his colleagues (1967, 1970a,b) in which circulating bovine serum albumin (BSA) labeled with [32P]phosphanilic acid (Baumgarten et al., 1968) serves as the "marker" of increased permeability. Since the emission from ^{32}P is confined to β particles whose radiation penetrates only 8 mm of water, radiation from subcutaneous tissues is absorbed before reaching the upper layers of the skin. Surface measurements of beta radiation therefore detect radioactivity emanating mainly from the skin but not the underlying tissues.

C. Increased Vascular Permeability in Inflammation

The vascular events comprising the early inflammatory process have been described in various chapters in Volumes I and II, and I have already referred to the complexity of the whole process, as well as of the individual vascular reactions. However, our awareness of this complexity, particularly for the permeability events, is comparatively recent and largely due to Sevitt's observation (1958) that distinct permeability responses are evoked by thermal injury of varying severity applied to the skin of guinea pigs.

1. Thermal Injury

With heating of skin sites at 55°C for 15–20 seconds, Sevitt (1958) observed that an early local exudation of dye begins within a few minutes and progresses for $\frac{1}{2}$–1 hour. With heating for 5 seconds, however, the exudation of dye is delayed for 2–3 hours, but subsides by the time the lesions are 5–6 hours old.

Sevitt's work on thermal injury was soon confirmed and extended in the guinea pig, rat, and rabbit (Allison and Lancaster, 1959; Spector and Willoughby, 1959b; Wilhelm and Mason, 1960). The studies of Sevitt (1958) and Spector and Willoughby (1959b) were made on the abdominal skin of anesthetized animals, but thermal lesions of the thicker skin of the dorsal trunk of unanesthetized animals (Wilhelm and Mason, 1960) reveal yet a third type of response which is immediate in appearance, transient in duration, and induced by relatively mild heating at 54°C for 5 seconds (Fig. 1). This immediate response appears in the first minute, reaches a peak in 5 minutes, and subsides within 10 minutes (Wilhelm and Mason, 1960). When the duration of heating at 54°C is increased to 20 seconds, a similar immediate response is evoked, but is now succeeded in $\frac{1}{2}$–1 hour by a second and prolonged response which corresponds to the delayed response of Sevitt (1958); see Fig. 2. With still stronger heating (e.g., 58°C for 20 seconds), the permeability response again becomes monophasic in pattern and early in onset (Wilhelm and Mason, 1960; cf. Sevitt, 1958).

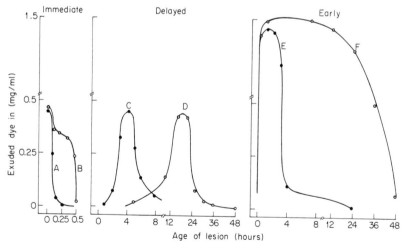

Fig. 1. Main types of vascular permeability responses evoked in guinea pig skin by thermal injury of varying intensity, by ultraviolet injury, and by the intracutaneous injection of compound 48/80. Immediate response: A, thermal injury (54°C for 5 seconds; Wilhelm and Mason, 1960); B, compound 48/80 (E. Comino, unpublished, 1972). Delayed response: C, thermal injury (54°C for 20 seconds; Wilhelm and Mason, 1960); D, ultraviolet injury (20 seconds; Logan and Wilhelm, 1966a). Early response: E, thermal injury (58°C for 20 seconds; Wilhelm and Mason, 1960); F, thermal injury (60°C for 60 seconds; extrapolated from Sevitt, 1958).

The immediate response in unanesthetized rats is feeble and in rabbits inconsistent. However, both species exhibit a prolonged delayed response similar to that in guinea pigs and forming the major reaction of the permeability effects (Wilhelm and Mason, 1960).

2. BACTERIAL INFECTION AND TOXINS

While Sevitt's work (1958) was in progress in Birmingham, England, Burke and Miles in London independently observed a diphasic permeability response in various types of bacterial infections. Figure 2, curve B, drawn from data of Burke and Miles (1958), illustrates some of their results. An initial phase of increased permeability begins soon after injecting $10^4 - 10^6$ organisms and lasts $\frac{1}{2}$–1 hour. However, it is at least partly due to substances in the culture media adsorbed to the bacteria, because washing the suspensions decreases the reaction. The initial response subsides in $\frac{1}{2}$–1 hour, and after a latent interval is followed by a delayed phase similar in time course to that in thermal injury. Similar results were also obtained with *Staphylococcus aureus*, *Streptococcus pyogenes*, *Clostridium welchii*, *Corynebacterium diphtheriae*, *Corynebacterium ovis*, *Listeria monocytogenes*, and *Pseudomonas pyocyanea*.

In earlier work, Petri et al. (1952) studied the effects of antihistamines on the accumulation of colloidal carbon at sites of staphylococcal infection in rabbit skin. Since the time course of accumulation of colloids at skin sites treated with permeability factors resembles that for exuded dye (Wilhelm et al., 1957), the results provide a useful index of the progressive permeability changes. Petri et al. (1952) observed a maximal histamine response in $\frac{1}{2}$–1 hour and a nonhistamine response beginning in 1 hour and maximal in 6 hours—a result remarkably similar in pattern to that found by Burke and Miles (1958).

In rats, the delayed response to staphylococci, streptococci, and clostridia appears more slowly than in guinea pigs and rabbits, becoming maximal in about 12 hours (A. A. Miles and D. L. Wilhelm, unpublished, 1957).

In summary, the work on thermal injury and bacterial infection has revealed that the pattern of the permeability response in the skin of laboratory animals is monophasic in mild or severe injury, being of immediate type in mild injury and of early type in severe injury (Fig. 1). With injury of intermediate intensity, the response becomes diphasic and consists of both immediate and delayed responses separated by a latent interval of normal low permeability. In some kinds of injury, however, an immediate phase cannot be discerned despite the presence of a delayed response, e.g., only a late or delayed phase is evident with *Clostridium oedematiens* toxin (Elder and Miles, 1957), the permeability effects being strikingly prolonged in duration

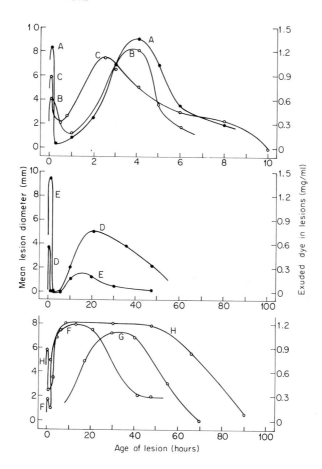

Fig. 2. Patterns of vascular permeability responses induced by various types of injury in the skin of the guinea pig. Open circles, mean lesion diameter (mm); closed circles, exuded dye (mg/ml). A, Thermal injury (54°C for 20 seconds; Wilhelm and Mason, 1960); B, acute bacterial infection (Burke and Miles, 1958); C, *Clostridium welchii* α toxin (Elder and Miles, 1957); D, delayed hypersensity (tuberculin reaction; Baumgarten and Wilhelm, 1969a); E, xylol injury (Steele and Wilhelm, 1966); F, *C. welchii*, type E, ι toxin (Craig and Miles, 1961); G. *C. oedematiens* toxin (Elder and Miles, 1957); H, *Vibrio cholerae* toxin (Craig, 1965b).

(Fig. 2). Other clostridial toxins, such as *C. welchii* and *C. septicum*, induce a diphasic permeability response (Fig. 2), but the initial or immediate phase is probably due to impurities in the preparations of toxin (Elder and Miles, 1957). The PF inducing the main response is an α toxin. In the case of *C. welchii*, it is a lecithinase (Macfarlane and Knight, 1941), but the toxin of *C. septicum*, although enzymic, attacks neither lecithin, cephalin, nor cerebrosides (Macfarlane, 1955).

Clostridium oedematiens toxins contain at least two lecithinases which are specifically neutralized by anti-γ and anti-β sera, respectively, and are immunologically distinct from *C. welchii* lecithinase. The α toxin of *C. oedematiens* has not been characterized (Macfarlane, 1955).

The ability to induce a prolonged increase of permeability appears to be exhibited by substances other than lecithinases. For example, *C. welchii* type E produces both α and ι toxins (Craig and Miles, 1961). In guinea pig skin, the ι toxin induces a late permeability response that begins in $1\frac{1}{2}$ hours and is sustained maximally for 6–18 hours before declining in the subsequent 18–30 hours (Fig. 2). The PF can be activated by trypsin from a nontoxic precursor in young cultures, but appears to have no lecithinase activity.

The prolonged increase of permeability provoked by the toxin of *C. oedematiens* is mimicked by the toxin in culture filtrates of *Vibrio cholerae* (Craig, 1965a,b). The prolonged effect with *V. cholerae* toxin is preceded by an initial permeability response lasting about 1 hour, but the pattern of response suggests that the initial phase is due to substances other than the toxin responsible for the later main PF response.

3. Other Types of Injury

Sevitt's report (1958) of variation in the pattern of permeability response with thermal stimuli of varying intensity and the independent report by Burke and Miles (1958) of a diphasic response in bacterial infection set the stage for renewed investigation of the inflammatory process and, in particular, of the characteristic increase of vascular permeability.

Ultrasonic injury (J. F. Burke, unpublished, 1961, cited by Wilhelm, 1962) provokes a diphasic response resembling that with moderate thermal injury (54°C for 20 seconds; see Fig. 2). Convenient doses of ultraviolet radiation (Logan and Wilhelm, 1966a,b) also provoke a diphasic response consisting of immediate and delayed phases (Fig. 3). However, the responses with ultraviolet injury differ in at least two respects from those with thermal injury; first, the delayed response has a later onset and longer duration, thereby resembling the pattern of response obtained with the ι toxin of *C. welchii* type E (Fig. 2); second, the ultraviolet stimulus needed to induce a strong immediate response has to be greater than that evoking a diphasic effect, whereas the reverse is true for thermal injury (Wilhelm and Mason, 1960; Logan and Wilhelm, 1963, 1966a; cf. Sim, 1965).

X Radiation (1000 rad to 6-cm^2 area) of rabbit skin induces a permeability response which is evident $\frac{1}{4}$–3 hours after injury (Jolles and Harrison, 1966), whereas, when 1500 rad is applied to 11 cm^2 of the abdominal wall of the rat, a permeability response in the underlying intestine takes 24 hours to become established and 72–96 hours to reach a maximum (Willoughby, 1960). With

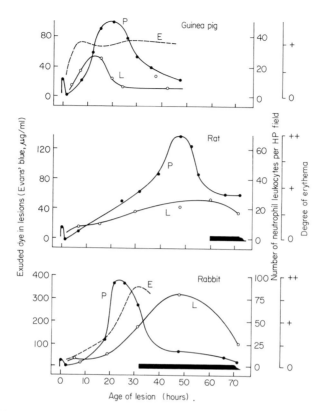

Fig. 3. The time course of erythema (E), increased vascular permeability (P), and tissue leukocytosis (L) induced by ultraviolet radiation in the skin of the guinea pig, rat, and rabbit. The horizontal bars in the middle and bottom blocks represent the formation and separation of a local slough. (From Logan and Wilhelm 1966a.)

β radiation of guinea pig skin from a $^{90}Sr-^{90}Y$ sealed source, a mild initial response is obtained at 3 hours, but the delayed response is maximal at 18 hours (Song *et al.*, 1966).

Chemical injury, applied superficially to the skin of guinea pigs, reveals yet a further pattern of permeability response in which an early response is combined with a delayed response. Such an effect is obtained with xylol, benzene, chloroform, or carbon tetrachloride applied for about 1 minute. The early response begins in a few minutes, reaches a peak in $\frac{1}{3}-\frac{1}{2}$ hour, and lasts $\frac{1}{2}-2$ hours. A latent interval of 3–8 hours then precedes a delayed phase, which reaches a peak in 15–20 hours (Steele and Wilhelm, 1966).

As with other types of injury, a stronger chemical stimulus enhances the initial early response, but the delayed effect is no longer obtained, i.e., the permeability response becomes monophasic and corresponds to a strong early effect. When a range of chemical elements is tested by intracutaneous injection, the pattern of permeability response varies considerably (Steele and Wilhelm, 1967). A number of elements induce a diphasic response consisting of an initial early effect which is stronger than the delayed effect, but many chemicals have only monophasic effects.

Surgical incision also provokes a monophasic response in rat skin. The response is strongest in the first 30 minutes, declines to less than one-third the initial intensity in the next 30 minutes, but does not disappear until the wounds are 3–5 hours old (Lykke and Cummings, 1969). Crush injury (10 kg/5 minutes) of rat skin produces a mild monophasic response lasting up to 4 hours. With stronger crushing (10 kg/10 minutes), the response becomes diphasic, but, as with stronger chemical stimuli, the initial early response overshadows the later delayed effect (Cummings and Lykke, 1970). Similar results are obtained with freezing (Cummings, 1971).

Various types of immunological reactions induce the same three principal types of permeability responses, *viz.*, immediate, delayed, and early (cf. Sevitt, 1964). For example, anaphylaxis evokes a typical immediate response (Craig and Wilhelm, 1963). On the other hand, delayed hypersensitivity induces a diphasic response consisting of early and delayed phases in chemical contact dermatitis (Baumgarten and Wilhelm, 1969b), but consisting of immediate and delayed phases in the tuberculin reaction (Inderbitzin, 1955; Voisin and Toullet, 1960, 1963). Furthermore, the diphasic response obtained in guinea pigs sensitized with live Bacille Calmette-Guérin in saline becomes triphasic when the animals are sensitized with killed *Mycobacterium tuberculosis* in a water-in-oil emulsion, with an early-type phase orrurring at $\frac{1}{2}$–2 hours, i.e., between the immediate and delayed responses (Baumgarten and Wilhelm, 1969a). An unusual permeability response is associated with skin allografts of rats. An initial permeability effect corresponds to the surgical incision, but is succeeded on the sixth to eighth days by a sharp response associated with impending rejection of the graft (Lykke and Cummings, 1970).

4. Vascular Lesions in Permeability Responses

The peripheral blood vessels involved in permeability responses are readily identified by the technique of intramural labeling with circulating colloidal carbon (Majno and Palade, 1961; Majno et al., 1961; Cotran et al., 1967). In immediate-type responses (e.g., in mild thermal injury; Fig. 1), the exuding plasma escapes from small venules up to 100 μm in diameter and particularly from venules 20–30 μm in diameter (Cotran, 1965). As illustrated elsewhere in this volume, the endothelium of the affected venules exhibits intercellular gaps which are considered by Majno et al. (1969) to result from contraction of adjacent endothelial cells. Circulating carbon passes through these gaps, but the relatively large particles of carbon cannot readily pass through the underlying basement membrane and come to lie in an intramural position between endothelial cells and basement membrane.

In delayed permeability responses (e.g., with heating of skin sites at 54° C for 20 seconds; Figs. 1 and 2), vascular lesions are not recognizable during the first 15 minutes, but the carbon-labeling technique reveals involvement of capillaries throughout the dermis in 1–5 hours (Wells and Miles, 1963; Cotran and Majno, 1964), as well as occasional small- and medium-sized venules. Again, the main ultrastructural lesion is an interendothelial gap (cf. Cotran, 1967b) as in immediate-type responses. Ultrastructural damage is inconspicuous, and endothelial necrosis is uncommon (Cotran, 1965). In delayed responses with an onset 2–10 hours after injury and a corresponding later peak and duration (Figs. 2 and 3, e.g., in ultraviolet injury, delayed hypersensitivity, and with bacterial toxins; Cotran and Pathak, 1968; Willms-Kretschmer et al., 1967; Cotran, 1967a), the vascular lesions in skin consist mainly of interendothelial gaps in small- and medium-sized venules and, to a lesser extent, in the subepidermal capillaries. Endothelial damage is variable in degree, usually infrequent, and mainly involves capillaries whose lumens are plugged by aggregates of carbon or which exhibit thrombosis (Cotran and Pathak, 1968).

In early-type responses (Figs. 1 and 2), as with strong thermal (60° C for 20 seconds) or chemical injury, the main vascular lesion damages venules, capillaries, and even occasional arterioles; some vessels, particularly capillaries, are occluded by plugs of fibrin, platelets, and carbon. Interendothelium gaps still occur, but are infrequent (Cotran and Majno, 1964; Cotran et al., 1967).

5. RELATIONSHIPS OF OTHER VASCULAR EVENTS

Little precise information is available about the time course of erythema in injury, but the emigration of neutrophil leukocytes is usually related to the delayed phase of increased permeability (see Miles, 1961; Spector and Willoughby, 1963; for further discussion, see Chapter 7).

Moderate heating of guinea pig skin at 54° C for 5 seconds induces initial blanching which is replaced by erythema in 30–40 seconds and which is succeeded in a further 10 seconds by edema or the exudation of dye. In the next 5 minutes, the erythema fades as exudation proceeds, but soon reappears and persists for some hours (Wilhelm and Mason, 1960). Ultraviolet injury of guinea pigs induces an initial faint erythema that disappears in the first minute, but reappears in 1–2 hours, reaching a maximal bright pink in 10–14 hours which persists for a further 24–48 hours (Fig. 3). In rats, erythema is inconspicuous or absent; in rabbits, moderate erythema is elicited by short exposures to radiation, although it does not appear until the lesions are at least 1 hour old (Logan and Wilhelm, 1966a; Fig. 3).

The absence of correlation between the time courses of erythema and increased permeability have been best demonstrated for superficial chemical injury of guinea pigs (Steele and Wilhelm, 1966). Within 1 minute of applying xylol, the sites become redder than the surrounding skin. Their color deepens for 5 minutes, then gradually fades so that in 30 minutes only the faintest blush remains. The color subsequently deepens, often becoming a bright red in 4 hours. At this stage, however, the permeability response is often minimal (Fig. 4). The erythema is brightest at 10–20 hours and then gradually fades to become indistinguishable from the surrounding skin in 70–100 hours. Perhaps the most convincing dissociation of erythema and increased permeability has been obtained with indium chloride injected intracutaneously in guinea pigs. Indium causes an unusually pronounced late erythema at the injection site, but at no stage is there increased vascular permeability (Steele and Wilhelm, 1967). Although the results for indium do not actually dissociate erythema from exudation, they indicate that intense erythema need not necessarily be associated with increased permeability.

Tissue leukocytosis is never prominent in thermal burns of guinea pig skin (Sevitt, 1957). In both guinea pigs and rats, ultraviolet radiation induces only mild leukocytosis that is confined to the superficial dermis (Logan and Wilhelm, 1966a). Nevertheless, the accumulation of neutrophils in the dermis several hours before the delayed permeability phase (Fig. 3) seems un-

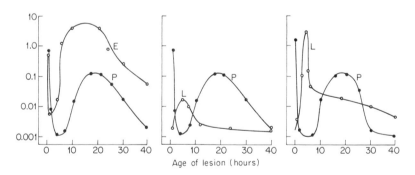

Age of lesion (hours)

Fig. 4.   The relationship of increased vascular permeability (P) to erythema (E, left block) and to tissue leukocytosis (L, middle block) after the application of xylol for 60 seconds to guinea pig skin, and the relationship of increased permeability (P) to tissue leukocytosis (L) after applying chloroform for 30 seconds (right block). On the ordinate, increased permeability (P) is recorded in terms of concentration of exuded dye in the lesions. The units on the ordinate for erythema (E) and tissue leukocytosis (L) are not recorded above, but correspond to the units in the original data of Steele and Wilhelm (1966, 1970). (Redrawn from Steele and Wilhelm, 1966, and Wilhelm, 1971a.)

related to the subsequent permeability events as judged by the inability of experimental neutropenia to suppress either the initial or the delayed permeability responses in ultraviolet injury. The nonrelation of the two events is further supported by the inability of whole neutrophil leukocytes or material liberated from disrupted neutrophils to induce permeability changes in the guinea pig (Miles, 1961).

The chronological dissociation of tissue leukocytosis from permeability responses is best illustrated with superficial chemical injury of the skin of guinea pigs (Steele and Wilhelm, 1970). Within 5 minutes of applying chemical irritants such as xylol (applied for 1 minute), neutrophils, accompanied by fewer monocytes and eosinophils, begin to accumulate in the mid-dermal veins. The number of neutrophils increases during the next 20 minutes, but at this stage most are intravascular. The proportion outside the vessels subsequently increases and often rises quite sharply 2 hours after injury, so that between 2 and 6 hours the tissues become heavily infiltrated by emigrated neutrophils (Fig. 4). The results with benzene or carbon tetrachloride resemble those with xylol except that the emigration of neutrophils into the tissues is less in the initial 2 hours, but is followed by a sudden increase to a peak at 6 hours with benzene (Fig. 4) and at 4 hours with carbon tetrachloride. But with these and other irritants which provoke a delayed phase of exudation, the neutrophil response reaches its peak between the two phases of increased permeability and is declining before the onset of the second phase (Steele and Wilhelm, 1970). Instead, the neutrophil response seems proportional to the extent of epidermal necrosis caused by the superficially applied irritant (cf. ultraviolet injury in Fig. 3).

The results illustrated in Fig. 4 might be interpreted to indicate that the accumulation of neutrophils is a necessary precursor for the subsequent development of the delayed permeability response (see also Janoff, 1970). Such an interpretation is not supported, however, by the events in dermal infection of guinea pigs with *Streptococcus pyogenes*, in which the tissue accumulation of neutrophils parallels the maturation of the delayed response, or with *Clostridium welchii* infection, in which neutrophil accumulation lags behind the response (see Burke and Miles, 1958). Further evidence of dissociation of the two events comes from the finding that in rats severely depleted of neutrophil leukocytes with methotrexate the permeability response is unaffected in chemical pleurisy, as well as in thermal injury of skin (Willoughby and Giroud, 1969).

6. SUMMARY

Increased vascular permeability in inflammation may be monophasic, diphasic, or even triphasic. These various patterns consist, in turn, of three main types of response, viz., (1) immediate, (2) delayed, and (3) early, which may occur alone or in combination. *Immediate* responses begin a minute or two after injury, usually last 10–15 minutes and no more than 30 minutes. *Delayed* responses exhibit two main patterns, either beginning $\frac{1}{2}$-1 hour after injury and reaching a peak in about 4 hours or beginning 2–10 hours after injury and usually reaching a peak at 12–24 hours, but occasionally as late as 48 hours. *Early* responses begin 10–30 minutes after injury, reach a peak in 20–60 minutes, and have a duration corresponding to the intensity of the stimulus.

In general, the pattern of permeability response is related to the intensity of stimulus rather than to the type of injury or species of test animal. Immediate responses are usually induced by mild stimuli, delayed responses by moderate, and early responses by strong stimuli.

Erythema is often diphasic and associated with both phases of increased permeability, particularly in guinea pigs, but less so in rabbits, and least so in rats. Nevertheless, erythema may be maximal when permeability is minimal, while the strong erythema induced by indium chloride is associated with no permeability response at all.

Tissue leukocytosis varies both in intensity and time course according to the type of injury and species of test animal. Leukocytosis is generally associated with no permeability response at all.

Tissue leukocytosis varies both in intensity and time course according to the type of injury and species of test animal. Leukocytosis is generally associated with the delayed permeability response, but does not appear to be responsible for its mediation.

III. Endogenous Mediators of the Vascular Events

There are four features of the permeability response which strongly suggest that chemical mediators rather than physical effects (see Cohnheim, 1882; Krogh, 1929; Landis, 1946) are responsible for the phenomenon. These have been summarized by Spector and Willoughby (1963) as follows: (1) the reversible nature of the inflammatory process which occurs only in living tissues; (2) the consistent nature and pattern of the response for a wide range of effective stimuli; (3) the suppression by drugs of at least part of the response; and (4) the existence of a latent period between the initial and delayed phases of increased permeability. Further support is afforded by the very presence of endogenous permeability factors in both normal and inflamed tissue. Not only are such substances able to reproduce the vascular events of inflammation, but at least some of their effects are suppressed by reasonably specific antagonists (see Wilhelm, 1962).

Many workers after Massart and Bordet (1890, 1891) have demonstrated that by-products from injured tissues increase vascular permeability as well as induce leukocytic emigration. Preparations of macerated or disrupted tissue, both normal and inflamed, of autolyzed tissue, or of protein by-products all yield permeability factors. Since normal tissue cells and blood both contain potent permeability factors (see below), however, practically any endogenous material is certain to contain permeability factors.

The preparations that have been reasonably characterized fall into two main groups: (a) vasoactive amines, e.g., histamine and 5-hydroxytryptamine, as well as their natural liberators, and (b) proteases and esterases concerned with the formation of polypeptides, particularly those known as *kinins*.

A. Vasoactive Amines

The vasoactive amines, histamine and 5-hydroxytryptamine (5-HT), are comparatively simple chemical substances which are widely distributed in plant and animal tissues. Histamine is the amine derivative obtained by de-carboxylation of histidine, and 5-HT is the amine derivative of tryptophan, which is first converted to 5-hydroxytryptophan before decarboxylation to 5-HT.

β-Iminazolylethylamine
(histamine)

5-Hydroxytryptamine
(serotonin)

1. HISTAMINE

After its synthesis as β-iminazolylethylamine by Windaus and Vogt (1907) and isolation from ergot (Kutscher, 1910; Barger and Dale, 1910a,b), histamine was soon identified in intestinal mucosa (Barger and Dale, 1911) and various other tissues of the body (Abel and Kubota, 1919; Best *et al.*, 1927). Its ability to increase vascular permeability was initially reported by Eppinger (1913) and Sollmann and Pilcher (1917), but the first detailed description of its ability to dilate capillaries, cause hypotension, and increase vascular permeability came from Dale and Richards (1918–1919). Then followed the well-known work of Lewis and his colleagues on the "triple response" (see Lewis, 1927) and the role of histamine in inflammation.

Lewis (1927) observed that firm stroking of the human forearm with a blunt edge applied to the skin evokes a characteristic triad of signs: initial dilation of small blood vessels along the line of the stroke followed by dilation of neighboring arterioles and, finally, a whealing of the line of the stroke. The initial vasodilation and the subsequent whealing in this so-called triple response are mediated by a locally released vasoactive substance, whereas the arteriolar dilation is due to a local axon reflex, which is itself possibly stimulated by the same vasoactive substance.

A similar response is evoked by mechanical, electrical, thermal, and chemical stimuli, as well as by pricking histamine into the skin. Lewis (1927) therefore concluded that the vasoactive substance was histamine itself or a closely related factor which he designated "H substance." The more prolonged responses provoked by ultraviolet or X radiation and by bacterial toxins or various chemicals (e.g., mustard gas, chloroform) were considered due to the slower, prolonged release of the same H-substance, possibly supplemented by "disintegration products" (Lewis, 1927). Although Lewis' histamine theory was later criticized when antihistamines were found not to suppress increased vascular permeability in experimental injury (Weeks and Gunnar, 1949), the misgivings were quite unwarranted because his critics had investigated the effects of the new antihistamines on severe injury, whereas Lewis' experiments were confined to the effects of mild stimuli. But before Lewis' work finally became accepted, the role of histamine in inflammation was reopened by the discovery of the histamine liberators among various classes of organic compounds (Feldberg and Paton, 1951; Feldberg and Schachter, 1952; Paton, 1957).

a. SOURCES AND RELEASE OF HISTAMINE. In higher animals, histamine is made available by two main processes: first, by synthesis and storage in tissues, particularly in mast cells; second, by synthesis of free histamine through controlled alterations in activity of an inducible form of histidine decarboxylase (Schayer, 1966b). Man probably cannot take up and store exogenous histamine. In fact, histamine absorbed from the bowel is efficiently broken down before it can reach the systemic circulation (Lindell and Westling, 1966). Although the evidence remains inconclusive that man can form histamine from L-histidine, Lindell and Westling (1966) nevertheless consider this to be the probable source of supply.

Histamine occurs in varying concentrations in most, if not all, tissues (Feldberg, 1956), a major portion in man being stored in mast cell granules (Riley and West, 1953) probably as a heparin–protein–histamine complex (Uvnäs, 1969). More than half the histamine in blood occurs in basophils (Graham et al., 1955), while much of the remainder resides in eosinophilic leukocytes.

The mechanism of release of histamine from tissues is poorly understood (see Paton, 1957; Mongar and Schild, 1962; Uvnäs, 1962, 1964, 1969). Histamine may be liberated (see Uvnäs, 1964) by mechanical trauma, radiant energy (e.g. X ray, ultraviolet radiation, heat), synthetic polymers (e.g., compound 48/80), dextran, biogenic polymers (eg., antigens, ovomucoid, bacterial toxins, tissue extracts), monomeric basic substances (e.g., alkylamines, alkaloids, basic organic compounds, and even antihistamines themselves), surface active agents (e.g., Tween 20, bile salts, lysolecithin), and proteolytic enzymes. Release of histamine is generally considered to involve at least four possible mechanisms: the splitting of a hypothetical bond linking histamine to protein; leakage of histamine through a cellular or subcellular membrane rendered permeable or even destroyed; an ion exchange reaction releasing histamine from its combination with an acidic intracellular site; or rupture of a polar linkage with protein or lipoprotein (Paton, 1957; Mongar and Schild, 1962).

Much of our information concerning the release of histamine from mast cells comes from studies with the synthetic polymer amine, compound 48/80, whose action resembles that of other basic polypeptides. Treatment of mast cells with compound 48/80 (Uvnäs, 1969) is followed after a latent period of 5–10 seconds by rapid expulsion of the cells' contents of granules through the cell membrane. The granules are capable of storing histamine when suspended in cation-free media, but readily release it when suspended in an isotonic solution of sodium chloride. Histamine seems to be stored in the granules in electrostatic linkage with carboxyl groups in the protein part of the granule complex (Åborg et al., 1967) from which it can be displaced by sodium or other basic radicles such as biogenic amines (Bergendorff and Uvnäs, 1967). Within the cell, the granules are probably shielded from cytoplasmic cations (e.g., potassium) by their covering of bilaminar membrane (Uvnäs, 1969).

The major routes for the catabolism of free histamine involve methylation and oxidation (Schayer, 1966a). Up to 80% of histamine administered to mammals is metabolized along two pathways whose importance varies with species. In man, as well for the dog, cat, and mouse, ring N-methylation accounts for most of the histamine loss, whereas an oxidative pathway to imidazoleacetic acid and its conjugated products is the main pathway in the rat. In other species, both pathways contribute about equally to the breakdown of histamine.

b. ANTIHISTAMINES. The antihistamines act by preventing histamine from combining with its receptors; the only effect of histamine which is resistant to such blockade is its ability to stimulate secretion of gastric acid. Almost all antihistamines are substituted ethylamines in which antihistaminic

TABLE I

<small>Inhibition of PF Potency of Histamine and Compound 48/80 by
Various Antihistamines Given Intravenously in
Guinea Pigs (0.1 mg/kg), Rats (0.5 mg/kg), and Rabbits (0.1 mg/kg)[a]</small>

	Factor of inhibition of PF				
	Guinea pig		Rat		Rabbit[b]
Antihistamine	Histamine	48/80	Histamine	48/80	Histamine
Triprolidine	1750	4	40	1.3	11
Chlorprophenpyridamine	530	5	13	1.8	2
Mepyramine	47	3	37	1.1	9
Promethazine	12	2	100	3.0	4
Tripelennamine	6	7	10	1.5	3
Chlorcyclizine	1.6	1.7	19	2.0	2
Diphenhydramine	1.4	1.5	8	3.0	2
Antazoline	1.1	3	3	2.0	3
Thenalidine	0.8	1.0	5	1.7	1.0

[a]From unpublished data by B. Mason and D. L. Wilhelm (1960). Doses of antihistamines
are cited as base.

[b]The susceptibility of compound 48/80 was not tested in the rabbit (see text).

activity appears when alkyl groups replace the hydrogen atoms on the nitrogen of the ethylamine chain.

Table I summarizes the activity of nine representative antihistamines
tested for suppression of the response lines to intracutaneous histamine and
compound 48/80 in guinea pigs, rats, and rabbits. Antihistaminic activity is
expressed as the factor of inhibition which is the ratio of PF potency of
histamine in control and treated animals. To minimize the nonspecific side-
effects of antihistamines, the intravenous test dose of antagonist was restricted to 0.1 mg of base per kilogram in the guinea pig. Substantial inhibition
in the rat requires a dose of 0.5 mg/kg, but doses exceeding 0.1 mg/kg cannot
be tested in the rabbit because such doses cause a slow and generalized
increase of vascular permeability.

Based on antihistaminic potency in all three test species, the antagonist
of choice is triprolidine in the guinea pig and triprolidine or mepyramine in
the rat and rabbit (Table I). But in the guinea pig and rat, both antihistamines
have little or no effect on the PF activity of compound 48/80. Comparable
results were obtained in the guinea pig by Logan and Wilhelm (1966b) when,
as in the above work, graded doses of intracutaneous histamine were given
promptly after intravenous dye and antihistamine. However, the effect of

the antihistamine is greatest 1 hour after administration, has decreased considerably in 2 hours, and has almost subsided in 3 hours (Logan and Wilhelm, 1966b).

2. 5-Hydroxytryptamine

The pharmacological characterization and isolation of 5-hydroxytryptamine (5-HT, serotonin, enteramine) resulted from independent studies by two groups of workers, *viz.*, first, Erspamer (1954) and his colleagues who investigated the "enteramine" that imparts the characteristic histochemical properties to the enterochromaffin cells of the gastrointestinal tract (Vialli and Erspamer, 1933); and, second, Rapport and his colleagues (1948a,b) who isolated and characterized a factor (serotonin) with vasoconstrictor and moderately hypertensive properties from serum and defibrinated blood. Erspamer and Asero (1952) subsequently identified enteramine as 5-HT, and the new preparation was synthesized by Hamlin and Fisher in 1954.

5-Hydroxytryptamine occurs in various plants and fruits, including the walnut, avocado pear, banana, tomato, and Australian pineapple (see Garattini and Valzelli, 1965). Among a wide variety of sources in animal tissues, 5-HT's most important localization in mammals is the gastrointestinal tract and brain (Erspamer, 1954). In the gastrointestinal tract, it is particularly associated with the enterochromaffin cells of the intestinal mucosa, and carcinoid tumors of these enterochromaffin cells may contain particularly high concentrations of 5-HT. Mast cells from the rat or mouse are also rich in 5-HT, whether the cells are normal or neoplastic. Its presence in blood is predominantly, if not exclusively, associated with platelets (Humphrey and Jacques, 1954; Stacey, 1957). High concentrations also occur in venoms and stings, e.g., venom of wasps or scorpions, stinging nettle (Collier, 1958).

The possible role of 5-hydroxytryptamine in the inflammatory response was suggested by the report of Rowley and Benditt (1956) that it had high PF activity in the rat (cf. Sparrow and Wilhelm, 1957; Spector and Willoughby, 1957). The low PF activity of histamine in this species had long been a major factor against a general acceptance of histamine as the "universal mediator" of the inflammatory response; but Rowley and Benditt's observation suggested that rather than histamine itself, the long-sought mediator may in fact be a family of amines whose members individually played major roles in the various species. However, no further amines with high PF activity have been identified, and, in any case, there is now general agreement that histamine and 5-HT play only a minor role in inflammation (see below).

a. STORAGE AND RELEASE OF 5-HYDROXYTRYPTAMINE. Hydroxytryptamine is stored intracellularly in a pharmacologically inactive form (Erspamer, 1954), but is possibly maintained at a high level in cells by an active transport mechanism (Brodie, 1958). In the intestinal mucosa, it is located mainly in large granules distinct from mitochondria, but analogous to the chromaffin granules of the adrenal medulla and the histamine-carrying granules of mast cells (Baker, 1959; see Garattini and Valzelli, 1965). The manner in which 5-HT is bound in its stored form remains unknown. In rabbit platelets, it is linked to none of the eight protein fractions present in these cells (Sano *et al.*, 1958).

5-Hydroxytryptamine is released by reserpine from its stores in the gastrointestinal tract, platelets, and brain, and is then rapidly metabolized by monoamine oxidase. A dose of 1 mg/kg of reserpine releases about 75% of the 5-HT in 30 minutes. Nevertheless, the release of the drug is subject to species differences, e.g. release from gastric mucosa is readily obtained in the guinea pig, but not in the rabbit (Brodie, 1958). Release of 5-HT by reserpine is not a simple chemical displacement from sites of binding, but a more complex activity that seems to be related to the mechanism by which the concentration of 5-HT is maintained in platelets (see Garattini and Valzelli, 1965). Nevertheless, the slow release of 5-HT from platelets contrasts markedly with the explosive liberation of histamine when compound 48/80 distrupts mast cells (Bhattacharya and Lewis, 1956).

5-Hydroxytryptamine is broken down or inactivated by a number of routes, the most important being degradation by monoamine oxidase to 5-hydroxyindoleacetaldehyde, most of which is oxidized to 5-hydroxyindoleacetic acid, the principle urinary metabolite of 5-HT. However, some of the indoleacetaldehyde in the tissues is reduced to 5-hydroxytryptophol; the reduction is reversible, but reconversion to the acetaldehyde is minimized by the conjugation of 5-hydroxytryptophol with glucuronic and sulfuric acids. A little 5-HT is excreted as conjugates and still less appears in the urine in free form (Udenfriend, 1958; Blaschko, 1958; Garattini and Valzelli, 1965).

b. ANTAGONISTS OF 5-HYDROXYTRYPTAMINE. Most antagonists of 5-HT have competitive activity, although different classes of antagonists maximally suppress its effects on either intestinal or other smooth muscles, respectively (Jacob, 1960). Several lysergic acid derivatives have strong effects, the best studied and most powerful being lysergic acid diethylamide (LSD), its bromo derivative (BOL), and 1-methyllysergic acid (butanolamide). Various antihistamines antagonize the effect of 5-HT on intestinal smooth muscle *in vitro*: in particular, promethazine (Garattini and Valzelli, 1965; Casenti and Galli, 1956; Levy and Michel-Ber, 1956), homochlorcyclizine (Kimura *et al.*, 1960), and cyproheptadine (Stone *et al.*, 1961). For *in vivo* tests of suppression of the PF response to 5-HT in the skin of the rat, the use of LSD is handicapped by its toxicity (Sparrow and Wilhelm, 1957). With the nontoxic bromo derivative, BOL 148, the PF response is decreased about 175-fold by pretreatment with 1 mg of BOL per kilogram intravenously (Wilhelm and Mason, 1960).

B. The Kinin System

The kinins are a family of straight chain polypeptides that resemble bradykinin in structure and pharmacological activity (Webster, 1966a). In addition to bradykinin, the family includes kallidin, methionyl-lysyl-bradykinin, glycine-bradykinin*, and phyllokinin. The prototype of the family is

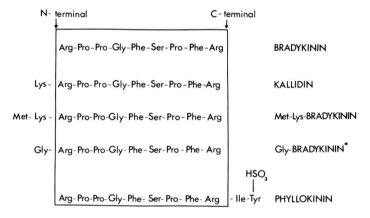

Fig. 5. Amino acid sequence of kinins, each of which contains the nonapeptide sequence of bradykinin (as indicated within the block). Bradykinin, kallidin, and methionyl-lysyl-bradykinin are released, respectively, by trypsin, kallikrein, and acidification from a substrate in mammalian plasma or serum. Of these three kinins, the first two have been prepared from human and other mammalian plasma and the third only from bovine plasma. Glycine-bradykinin is released by trypsin from an octadecapeptide in wasp venom. Phyllokinin has been isolated from amphibian skin. (Redrawn and modified from Kellermeyer and Graham, 1968, and Schachter, 1969. From Wilhelm (1971b) reproduced by permission of *Annual Review of Medicine*.)

*The Report of the Committee on Nomenclature for Hypotensive Peptides (see Webster, 1966a) states that "the committee was unable to agree on a uniform policy for naming derivatives of bradykinin or kallidin. It was recommended that this decision be reserved to the author who first identified or synthesized the structure. Thus methionylkallidin should be referred to as methionyllysylbradykinin. [(Met-Lys-Arg)[1]-bradykinin] (Elliot and Lewis, 1965) and the derivative obtained by the action of trypsin on wasp kinin should be referred to as glycine[1]-kallidin (Gly[1]-kallidin) (Schröder and Hempel, 1964; Pisano et al., 1965)." What the Committee decided to call "glycine-kallidin" is here referred to as "glycine-bradykinin."

bradykinin, a nonapeptide with the structure indicated in Fig. 5. The other members of the family all have this nonapeptide sequence and differ only in having additional amino acid residues at the N- or C-terminal. Kallidin would be better called lysyl-bradykinin, but popular usage perpetuates the former name.

Kinins are produced by the enzymic activity of proteolytic and esterolytic enzymes (collectively termed kininogenases) on glycoprotein substrates (kininogens) which are associated with α_2-globulins and plasma. The kinins are finally broken down to inactive peptides by enzymes collectively known as kininases (Fig. 6).

Proteases, particularly those of plasma, first received attention as possible mediators of increased permeability and other vascular responses during the early studies on anaphylatoxin (Friedberger, 1909; Jobling and Peterson, 1914). I have referred earlier in this chapter to the interest in histamine as a PF and as a mediator of the triple response. The consequent overshadowing of the proteases by histamine came to an end with the advent of the antihistaminic drugs and their failure to suppress increased permeability in experimental injury (Weeks and Gunnar, 1949). Meanwhile, the protease theory gained fresh support from Menkin's work (1938, 1940) on leukotaxine and from the report of Beloff and Peters (1945) on the activation by thermal injury of a protease in skin.

After observing that pleural effusions in turpentine- induced pleurisy increased vascular permeability, Menkin (1938, 1940) fractionated such preparations by a pyridine–acetone technique to obtain an alleged polypeptide which he named "leukotaxine" and considered a primary mediator in inflammation. Menkin's work has since been criticized because his technique really consisted of the precipitation of protein with acetone, the pyridine acting as a buffer to prevent adsorption of peptides on the precipitated protein (Spector, 1958) and because he failed to remove turpentine byproducts during fractionation (Harris, 1954). The leukotaxine theory has now been discarded, but the stimulus of Menkin's work has nevertheless been an important factor in the study of inflammation.

In any case, it soon became clear that the permeability effects claimed for leukotaxine were also exhibited by various polypeptide preparations. For example, leukotaxine-like substances were obtained from suppurative exudates, succus entericus, and the fluid from blisters or pulmonary edema (Cullumbine and Rydon, 1946). The digestion of albumin, globulin, and

KININOGEN $\xrightarrow{\text{Kininogenase}}$ KININ $\xrightarrow{\text{Kininase}}$ INACTIVE PEPTIDES

Fig. 6. Simplified scheme for the formation and breakdown of kinins.

fibrin with proteases also yielded PF preparations with higher potency when digestion was partial rather than prolonged (Duthie and Chain, 1939; Cullumbine and Rydon, 1946). Finally, Spector (1951) observed that tryptic and peptic digests of human fibrin also mimicked the permeability and leukocytic effects of leukotaxine, as well as evoking swelling of the capillary endothelial cells. Polypeptides with eight to fourteen amino acid chains induced all three effects, those with five amino acid chains only the first two. Even a crystalline peptide such as pancreatic trypsin inhibitor elicited the effects of peptides containing eight to fourteen amino acid chains.

1. UNGAR'S HYPOTHESIS

Despite the criticism that Menkin's work received, leukotaxine continued to attract attention, particularly because its permeability and leukocytic effects were insusceptible to antihistamines. Then in 1952, Ungar attempted to unite the histamine and leukotaxine theories by proposing that the proteolytic activity of plasmin possibly released both histamine and leukotaxine, which were responsible for increased permeability and tissue leukocytosis, respectively. Ungar's proposals were supported by evidence (see Miles and Wilhelm, 1960a) that proteolytic enzymes liberate histamine and that histamine release is accompanied by proteolytic activity. But he later abandoned his theory (Ungar, 1956) when it was demonstrated that protease inhibitors do not suppress histamine release and that proteolysis ceases before the release of tissue histamine is completed.

2. DISCOVERY OF THE KININ SYSTEM

In retrospect, it seems ironic that while Menkin's work on leukotaxine attracted so much attention in the 1940's and 1950's other relevant investigation were being pursued unnoticed on the Continent by Frey (1925, cited by Frey, 1963), Frey and Kraut (1926), and later Werle et al. (1937) who isolated a vasodepressor substance from urine. Since pancreatic extracts and juice contained a similar vasodepressant, it appeared that "kallikrein" (*kallikreas* = pancreas; Kraut et al., 1930) was released by the pancreas into the blood stream where it formed an inactive complex and was finally excreted by the kidney (Frey et al., 1930).

The next link in the kinin chain came from South America. In 1949, Rocha e Silva and his colleagues reported the release of a "polypeptide-like" factor from pseudoglobulin fractions treated with trypsin or snake venom. The factor, which they named "bradykinin," induced hypotension as well as slow and prolonged contraction of smooth muscle. Rocha e Silva's work, in turn, suggested that kallikrein had effects similar to those of trypsin and snake venom, and the substance described by Werle and his colleagues

(1937) as "factor DK" was finally identified as the polypeptide now known as "kallidin."

As the probable importance of pharmacologically active polypeptides became apparent, Elliott et al.. (1960a,b) began investigating the amino acid sequence of natural bradykinin. This work, in turn, prompted other investigations by a team led by Boissonnas, and resulted in the synthesis of a nonapeptide (Boissonnas et al., 1960; see also Nicolaides and DeWald, 1961), with the structure proposed by Elliott et al. (1960c,d) for the natural product. The structure is indicated in Fig. 5.

Webster and Pierce (1963) subsequently demonstrated that the kallikrein in human urine liberated two kinins from human plasma treated with acid, viz., kallidin-9 (kallidin I), which was indistinguishable from bradykinin, and kallidin-10 (kallidin II), a decapeptide differing from kallidin-9 in having an additional N-terminal lysine residue (Fig. 5). Synthetic kallidin-10, subsequently prepared by Nicolaides and DeWald (1961), could not be distinguished chromatographically from the natural product, but had only 60–70% of its biological activity. The lesser activity of the synthetic product was possibly due to racemization of the peptide during synthesis.

The next evidence came from England. While investigating the permeability effects of histamine, compound 48/80, and leukotaxine, Miles and Miles (1952) observed that the intracutaneous injection of histamine, for example, rendered the treated site refractory to a subsequent injection. The lowered reactivity persisted for about 4–5 hours and was nonspecific, in that each of the above three preparations induced refractoriness against itself or the other factors. Although itself not a PF, fresh guinea pig serum induced similar refractoriness, suggesting that serum contained a masked permeability factor. The inert precursor of the PF was demonstrated by Miles to be activated by dilution in saline of fresh guinea pig serum or plasma (PF/dil; Mackay et al., 1953; Miles and Wilhelm, 1955), the active factor being isolable as an α_2-globulin (Wilhelm et al., 1955, 1957).

With a natural plasma inhibitor (IPF) of the PF, the globulin PF constitutes a PF/IPF system that has been demonstrated in the guinea pig, rat, and rabbit, as well as in man (see Miles, 1958–1959; Miles and Wilhelm, 1960a,b). Subsequent evidence suggested that PF/dil from the guinea pig was an activator of the inert precursor of plasma kallikrein (Miles, 1964; Webster, 1968).

Against the background of this brief historical introduction, various features of the kinin system will now be considered in greater detail.

a. Kinin Formation—Kallikreins. Enzymes capable of forming kinins from appropriate substrates (kininogens) are collectively termed kininogenases, and include various kallikreins, as well as trypsin, pepsin, and proteases in snake venoms and bacterial products. The kininogenases are proteolytic and esterolytic enzymes, most of which share with trypsin the ability to hydrolyze peptide bonds having the carboxyl group contributed by arginine (Webster, 1966b). Of the kininogenases, the kallikreins have the greatest hydrolytic activity and substrate specificity. Kallikreins are widely distributed in the body, occurring as inactive precursors which are readily activable or, alternatively, as active substances. They can be divided into *tissue* and *plasma* kallikreins.

Various tissues, particularly of glandular organs, contain kallikreins which are often found in the corresponding secretions or excretions in active form, e.g., saliva (Werle and von Roden, 1936), pancreatic juice (Frey *et al.*, 1930), sweat (Fox and Hilton, 1958), tears (Lewis, 1959), feces (Werle and Vogel, 1961; Werle *et al.*, 1963), and urine (Werle and Vogel, 1961; De Carvalho and Diniz, 1964; Frey *et al.*, 1968). In fact, pancreas (Fielder and Werle, 1967) and submaxillary gland (Ekfors *et al.*, 1967) both contain several kallikreins. The tissue kallikreins are closely related, but nevertheless distinct. For example, the molecular weights of homogeneous kallikreins from the pancreas, urine, and submaxillary gland are 33,300, 36,300, and 32,800, respectively (Fritz *et al.*, 1967). Their distinction is also indicated by varying susceptibility to protease inhibitors, and by differing physiochemical and immunological characteristics (see Webster, 1968; Schachter, 1969).

Compared with tissue kallikreins, plasma kallikrein is a larger molecule (molecular weight, 97,000; Habermann and Klett, 1966) which is physicochemically and immunologically distinct and is probably elaborated as an inert precursor (prekallikrein) by the liver (Werle *et al.*, 1963; Forell, 1957).

b. PREKALLIKREINS AND THEIR ACTIVATION. Tissue kalikreins are found in active form in urine, sweat, saliva, and feces, but in the corresponding parent tissues they usually occur as the inactive precursors, *viz.*, prekallikreins (Webster, 1966b). In pancreas, the prekallikrein is probably contained in the zymogen granules of the acinar cells (Frey *et al.*, 1968), whereas tissue kallikrein occurs in active form in salivary gland, though the enzyme is similarly confined in secretory granules lying mainly at the apex of the serous cells. Salivary kallikrein may, therefore, be an exocrine enzyme with a primary function in saliva (Bhoola and Heap, 1970).

Activation of a tissue prekallikrein (e.g., pancreatic) is best obtained with trypsin (Werle *et al.*, 1955). Activation seems to involve only minor molecular modification that is possibly produced by removal of a steric hindrance of the active site for its substrate (see Schachter, 1969).

Recent views on the activation of plasma prekallikrein stem from earlier observations (Margolis, 1957, 1958; Margolis and Bishop, 1963; Webster and Ratnoff, 1961) that the generation of bradykinin in human plasma is initiated by activation of Hageman factor (Factor XII of blood clotting). Activation of Hageman factor was initially obtained by contact with a glass surface, but has since been demonstrated with numerous insoluble substances such as kaolin, charcoal, diatomaceous earth, ellagic acid, sodium urate crystals, collagen, and skin (Webster 1968). The presence of Hageman factor was subsequently shown to be necessary for the activation of the inert precursor of PF/dil, and the latter, in turn, seemed to be the final activator of the inert precursor of kallikrein. It was, therefore, considered that the derivation of active kallikrein probably stemmed from a sequential enzymic activation of pre-enzyme to active enzyme, the latter activating the next preenzyme in the system (Fig. 7). In fact, chromatography of acetone-activated human plasma on DEAE-cellulose reveals five peaks, each with kinin-forming activity, which have been designated enzymes I, II, III, IV, and V (Webster, 1968). Peak I probably corresponds to kallikrein, peak II to PF/dil, and peak IV to Hageman factor (Fig. 7).

Kaplan and Austen (1970) have confirmed Webster's results (1968) for DEAE-cellulose chromatography, but consider that the ability of the substance in each peak to directly activate a partially refined prekallikrein suggests that the individual peaks do not correspond to distinct enzymes in the serial activation of prekallikrein. Instead, Kaplan and Austen (1970) suggest that the peaks probably correspond to "different molecular forms" of the same prekallikrein activator in serum and, in fact, have produced convincing evidence that the activator of prekallikrein is a derivative of active Hageman factor itself. Later work by Kaplan and Austen (1971) suggests that activated Hageman factor and fragments of activated factor resulting from digestion by fibrinolysin are responsible for the conversion of prekallikrein to active kallikrein. The primary activator of prekallikrein seems to be the smallest of the fragments from Hageman factor, the fragment being stable, having a molecular weight of 30,000–35,000, and being a sixfold stronger activator for prekallikrein than the parent Hageman factor molecule. By disc gel electrophoresis, Kaplan and Austen (1970) have shown that the prekallikrein

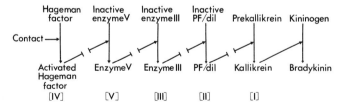

Fig. 7. Sequential activation of human plasma kallikrein according to Webster (1968, 1969). The Roman numerals in brackets refer to the kininogenases isolated by Webster (1968). (Redrawn and modified from Webster, 1969, by Wilhelm, 1971b, and reproduced by permission of *Annual Review of Medicine*.)

activator has the electrophoretic mobility of prealbumin. Movat and his colleagues have also reported a prekallikrein activator with the electrophoretic mobility of prealbumin in man (Movat *et al.*, 1971; Soltay *et al.*, 1971) and in the guinea pig (Teloar and Movat, 1970).

In still other independent and concurrent work, Cochrane and his colleagues have investigated the components of the kinin system in rabbit and human plasma (Wuepper *et al.*, 1969, 1970; Cochrane and Wuepper, 1971; Wuepper and Cochrane, 1972). They have isolated but a single kininogen from rabbit plasma (cf. Spragg and Austen, 1971) and only a single prekallikrein from both rabbit and human preparations. Prekallikrein is a glycoprotein with a molecular weight of 99,900 (rabbit) or 107,000 (man) and is selectively activated by an acidic enzyme (prekallikrein activator) which owes its effects to "limited proteolysis" (Fig. 8). In agreement with Kaplan and Austen (1971), the activator of prekallikrein has been identified as a fragment (MW 32,000) of Hageman factor (MW 110,000) with the electrophoretic mobility of prealbumin (Cochrane and Wuepper, 1971). Activation of prekallikrein involves enzymic cleavage into two polypeptide fragments with molecular weights of 88,000 and 11,000, respectively, the larger fragment being kallikrein.

In summary, the identification by Kaplan and Austen of prekallikrein activator as a one-stage cleavage product from its precursor, Hageman

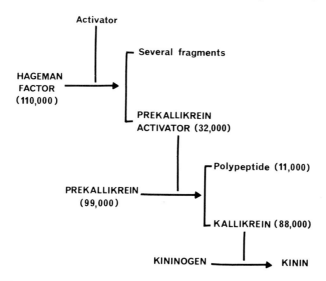

Fig. 8. Diagrammatic summary of the formation of kinins in rabbit plasma, according to Cochrane and Wuepper (see text), and Kaplan and Austen (1970, 1971). The numbers in parentheses refer to the reported molecular weights of the corresponding substances. (Redrawn and modified from Cochrane and Wuepper, 1971.)

factor, is supported by Cochrane and his colleagues (Fig. 8). Judged by the further results of Cochrane and his colleagues, as well as of Spragg and Austen (1971), the rest of the plasma kinin system is correspondingly simple, with but a single kallikrein and a single kininogen.

c. KALLIKREIN ANTAGONISTS. Of various antagonists reported in animal and plant tissues (Vogel et al., 1966), the best known is "Trasylol," a polyvalent protease inhibitor (MW 6511) which occurs in bovine parotid, pancreas, and lung (see Schachter, 1969). Based on recent work with highly purified components of the kinin system, Wuepper and Cochrane (1972) report that kallikrein is antagonized by Trasylol, soya bean trypsin inhibitor, and diisopropyl fluorophosphate (DFP), but not by the trypsin inhibitors in lima bean or ovomucoid, tolsyllysinechromomethyl ketone (TLCK), or phenylmethylsulfonyl fluoride (PMSF).

d. KININOGENS. Margolis and Bishop (1963) considered that plasma kininogens comprised two substrates associated with α_2-globulins and corresponding, respectively, to the decapeptide, kallidin, and the nonapeptide, bradykinin. Further work by Pierce and Webster (1966), Pierce (1968), and Habermann (1966) identified two groups of kininogens, I and II, which are glycoproteins with a molecular weight of about 50,000 and which represent the main kininogen content of plasma. These low molecular weight (LMW) kininogens yield kallidin when treated with human urinary kallikrein, and yield bradykinin when treated with trypsin (Fig. 9).

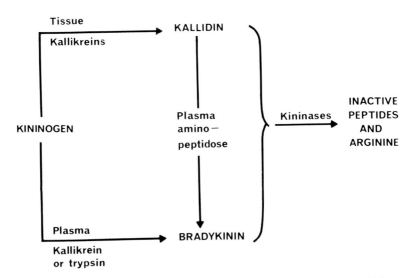

Fig. 9. Diagrammatic summary of the interrelationships between kininogens, kinins, and their breakdown products. (Redrawn from Wilhelm, 1971c.)

Two other classes of kininogens, a and b, have high molecular weights (HMW). Those designated HMW-a have a molecular weight of about 200,000 and, like LMW kininogens, yield kallikrein when treated with human urinary kallikrein, but bradykinin when treated with trypsin or plasma kallikrein. The HMW-b kinogens (Webster *et al.*, 1969) have not been characterized, but seem to be hydrolyzed by trypsin alone. However, Spragg and Austen (1971) have recently suggested that the multiple human kininogens reported from other laboratories may represent modifications of a single plasma kininogen, a proposal which arises from their own work and which is supported by that of Cochrane and Wuepper (see above).

e. KININ BREAKDOWN. In tests with the blood-bathed organ technique, kinins have a half-life of < 15 seconds (Ferreira and Vane, 1967). Human plasma contains two known kininases of which the first, carboxypeptidase N, cleaves the C-terminal arginine residue (Fig. 5) from bradykinin and kallidin, whereas the second is a peptidase that splits off both the C-terminal arginine and the adjacent phenylalanine residues (Erdös and Sloane, 1962; Yang and Erdös, 1967). Human plasma also contains one, or possibly two, aminopeptidases that rapidly convert kallidin to bradykinin (Fig. 9; see Schachter, 1969). Kinins are destroyed more effectively in the pulmonary than in the extrapulmonary circulation (Ferreira and Vane, 1967), and tissue kininases also include cathepsins from the spleen (Greenbaum and Yamafuji, 1966), kidney (Erdös and Yang, 1965), and intestinal mucosa (Amunsden and Nustad, 1965). Of two carboxypeptidases (A and B) in pancreas, B from hog pancreas has the highest kininase activity which has been identified (Skinner and Webster, 1968).

C. Other Endogenous Permeability Factors

Three other groups of permeability factors have been proposed as natural mediators in the inflammatory response, *viz.*, (1) substances with relatively prolonged permeability effects in the rabbit; (2) the complement system; and (3) prostaglandins.

1. SUBSTANCES WITH PROLONGED PERMEABILITY EFFECTS IN THE RABBIT

Vasoactive amines and kinins induce permeability responses that usually last about 10 minutes, and not more than 15–20 minutes, in both guinea pigs and rats. In the rabbit, the effects of histamine, for example, have a similar short duration in about half the test animals. In the other half, however, the permeability response may last an hour or more (Logan and Wilhelm, 1966b).

The short-term effects of amines and kinins, particularly in the guinea pig and rat, have aroused some interest in a group of permeability factors with effects lasting 1–2 hours, thereby coming closer in duration to the major response in moderate or severe injury. These factors include various proteins or large peptides (Table II) which, except Hageman factor, have been obtained from the cells or plasma of the rabbit. However, for all these factors, including Hageman factor, the prolonged effects are only demonstrable when tested in rabbit skin. Exogenous factors, such as various bacterial toxins (Table II), may have remarkably prolonged permeability effects in

TABLE II

ENDOGENOUS SUBSTANCES WITH PROLONGED PERMEABILITY EFFECTS
ONLY IN THE RABBIT AND BACTERIAL TOXINS WITH
PROLONGED EFFECTS IN BOTH THE GUINEA PIG AND RABBIT

Permeability factor	Age of lesion at maximal permeability response (hours)
Endogenous substances	
Rabbit granulocytic substance[a,b]	$1\frac{1}{2}$–2
Rabbit neutrophil granules[c]	2
Pseudoglobulin fraction of rabbit skin in thermal injury and Arthus reaction[d]	1
Rabbit globulin PF[e]	$1\frac{1}{2}$–$2\frac{1}{2}$
Hageman factor[f]	$1\frac{1}{2}$–2
Bacterial toxins	
C. welchii type A, α toxin[g,h]	3–4
C. welchii type E, ι toxin[i]	12–18
C. septicum, α toxin[g]	$\frac{3}{4}$–4
C. oedematiens, α toxin[g,j]	20–35
V. cholerae toxin[k]	16–24

[a]Moses et al. (1964).
[b]Muller et al. (1968).
[c]Golub and Spitznagel (1966).
[d]Hayashi et al. (1964).
[e]Wilhelm et al. (1958).
[f]Graham et al. (1965).
[g]Elder and Miles (1957).
[h]Logan and Wilhelm (1966c).
[i]Craig and Miles (1961).
[j]Cotran and Pathak (1968).
[k]Craig (1965a, b).

several species, but the endogenous factors listed in Table II are among the few that evoke reasonably prolonged permeability responses. However, their effects are peculiar to the rabbit and recall the fact that even histamine evokes a permeability response lasting longer in this species than in the guinea pig or rat.

2. THE COMPLEMENT SYSTEM

The evidence for derivatives of the complement system as potent chemotactic factors is dealt with elsewhere in this volume. In addition, the complement system has recently been proposed for a significant role in the permeability response in inflammation. Dias da Silva and Lepow (1967) have isolated a polypeptide which is dissociated from $C'3$ by the action of $C'1$ esterase on $C'2$ and $C'4$ in the presence of magnesium ions. The polypeptide, designated $F(a)$ $C'3$, has the properties of an anaphylatoxin that liberates histamine from mast cells of rat peritoneum and whose strong permeability effects in man are suppressed by antihistamine (Lepow et al., 1970). On the other hand, Jensen (1967) related the production of anaphylatoxin activity to $C'5$ and not $C'3$, while Cochrane and Müller-Eberhard (1968) reported that both $C'3$ and $C'5$ may serve as parent molecules for two distinct anaphylatoxins, as well as from the guinea pig counterpart. Whatever the final answer on these anaphylatoxins, however, the dependence of their permeability effects on the liberation of histamine seems to be a major argument against their role as prime mediators of increased vascular permeability in inflammation (see below).

3. PROSTAGLANDINS

Prostaglandins are widely distributed in the body (Horton, 1969), and both prostaglandins E_1 and E_2 increase vascular permeability in rat skin (Crunkhorn and Willis, 1971). Prostaglandin E_1 disrupts mast cells (Horton, 1963). Although the prostaglandins have substantial PF activity in the rat (Arora et al., 1970), their role is open to the same criticism as that for anaphylatoxin, viz., that PF activity is due to the liberation of histamine.

IV. Evidence for the Natural Role of Amines, Polypeptides, and Proteases in the Inflammatory Process

The criteria for identifying the mediators in inflammation can be considered in two categories: (1) those supporting the plausibility of a substance's natural role, and (2) those proving its actual participation (Miles and Wilhelm, 1960a).

A. Criteria Supporting Plausibility

Briefly, the criteria supporting plausibility include the distribution of a factor both in the various tissues of the same animal and between different species; its availability and activability; its induction of the appropriate vascular response and its potency in this respect; and, finally, the presence of natural antagonists. The criteria were discussed in detail by Miles and Wilhelm (1960a) who concluded that on these grounds all the above factors may possibly play a natural role in inflammation.

Table III summarizes the PF potencies of various factors in the skin of laboratory animals. Of the amines, histamine has high PF potency in the guinea pig and rabbit, but low activity in the rat, whereas 5-HT has strong

TABLE III

PF POTENCY (EBD[a]/MG) OF VARIOUS PERMEABILITY FACTORS—VASOACTIVE AMINES AND THEIR LIBERATORS (GROUP I), KININS (GROUP II), AND VARIOUS OTHER PROTEOLYTIC AND ESTEROLYTIC SUBSTANCES (GROUP III) IN THE GUINEA PIG, RAT AND RABBIT

Permeability factor		EDB[a]/mg when tested in		
Group	Substance[b]	Guinea pig	Rat	Rabbit
I	Histamine (1)	32,200	1,400	37,000
	5-Hydroxytryptamine (1)	60	16,200	< 20
	Compound 48/80 (1)	3,500	6,800	30
	Polymyxin B (2)	1,120	14,900	< 20
II	Bradykinin (3)	2,700,000	9,720	2,330,000
	Kallidin (3)	2,133,000	5,820	769,000
	Leukotaxine (2)	65	nt[c]	nt[c]
	"Leucotaxine" (2)	320	120	80
	Eledoisin (3)	1,780,000	168,000	< 20
III	Guinea pig globulin PF (2)	38,700	1,100	130
	Rat globulin PF (2)	1,400	620	400
	Rabbit globulin PF (2)	930	120	22,000
	Guinea pig TAM esterase (4)	50,000	50	600,000
	Kallikrein (hog) (2)	240	70	1,130
	Trypsin (bovine) (5)	2,560	900	600

[a]EBD, Effective blueing dose (see Wilhelm *et al.*, 1958).
[b]Parenthetical numbers refer to reference sources:
(1), data from Sparrow and Wilhelm (1957); (2), data from Miles and Wilhelm (1960a); (3), the above results are calculated from data from Carr and Wilhelm (1965); (4), data from Freund *et al.* (1958); (5), data from D. L. Wilhelm (unpublished, 1957).
[c]nt, Not tested.

activity in the rat, but low in the other two species. Compound 48/80 and polymyxin B have comparable activities in the rat as liberators of histamine, but both preparations also release 5-HT (Bushby and Green, 1955; Bhattacharya and Lewis, 1956; Parratt and West, 1957).

Similar interspecies differences in PF activity are also exhibited by the kinins. Bradykinin has outstanding PF activity in the guinea pig and rabbit (Konzett and Boissonas, 1960; Elliott *et al.*, 1960e, 1961), but relatively low PF potency in the rat (Carr and Wilhelm, 1965). Kallidin differs from bradykinin only in possessing an N-terminal lysine residue (Fig. 5), but, in all three species, it has rather less activity than bradykinin. Structural studies of bradykinin indicate that the arginines at either terminal (Fig. 5) have equal importance for biological activity (Schröder and Hempel, 1964; Stewart and Woolley, 1967; Melrose *et al.*, 1970), whereas the glycine and serine residues probably act as "spacers" which provide appropriate separation of the important functional groups (Stewart and Woolley, 1967).

High vasoactivity may also be exhibited by straight chain polypeptides in which the nature and arrangement of the amino acids differ substantially from those in kinins. For example, eledoisin is a peptide obtained from the posterior salivary gland of *Eledone*, a close relative of the genus *Octopus*. Its eleven amino acid residues differ substantially in both nature and arrangement from the nine residues of bradykinin (Erspamer and Anastasi, 1962).

Bradykinin: Arg-Pro-Pro-Gly-Phe-Ser-Pro-Phe-Arg

Eledoisin: Pyr*-Pro-Ser-Lys-Asp(OH)-Ala-Phe-Ileu-Gly-Leu-Met-NH₂

*Pyr = pyroglutamyl

Eledoisin has high PF activity in both the guinea pig and rat, but negligible activity in the rabbit (Table III). In the guinea pig, eledoisin's potency matches that of bradykinin and kallidin, but, in the rat, it outstrips that of any other permeability factor that has been tested in this species (Carr and Wilhelm, 1965).

Of various proteases that have been tested, most have relatively low PF activity. However, the varying activity of a guinea pig TAM esterase in the rabbit, guinea pig, and rat (Freund *et al.*, 1958; Table III) illustrates still again how the potency of permeability factors may vary among different species and the importance, therefore, of testing PF's in the homologous species.

An important criterion contributing to the plausibility of the natural role of a permeability factor concerns the duration of its effects. The endogenous PF's as a group characteristically increase permeability maximally in about 3 minutes, but the effects last only 10–15 minutes and at the most about 20 minutes. The main exception to this generalization is provided by a group of endogenous susbtances with relatively prolonged effects in rabbit skin (Table II), which are similar to those obtained in bacterial infection and thermal injury. With the exception of Hageman factor, however, both the PF's and their prolonged effects are peculiar to the rabbit.

The majority of endogenous PF's evoke a response similar in duration to the immediate phase of the permeability response in injury, and histamine and 5-HT, in fact, are often responsible for these immediate events (see below).

It remains to be demonstrated, however, whether or not delayed and prolonged permeability responses can be mediated by short-acting substances. Such a proposal requires that (1) adequate PF is locally available to initiate and maintain the response, (2) the release of PF is continuous and prolonged, and (3) the blood vessels in the injured site can respond adequately for a relatively long period.

The first and second requirements might reasonably be obtained. For example, although the amount of histamine in guinea pig skin (see Feldberg, 1956) appears inadequate to maintain the late response in, e.g., thermal injury, the local supply of histamine could well be replenished by activation of histidine decarboxylase (Schayer, 1963). On the other hand, the large reservoir of plasma proteins would ensure adequate supplies of kinins.

Similarly, all the endogenous PF's are activated or liberated with comparative ease *in vitro* and, hence, if available in sufficient amounts, could well be released *in vivo* for periods equal to the duration of the delayed response.

The third requirement—that the blood vessels are able to respond to repeated and prolonged stimulation—has been a major stumbling block to accepting the amines as relevant mediators. Histamine, for example, induces refractoriness of the test site to subsequent injections of histamine or histamine liberators (Miles and Miles, 1952). The combination of short-term effects with induction of refractoriness to further increase of vascular permeability therefore makes it hard to accept that histamine, for example, could play anything but a minor role in permeability responses in inflammation.

On the other hand, the situation concerning kinins has been substantially changed by Greaves and Shuster's (1967) observation that, for the dermal vessels of the human forearm, histamine or 5-HT induces tachyphylaxis to wealing, whereas bradykinin does not. Intracutaneous injections of all three factors initially evoke both wealing and erythema, whereas arterial occlusion applied prior to injection of PF suppresses wealing, but not erythema. When the circulation is restored 30 minutes after injection of PF, wealing with all three PF's is absent or minimal.

This ingenious application of Lewis' earlier experiments (1927) was then employed by Greaves and Shuster (1967) to test the response of dermal vessels at sites where one of the PF's had been previously injected. After 100 μg of histamine had been initially injected in skin rendered ischemic by occlusion, a further injection in the same site of 100 μg of histamine 5 minutes after restoration of the circulation resulted in no wealing in six of eight subjects and markedly reduced wealing in the other two. Similar results were obtained with 5-HT.

When bradykinin (10 μg) was the initial test substance, wealing was again absent when the circulation was restored 30 minutes later. But a second dose of 10 μg of bradykinin elicited weals having dimensions comparable to those at control sites receiving an initial dose of bradykinin. In contrast to histamine or 5-HT, bradykinin therefore does not induce tachyphylaxis. In further tests, Greaves and Shuster (1967) also demonstrated that bradykinin does not induce tachyphylaxis to histamine, nor histamine to bradykinin. The specificity of tachyphylaxis, as well as the failure of an antihistamine to antagonize wealing with bradykinin, prompted Greaves and Shuster (1967) to conclude that bradykinin and histamine act on separate vascular receptors. Similar results for bradykinin have been observed in rabbits, guinea pigs, and rats by Oyvin *et al.* (1967).

At the time that the report of Greaves and Shuster (1967) was published, Baumgarten and his colleagues (Baumgarten *et al.*, 1967, 1970b) were developing a technique for the continuous recording of permeability responses in guinea pig skin. The indicator of increased permeability was ^{32}P since this isotope emits only β particles with short penetrating power (8 mm in water; Levi, 1959). ^{32}Phosphorous is therefore suitable for the scanning of skin because radiation from the underlying tissues is absorbed. [^{32}Phosphorous] phosphanilic acid (Baumgarten *et al.*, 1968) was coupled to bovine serum albumin (BSA) and the complex given intravenously to unanesthetized guinea pigs.

Baumgarten and his colleagues (1970b) then used the above test system to demonstrate that the results of Greaves and Shuster (1967) for man were also applicable to the guinea pig. Histamine induced refractoriness to a subsequent permeability response of the same PF injected 30–60 minutes later, with refractoriness subsequently subsiding by half in $3\frac{1}{2}$ hours (cf. Miles and Miles, 1952). Contrary to Greaves and Shuster's (1967) results in man, however, Baumgarten *et al.* (1970b) observed that initial treatment with histamine did not affect the subsequent response to bradykinin. Initial injection of bradykinin, in turn, had no effect on the subsequent response to further bradykinin or equipotent doses of histamine.

Refractoriness of permeability responses induced by histamine or its liberators to subsequent doses of the same PF's increases in degree for periods up to 2 hours, but declines after 4 hours (Miles and Miles, 1952). Nevertheless, Miles (see Miles and Wilhelm, 1960a) has considered that short-acting PF's might well mediate prolonged permeability responses.

The above results of Greaves and Shuster (1967) and Baumgarten *et al.* (1970b) now make Miles' forecast a distinct possibility.

B. Criteria Proving Mediation

Proof that a PF is a natural mediator may be obtained (1) by isolating the PF at the relevant period of the inflammatory process, or (2) by suppressing the response in animals that are treated with specific antagonists or analogs of PF's, or that are depleted of a particular PF.

The isolation of a factor clearly has prime importance not only in identifying the mediator, but also in guiding tests of inhibition or depletion. Nevertheless, the attempted isolation of a relevant PF is complicated both by the simple release of histamine in practically any tissue manipulation as well as by the presence of the globulin PF in normal tissue fluid (Miles and Wilhelm, 1958).

Most of the available antagonists are not sufficiently specific to permit a confident assessment of their effects. For example, antihistamines are well known to be anticholinergic, and the trypsin inhibitors of vegetable origin usually antagonize plasmin, kallikrein, and globulin PF. The few antagonists with substantial effects on kinins often suppress other PF's such as histamine (Rocha e Silva, 1964).

On the other hand, the mediator may never be released in a free state, but as Dale's (1948) "intrinsic histamine," it may instead be produced in the cells responding to it and hence be pharmacologically inaccessible (Miles and Wilhelm, 1960a). The use of analogs promises to have greatest relevance for kinins, but satisfactory analogs are not yet available.

Although the depletion of amines in rats has provided evidence of their role in the early stages of chemical and thermal injury (Spector and Willoughby, 1959a,b), the process of depletion itself induces nonspecific suppression of reactivity to various permeability factors (Wilhelm *et al.*, 1958). Depletion of potential kinin reservoirs is obviously not feasible.

In summary, the criteria proving mediation seem difficult to attain. The isolation of factors must remain of prime importance, but the use of inhibitors seems preferable to depletion procedures.

C. Susceptibility of Permeability Responses in Inflammation to Various Antagonists

Three groups of inhibitors have been investigated for their effects on the permeability response in injury: (1) antihistamines and 5-HT antagonists, (2) inhibitors of kinins, proteases, and esterases, and (3) various other preparations, some of which appear to have nonspecific activity.

Since the permeability response in injury may be immediate, delayed, or early in type, or various combinations of these main types (see Section II,C, 3), it is convenient to discuss the effects of antagonists on each main type of permeability response.

1. SUSCEPTIBILITY OF THE IMMEDIATE PERMEABILITY RESPONSE

If the time course of the permeability responses and the refractoriness which are induced by endogenous mediators are reliable guides to their role in injury, we might anticipate that the vasoactive amines do no more than induce the immediate phase of the permeability response in inflammation. This conclusion is fully supported by tests with appropriate antagonists which indicate that immediate-type responses are mediated by histamine or 5-HT in thermal and ultraviolet injury, hypersensitivity, and bacterial infection.

The immediate response in thermal injury in guinea pigs, rabbits (54°C for 5 seconds; Wilhelm and Mason, 1960), and rats (55°C for 27 seconds; Spector and Willoughby, 1959b; cf. Wilhelm and Mason, 1960) is suppressed by relatively small doses of antihistamines such as triprolidine or mepyramine, injected intravenously or locally in the test site. When an immediate response is the initial event in a diphasic response in skin sites heated to 54°C for 20 seconds (Fig. 2), the immediate phase retains its susceptibility to antihistamine, but its suppression in no way affects the onset or maturation of the subsequent delayed phase.

In ultraviolet injury, tests with pharmacological antagonists indicate that the immediate response is usually abolished in guinea pigs by antihistamine, and in rats by a 5-HT antagonist, but the mediator of the immediate response in rabbits remains unidentified (Logan and Wilhelm, 1966a,b).

Cutaneous anaphylaxis evokes a typical immediate-type permeability response which is variously reported to have strong, slight, or no susceptibility to antihistamine drugs (Ovary, 1958; Craig and Wilhelm, 1963; Brocklehurst et al., 1955). In our own experience, suppression in the guinea pig is variable and usually slight. It seems noteworthy, however, that the absence of suppression by antihistamine reported by Brocklehurst et al. (1955) was observed in the rat. The immediate phase of the diphasic response in the tuberculin reaction in guinea pigs has moderate susceptibility to antihistamine (Baumgarten and Wilhelm, 1969a). In staphylococcal infection of rabbit skin, the initial permeability response is also suppressed by antihistamine (Petri et al., 1952).

In summary, the results with relatively small doses of antagonists of histamine or 5-HT indicate that these vasoactive amines are the relevant mediators of most examples of immediate-type permeability responses. This conclusion is supported by the demonstration that the ultrastructural vascular lesion in immediate-type responses resembles the lesion with local histamine or 5-HT, i.e., the formation of endothelial gaps in venules, particularly in medium-sized venules, 20–30 μm in diameter (Majno and Palade, 1961; Cotran and Majno, 1964; Cotran and Remensnyder, 1968).

2. Evidence Concerning the Delayed Permeability Response

Although the mediation of the immediate response seems to be established, opinions on the late response conflict. There is agreement, however, that the late response does not appear to be evoked by vascoactive amines (see Wilhelm, 1962; Spector and Willoughby, 1963) since antihistamines or 5-HT antagonists in no way affect the delayed events. This is equally true whether the drugs are given before injury and hence suppress the immediate response or during the maturation of the response.

The role of histamine in mediating the early permeability response has been interpreted as one of initiating but not sustaining the vascular sequelae of injury (Spector, 1958). On the other hand, the results with antihistamines might equally indicate that the early permeability response is not a necessary precursor of the late events, but simply reflects the ease with which histamine can be liberated from tissues by practically any type of manipulation. Nevertheless, Schayer's demonstration (1961) that the rise and fall of histidine decarboxylase activity in injured sites parallels the maturation and decline of the delayed response means that histamine cannot be entirely dismissed as the mediator; but the consensus favors kinins for this role rather than histamine.

Suppression of edema evoked in the rat's paw by injecting kaolin has been accomplished by relatively large doses (50 mg/kg intraperitoneally) of trypsin and esterase inhibitors from soybean, potato, and pancreas (Hladovec et al., 1958). Similar suppression of the delayed response in thermal or ultraviolet injury has not been obtained with these drugs (Wilhelm and Mason, 1960; Logan and Wilhelm, 1966b), but conflicting results have been reported with an esterase inhibitor, diisopropyl fluorophosphorate (DFP). This is an organophosphorus compound that decreases both edema and dye exudation in thermal injury and X irradiation in rats (Spector and Willoughby, 1959b; Willoughby, 1960)—a conclusion supported by the effects on thermal injury of various other esterase antagonists (Spector and Willoughby, 1960). Nevertheless, DFP has high toxicity (Aldridge, 1956), and, judged by its suppression of nonprotease PF's (Spector and Willoughby, 1960), the drug's effects in injury may be largely nonspecific. The problem is further complicated becasue other workers (Wilhelm and Mason, 1960) have failed to suppress the late response in thermal injury with DFP, and the role of esterases remains unsettled (cf. Spector and Willoughby, 1963).

Evidence from the use of antagonists of kallikreins and other proteases has yielded no convincing evidence to support the role of the kinin system in mediating delayed permeability responses in inflammation. On the other hand, increased levels of bradykinin itself have been reported in blister fluid, serum, and urine from patients with burns (Goodwin et al., 1963). In experimental thermal injury (44°–45°C for 30 minutes) of the rat's paw, Rocha e Silva (9164) has also demonstrated that edema is accompanied by release of kinin, the formation of edema being strongly suppressed by cyproheptadine, imipramine, dibenzyline, and reserpine, less so by chlorpromazin and dibenamine. Although these drugs suppress the vasoactivity of kinins, they also antagonize that of histamine, 5-HT, epinephrine, and acetylcholine. Similarly, intraperitoneal cellulose sulfate or carrageenan moderately depresses the level of plasma kininogen (Leme et al., 1967), but such treatment seems certain to have other nonspecific effects so that the suppression of thermally induced edema lacks conviction correspondingly (cf. Rocha e Silva, 1964). As with thermal injury, there is some evidence to suggest that kinins might be involved in the later stages of the permeability responses evoked by chemical and crush injury (Lykke et al., 1967; Cummings and Lykke, 1970), but the various authors themselves point out that their evidence is inconclusive.

In summary, of the established permeability factors, the kinins seem most likely to be the final mediators of the delayed permeability response. Repeated doses of bradykinin do not induce refractoriness of the vascular permeability response, and the main ultrastructural lesion is the interendothelial gap, which by analogy with immediate-type responses is consistent with increased permeability induced by biochemical mediation. Nevertheless, a satisfactory pharmacological evaluation of the role of kinins is currently restricted by the absence of appropriate antagonists.

3. EVIDENCE CONCERNING THE EARLY PERMEABILITY RESPONSE

The ultrastructural lesion in peripheral blood vessels involved in the early response is mainly endothelial damage. However, the basement membrane remains surprisingly intact, even in capillaries exhibiting substantial damage. Pharmacological antagonists, as expected, have little effect on early responses. Antihistamines slow the onset and early development of superficial chemical lesions in guinea pigs (Miles and Wilhelm, 1960a), but the suppression is slight and not detectable in the fully developed response. In turpentine pleurisy of rats, antihistamine also suppresses the initial permeability effects (Spector and Willoughby, 1959b), although it has not been established whether or not these initial events correspond to an immediate-type response or to the preliminary stages of an early-type response.

If the occasional interendothelial gap seen in early-type lesions reflects pharmacological activity, the mediator might be vasoactive amine and/or kinin. Nevertheless, the contribution by either type of permeability factor is probably small.

4. THE HISTAMINE CONTROVERSY

Earlier reference has been made in this chapter to the conclusions of Lewis (1927) concerning the role of histamine in the triple response and the subsequent controversy aroused by the demonstration that antihistamines failed to suppress the permeability response in experimental injury. Nevertheless, the two sets of results are explainable in terms of variation in technique, particularly from more recent work in guinea pigs.

Briefly, the immediate permeability response induced by mild heating (54°C for 5 seconds) and the initial immediate phase in the diphasic response evoked by 54°C for 20 seconds in guinea pigs are suppressed by antihistamines, whereas the delayed phase with 54°C for 20 seconds and the early response with stronger heating are unaffected. When the heating is increased 2°–6°C above 54°C, the initial immediate response becomes progressively less noticeable, and the delayed phase becomes stronger as well as quicker in development; at 58°C for 20 seconds, the diphasic pattern is replaced by a monophasic "early" response, insusceptible to antihistamine (Wilhelm and Mason, 1960).

The evidence from work in guinea pigs seems relevant to that in both man and the rabbit, because in all three species histamine has high PF activity, and it explains why heating at 43°–52°C for 5–180 seconds in man (Lewis and Love, 1926) induces only a histamine response, whereas stronger heating —60°C for 15 seconds in man (Sevitt *et al.*, 1952) or 96°C for 10 seconds in the rabbit (Weeks and Gunnar, 1949) evokes a susbtantial response insusceptible to antihistamine.

5. EVIDENCE CONCERNING VASODILATION

Lewis' work (1927) on the triple response suggests that capillary dilation is mediated by histamine, and arteriolar dilation by an axon reflex, which is itself perhaps stimulated by histamine. No further progress on the mechanisms of vasodilation ensued until evidence was forthcoming that kinins induce vasodilation in mild thermal stimulation (Fox and Hilton, 1958) and functional activity of the salivary gland (Hilton and Lewis, 1955, 1956), although not in other tissues (see Hilton, 1963). Experimentally, kinins have outstanding activity as vasodilator substances and occur in significant amounts in conditions that exhibit prominent vasodilation, although their role as natural vasodilators under physiological or pathological circumstances nevertheless remains in doubt (see Schachter, 1966; Webster, 1966b; Skinner and Webster, 1968).

Falling between the kinin and histamine theories are the observations of Wilhelm and Domenjoz (1951) that various butazone and salicylate preparations suppress ultraviolet erythema in guinea pigs, while Winder *et al.* (1958) observed that aminopyrine strikingly antagonizes the early erythema in ultraviolet injury, but not that at 24 hours.

Results with pharmacological antagonists in thermal and ultraviolet injury (Wilhelm and Mason, 1960; Logan and Wilhelm, 1966b) indicate that erythema is unaffected by treatment of laboratory animals with antihistamines or antagonists of proteases and esterases. The time course of erythema roughly corresponds to that of increased permeability in experimental inflammation, but, under particular circumstances in chemical injury of skin, erythema may be strong when the permeability response has subsided. Such a dissociation of these two responses may possibly be due to diversion of blood flow from superficial to deep vessels of the skin during the progression of the inflammatory response at the site of injury (Steele and Wilhelm, 1966, 1970). However, the peripheral mechanisms that control vasodilation and changes in blood flow remain poorly understood; two aspects which require further investigation are the role of kinins and of the nervous system (Steele, 1969).

6. EVIDENCE CONCERNING TISSUE LEUKOCYTOSIS

Tissue leukocytosis varies in relation to the main permeability response in inflammation according to the type of injury and species of test animal. In ultraviolet lesions, leukocytosis into injured skin sites reaches its peak in guinea pigs (Fig. 3) as the delayed permeability response is developing, but a relevant role for the emigrating leukocyte as mediator of increased permeability is not supported by testing the exudative response in animals rendered neutropenic with nitrogen mustard (Logan and Wilhelm, 1966a). More effective neutropenia is obtained with methotrexate, but again without affecting the permeability response in thermal or chemical injury in rats (Willoughby and Giroud, 1969). Although tissue leukocytosis also chronologically accompanies increased vascular permeability in bacterial infection (Burke and Miles, 1958) and the Arthus phenomenon (Stetson and Good, 1951; Humphrey, 1955), the emigration of neutrophils precedes the delayed permeability response in superficial chemical injury of guinea pig skin (Steele and Wilhelm, 1970) or follows the permeability response by an interval of 24 hours in ultraviolet lesions of rabbit skin (Fig. 3). However, despite the frequent lack of correlation between tissue leukocytosis and the main permeability response in experimental inflammation, this approach to the problem of mediation of vascular exudation requires much more information concerning the accumulation in injured tissues of both neutrophils and monocytes.

Chemotactic factors responsible for leukocytic emigration are considered elsewhere in this treatise. In the present context, it only remains to add that proposed mediators of tissue leukocytosis have not been assessed *in vivo* by the use of pharmacological antagonists.

V. Inflammatory Response in Various Organs

Practically all our knowledge of the inflammatory response is confined to the events in experimental injury of skin and to lesser extent, of muscle and the pleural cavity. But what of the response in other organs? Skin is peculiar in having a complicated network of venules in the dermis, but a striking lack of capillaries which are confined to the dermal papillae (Spalteholz, 1893; Majno, 1964). At the ultrastructural level, vascular endothelium varies considerably from organ to organ (Majno, 1965), so that the inflammatory response might be expected to exhibit corresponding heterogeneity.

In the lung, histamine, either inhaled as a nebule or injected subpleurally, causes exudation through interendothelial gaps in venules along the entire bronchial tree (Pietra *et al.*, 1971). Intraperitoneal injection of α-naphthylthiourea or ammonium sulfate provokes pulmonary edema that, in each case, occurs 60 minutes after treatment, but the technique of carbon labeling reveals that the effects of naphthylthiourea occur mainly in venules and less so in capillaries, whereas with ammonium sulfate the leaking vessels are capillaries (Böhm, 1966). In pulmonary edema provoked with nephrotoxic serum, carbon labeling predominates in capillaries (Böhm and Laus-Filho, 1968). Nevertheless, the progression and extent of the exudation of plasma in pulmonary edema have yet to be established.

Investigations of the inflammatory process in the intestine have been no less sporadic than in lung. Northover (1963, 1964) observed that intraperitoneal histamine, 5-HT, and bradykinin all induce an accumulation of peritoneal fluid, while Buckley and Ryan (1969) have reported that topical applications of histamine or 5-HT cause circulating carbon to accumulate in venules of rat mesentery without affecting their caliber. X Radiation of the abdomen evokes a delayed permeability response of the underlying bowel which commences at 24 hours and reaches a peak 72–96 hours after injury (Willoughby, 1960).

Studies of traumatic injury of internal organs have been complicated by exposure of the organs for surgical incision as the test stimulus. One of the few such studies made was that of Carscadden (1927) who investigated the inflammatory response in incisional injury of the liver. Plasma exudation commenced in 3 minutes, and the accumulation of fibrinogen became noticeable in $\frac{1}{2}$ hour, with leukocytic emigration being well established by the end of the first hour. Incisional wounds of the rabbit kidney and spleen also exhibited a ready accumulation of leukocytes, but for uterine wounds the cellular response was delayed until about 3 hours after injury (Carscadden, 1927). Needle biopsy wounds of the rat kidney induce a biphasic permeability response consisting of initial exudation due to the puncture wound, succeeded, in turn, by a delayed phase of exudation which is exhibited by lesions 3–6 hours old (R. N. Shute and A. W. J. Lykke, unpublished, 1970).

A striking example of chemical injury is provided by the subsceptibility of the mammalian testis to cadmium salts (Parizek and Zahor, 1956; Parizek, 1960). Subcutaneous cadmium chloride causes acute damage of the seminiferous tubules and interstitial tissue of the rat testis, with progression to necrosis of all seminiferous elements, and, finally, to fibrosis. In the initial 36 hours after giving subcutaneous cadmium chloride, there is progressive and, finally, intense engorgement of the testis and the proximal aspect of the head of the epididymis, corresponding to the tissues supplied by the internal spermatic artery, its testicular and epididymal branches, and the pampiniform plexus (Gunn et al., 1963). The same vascular bed exhibits a strong permeability response with extravasation of circulating Evan's blue from capillaries and venules beginning in 10 minutes, becoming substantial by 2 hours, maximal in 6 hours, and reported to involve even arterioles and small arteries (Clegg and Carr, 1967).

A similar vascular lesion and cellular necrosis are provoked by cadmium salts in the Gasserian ganglion and spinal sensory ganglia of the rat and other species of laboratory animals (Gabbiani, 1966). But the most exciting aspect of this unexpected involvement of both testis and Gasserian ganglion is that the small blood vessels in both sets of tissues have an endothelium exhibiting numerous luminal microvilli, arranged singly or in small groups (Gabbiani and Majno, 1969). The susceptibility of this unique endothelium to cadmium strongly suggests an enzymic lesion. Cadmium strongly inhibits sulfhydryl enzymes (Simon et al., 1947), but Gabbiani (1966) considers it unlikely that this is the mechanism involved in the effects of cadmium on nerve ganglia.

A more common model of chemical toxicity is provided by the effect of carbon tetrachloride on the parenchyma of the liver. McClugage and McCuskey (1971) consider that the initial lesion is microvascular, but the fenestrated endothelium that lines the hepatic sinusoids makes it unlikely that there would be exudation in the usual context—a conclusion that is supported by the results for carbon tetrachloride lesions in the guinea pig liver (T. N. Borody and D. L. Wilhelm, unpublished, 1971). Instead, the inflammatory response seems to be mainly characterized by adherence of neutrophils and monocytes to sinusoidal endothelium and migration of these leukocytes into the injured liver (McClugage and McCuskey, 1971; T. J. Borody and D. L. Wilhelm, unpublished, 1971).

The above references to inflammation in tissues other than skin and muscle by no means cover all the work on this subject. But the relatively few studies already made strongly suggest that the inflammatory response varies considerably among different organs and tissues. As Majno (1964) has forecast: "It may well turn out, in the end, that each organ is a special case of its own. This means that we will soon have to revise our stereotyped notion of acute inflammation, by adapting it to the particular environment of each organ."

VI. Conclusions

Half a century of work on the identification of substances increasing vascular permeability and the other vascular events in the inflammatory process has resulted in little reliable information concerning the relevant chemical mediators. Work in the last decade has established that the permeability response of skin or striated muscle is usually monophasic in mild or severe injury and diphasic in injury of moderate intensity, and that the pattern of the response is probably related to the severity of the stimulus rather than to the type of injury. Histamine or 5-hydroxytryptamine usually mediates the transient immediate phase of increased vascular permeability involving venules in mild injury or the same phase when it contributes the initial effect in diphasic responses that characterize moderate injury. Chemical mediation seems likely to be responsible for the delayed effects in diphasic responses, but it makes only a minor contribution to the strong permeability response evoked by severe injury. To date, however, the corresponding mediators have not been identified among kinins or vaso-active amines.

References

Abel, J., and Kubota, S. (1919). *J. Pharmacol. Exp. Ther.* **13**, 243.
Åborg, C.-H., Novotný, J., and Uvnäs, B. (1967). *Acta Physiol. Scand.* **69**, 276.
Aldridge, W. N. (1956). *Annu. Rep. Chem. Soc.* **53**, 294.

Allison, F., and Lancaster, M. G. (1959). *Brit. J. Exp. Pathol.* **40**, 324.
Amunsden, E., and Nustad, K. (1965). *J. Physiol. (London)* **179**, 479.
Arora, S., Lahiri, P. K., and Sanyal, R. K. (1970). *Int. Arch. Allergy Appl. Immunol.* **39**, 186.
Baker, R. V. (1959). *J. Physiol. (London)* **145**, 473.
Barger, G., and Dale, H. H. (1910a). *J. Physiol. (London)* **40**, 38P.
Barger, G., and Dale, H. H. (1910b). *J. Chem. Soc., (London)* **97**, 2592.
Barger, G., and Dale, H. H. (1911). *J. Physiol. (London)* **41**, 499.
Bhattacharya, B. K., and Lewis, G. P. (1956). *Brit. J. Pharmacol. Chemother.* **11**, 411.
Baumgarten, A., and Wilhelm, D. L. (1969a). *Pathology* **1**, 301.
Baumgarten, A., and Wilhelm, D. L. (1969b). *Pathology* **1**, 317.
Baumgarten, A., Melrose, G. J. H., and Vagg, W. J. (1967). *Experientia* **23**, 884.
Baumgarten, A., Melrose, G. J. H., and Vagg, W. J. (1968). *Anal. Biochem.* **24**, 243.
Baumgarten, A., Melrose, G. J. H., and Vagg, W. J. (1970a). *Dermatologica* **140**, 219.
Baumgarten, A., Melrose, G. J. H., and Vagg, W. J. (1970b). *J. Physiol. (London)* **208**, 669.
Beloff, A., and Peters, R. A. (1945). *J. Physiol. (London)* **103**, 461.
Bergendorff, A., and Uvnäs, B. (1967). *Acta Pharmacol. Toxicol.* **25**, Suppl. 4, 32.
Best, C. H., Dale, H. H., Dudley, H. W., and Thorpe, W. V. (1927). *J. Physiol. (London)* **62**, 397.
Bhattacharya, B. K., and Lewis, G. P. (1956). *Brit. J. Pharmacol. Chemother.* **11**, 411.
Bhoola, K. D., and Heap, P. F. (1970). *J. Physiol. (London)* **210**, 421.
Blaschko, H. (1958). *In* "5-Hydroxytryptamine" (G. P. Lewis, ed.), pp. 50–57. Pergamon, Oxford.
Böhm, G. M. (1966). *J. Pathol. Bacteriol.* **191**, 151.
Böhm, G. M., and Laus-Filho, J. A. (1968). *J. Pathol. Bacteriol.* **95**, 489.
Boissonas, R. A., Guttmann, St., Jaquenona, P. A., Konzett, H., and Sturmer, E. (1960). *Experientia* **16**, 326.
Brocklehurst, W. E., Humphrey, J. H., and Perry, W. L. (1955). *J. Physiol. (London)* **129**, 205.
Brodie, B. B. (1958). *In* "5-Hydroxytryptamine" (G. P. Lewis, ed.), pp. 64–83. Pergamon, Oxford.
Buckley, I. K., and Ryan, G. B. (1969). *Amer. J. Pathol.* **55**, 329.
Burke, J. F., and Miles, A. A. (1958). *J. Pathol. Bacteriol.* **76**, 1.
Bushby, S. R. M., and Green, A. F. (1955). *Brit. J. Pharmacol. Chemother.* **10**, 215.
Carr, J., and Wilhelm, D. L. (1964). *Aust. J. Exp. Biol. Med. Sci.* **42**, 511.
Carr, J., and Wilhelm, D. L. (1965). *Nature (London)* **208**, 653.
Carscadden, W. G. (1927). *Arch. Pathol.* **4**, 329.
Casenti, S., and Galli, G. (1956). *Boll. Soc. Ital. Biol. Sper.* **32**, 1640.
Chambers, R., and Zweifach, B. W. (1940). *J. Cell. Comp. Physiol.* **15**, 255.
Chambers, R., and Zweifach, B. W. (1947). *Physiol. Rev.* **27**, 436.
Clark, E. R., and Clark, E. L. (1935). *Amer. J. Anat.* **57**, 385.
Clark, E. R., and Clark, E. L. (1936). *Amer. J. Anat.* **59**, 123.
Clegg, E. I., and Carr, I. (1967). *J. Pathol. Bacteriol.* **94**, 317.
Cochrane, C. G., and Müller-Eberhard, H. J. (1968). *J. Exp. Med.* **127**, 371.
Cochrane, C. G., and Wuepper, K. D. (1971). *J. Exp. Med.* **134**, 986.
Cohnheim, J. (1882). "Vorlesungen," 2nd ed. Leipzig (translated by A. B. McKee, New Sydenham Society, London, 1889).
Collier, H. O. J. (1958). *In* "5-Hydroxytryptamine" (G. P. Lewis, ed.), pp. 5–19. Pergamon, Oxford.
Cotran, R. S. (1965). *Amer. J. Pathol.* **46**, 589.
Cotran, R. S. (1967a). *Lab. Invest.* **17**, 39.
Cotran, R. S. (1967b). *Exp. Mol. Pathol.* **6**, 143.
Cotran, R. S., and Majno, G. (1964). *Amer. J. Pathol.,* **45**, 261.

Cotran, R. S., and Pathak, M. A. (1968). *J. Invest. Dermatol.* **51**, 155.

Cotran, R. S., and Remensnyder, J. P. (1968). *Ann. N.Y. Acad. Sci.* **150**, 495.

Cotran, R. S., Suter, E. R., and Majno, G. (1967). *Vasc. Dis.* **4**, 107.

Craig, J. P. (1965a) *Nature (London)* **207**, 614.

Craig, J. P. (1965b). *In* "Proceedings of The Cholera Research Symposium" (O. A. Bushnell, and C. S. Brookhyser, eds.), pp. 153–158. U.S. Government Printing Office, Washington, D.C.

Craig, J. P., and Miles, A. A. (1961). *J. Pathol. Bacteriol.* **81**, 481.

Craig, J. P., and Wilhelm, D. L. (1963). *J. Immunol.* **90**, 43.

Crunkhorn, P. and Willis, A. L. (1971). *Brit. J. Pharmacol.* **41**, 49.

Cullumbine, H., and Rydon, H. N. (1946). *Brit. J. Exp. Pathol.* **27**, 33.

Cummings, R. (1971). M.D. Thesis, pp. 142–169. University of New South Wales.

Cummings, R., and Lykke, A. W. J. (1970). *Brit. J. Exp. Pathol.* **51**, 19.

Dale, H. H. (1948). *Brit. Med. J.* **2**, 281.

Dale, H. H., and Richards, A. N. (1918–1919). *J. Physiol. (London)* **52**, 110.

De Carvalho, I. F., and Diniz, C. R. (1964). *Ann. N.Y. Acad. Sci.* **116**, 912.

Dias da Silva, W., and Lepow, I. H. (1967). *J. Exp. Med.* **125**, 921.

Duthie, E. S., and Chain, E. (1939). *Brit. J. Exp. Pathol.* **20**, 417.

Ekfors, T. O., Riekkinen, P. J. Malmiharju, T., and Hopsu-Havu, V. K. (1967). *Hoppe-Seyler's Z. Physiol. Chem.* **348**, 111.

Elder, J. M., and Miles, A. A. (1957). *J. Pathol. Bacteriol.* **74**, 133.

Elliott, D. F., and Lewis, G. P. (1965). *Biochem. J.* **95**, 437.

Elliott, D. F., Lewis, G. P., and Horton, E. W. (1960a). *In* "Polypeptides which Affect Smooth Muscles and Blood Vessels" (M. Schachter, ed.), p. 266. Pergamon, Oxford.

Elliott, D. F., Lewis, G. P., and Horton, E. W. (1960b). *Biochem. J.* **74**, 15P.

Elliott, D. F., Lewis, G. P., and Horton, E. W. (1960c). *Biochem. J.* **76**, 16P.

Elliott, D. F., Lewis, G. P., and Horton, E. W. (1960d). *Biochem. Biophys. Res. Commun.* **3**, 87.

Elliott, D. F., Horton, E. W., and Lewis, G. P. (1960e). *J. Physiol. (London)* **153**, 473.

Elliott, D. F., Horton, E. W., and Lewis, G. P. (1961). *Biochem. J.* **78**, 60.

Eppinger, H. (1913). *Wien. Med. Wochenschr.* **63**, 1413.

Erdös, E. G., and Sloane, E. M. (1962). *Biochem. Pharmacol.* **11**, 585.

Erdös, E. G., and Yang, H. Y. T. (1965). *Biochem. Pharmacol.* **14**, 1391.

Erspamer, V. (1954). *Pharmacol. Rev.* **6**, 425.

Erspamer, V., and Anastasi, A. (1962). *Experientia* **18**, 58.

Erspamer, V., and Asero, B. (1952). *Nature (London)* **169**, 800.

Faulk, W. P., Snippe, H., and Pondman, K. W. (1971). *Immunology* **21**, 489.

Feldberg, W. (1956). *Histamine, Ciba Found. Symp., 1955* pp. 4–13.

Feldberg, W., and Paton, W. D. M. (1951). *J. Physiol. (London)* **114**, 490.

Feldberg, W., and Schachter, M. (1952). *J. Physiol. (London)* **118**, 124.

Ferreira, S. H., and Vane, J. R. (1967). *Brit. J. Pharmacol.* **30**, 417.

Fiedler, F., and Werle, E. (1967). *Hoppe-Seyler's Z. Physiol. Chem.* **348**, 1087.

Florey, H. (1970). "General Pathology," 4th ed., pp. 21–127. Lloyd-Luke, London.

Florey, H. W., and Grant, L. H. (1961). *J. Pathol. Bacteriol.* **82**, 13.

Forell, M. M. (1957). *Schweiz. Med. Wochenschr.* **87**, 828.

Fox, R. H., and Hilton, S. M. (1958). *J. Physiol. (London)* **142**, 219.

Freund, J., Miles, A. A., Mill, P. J., and Wilhelm, D. L. (1958). *Nature (London)* **182**, 174.

Frey, E. K. (1963). *Ann. N.Y. Acad. Sci.* **104**, 90.

Frey, E. K., and Kraut, H. (1926). Naunyn-Schmiedebergs Arch. Exp. Pathol. Pharmakol. **133**, 1.

Frey, E. K., Kraut, H., and Schultz, F. (1930). Naunyn-Schmiedebergs Arch. Exp. Pathol. Pharmakol. **158**, 334.

Frey, E. K., Kraut, H., and Werle, E. (1968). "Das Kallikrein-Kinin-System und Sein Inhibitoren." Enke, Stuttgart.

Friedberger, E. (1909). Z. Immunforsch. Exp. Ther. **2**, 208.

Fritz, H., Eckert, I., and Werle, E. (1967). Hoppe-Seyler's Z. Physiol. Chem. **348**, 1120.

Gabbiani, G. (1966). Experientia **22**, 261.

Gabbiani, G., and Majno, G. (1969). Z. Zellforsch. Mikrosk. Anat. **97**, 111.

Garattini, S., and Valzelli, L. (1965). "Serotonin." Elsevier, Amsterdam.

Golub, E. S., and Spitznagel, J. K. (1966). J. Immunol. **95**, 1060.

Goodwin, L. G., Jones, C. R., Richards, W. H. G., and Kohn, J. (1963). Brit. J. Exp. Pathol. **44**, 551.

Graham, H. T., Lowry, O. H., Wheelwright, F., and Lenz, M. A. (1955). Blood **10**, 467.

Graham, R. C., Ebert, R. H., Ratnoff, O. D., and Moses, J. M. (1965). J. Exp. Med. **121**, 807.

Greaves, M., and Shuster, S. (1967). J. Physiol. (London) **193**, 255.

Greenbaum, L. M., and Yamafuji, K. (1966). In "Hypotensive Peptides" (E. G. Erdös, N. Back, and F. Sicuteri, eds.), pp. 252–260. Springer-Verlag, Berlin and New York.

Gunn, S. A., Gould, T. C., and Anderson, W. A. D. (1963). Amer. J. Pathol. **42**, 685.

Habermann, E. (1966). In "Hypotensive Peptides" (E. G. Erdös, N. Back, and F. Sicuteri, eds.), pp. 116–128. Springer-Verlag, Berlin and New York.

Habermann, E., and Klett, W. (1966). Biochem. Z. **346**, 133.

Hamlin, K. E., and Fisher, F. E. (1954). J. Amer. Chem. Soc. **73**, 5007.

Harris, H. (1954). Physiol. Rev. **34**, 529.

Hayashi, H., Yoshinaga, M., Koono, M., Miyoshi, H., and Matsumura, M. (1964). Brit. J. Exp. Pathol. **45**, 419.

Hilton, S. M. (1963). Ann. N.Y. Acad. Sci. **140**, 275.

Hilton, S. M., and Lewis, G. P. (1955). J. Physiol. (London) **129**, 253.

Hilton, S. M., and Lewis, G. P. (1956). J. Physiol. (London) **134**, 471.

Hladovec, J., Mansfeld, V., and Horakova, Z. (1958). Experientia **14**, 146.

Horton, E. W. (1963). Nature (London) **200**, 892.

Horton, E. W. (1969). Physiol. Rev. **49**, 112.

Humphrey, J. H. (1955). Brit. J. Exp. Pathol. **36**, 268.

Humphrey, J. H., and Jacques, R. (1954). J. Physiol. (London) **124**, 305.

Inderbitzin, T. (1955). Int. Arch. Allergy Appl. Immunol. **7**, 140.

Jacob, J. (1960). "Les antagonistes de la sérotonine. Actualités pharmacologiques," p. 131. Masson, Paris.

Janoff, A. (1970). Ser. Haematol. **3**, 96.

Jensen, J. (1967). Science **155**, 1122.

Jobling, J. W., and Peterson, W. (1914). J. Exp. Med. **19**, 480.

Jolles, B., and Harrison, R. G. (1966). Brit. J. Radiol. **39**, 12.

Judah, J. D., and Willoughby, D. A. (1962). J. Pathol. Bacteriol. **83**, 567.

Kaplan, A. P., and Austen, K. F. (1970). J. Immunol. **105**, 802.

Kaplan, A. P., and Austen, K. F. (1971). J. Exp. Med. **133**, 696.

Kellermeyer, R. W., and Graham, R. C. (1968). New Engl. J. Med. **279**, 754.

Kimura, E. T., Young, P. R., and Richards, R. K. (1960). J. Allergy **31**, 237.

Konzett, H., and Boissonas, R. A. (1960). Experientia **16**, 456.

Kraut, H., Frey, E. K., and Werle, E. (1930). Hoppe-Seyler's Z. Physiol. Chem. **189**, 97.

Krogh, A. (1929). "The Anatomy and Physiology of Capillaries", 2nd ed., p. 317. Yale Univ. Press, New Haven, Connecticut.

Kutscher, F. (1910). *Zentralbl. Physiol.* **24**, 163.

Landis, E. M. (1946). *Ann. N.Y. Acad. Sci.* **46**, 679.

Leme, J. G., Schapoval, E. E. S., and Rocha e Silva, M. (1967). *In* "Vaso-active Polypeptides: Bradykinin and Related Kinins" (M. Rocha e Silva and H. A. Rothschild, eds.), pp. 213–221. Edart Livraria Editora Ltda., Sao Paulo.

Lepow, I. H., Willms–Kretschmer, K., Patrick, R. A., and Rosen, F. S. (1970). *Amer. J. Pathol.* **61**, 13.

Levi, H. (1959). *In* "Documenta Geigy Scientific Tables" (K. Diem, ed.), 5th ed., p. 98. Geigy Pharmaceuticals, Basle.

Levy, J., and Michel-Ber, E. (1956). *J. Physiol. (Paris)* **48**, 1051.

Lewis, G. P. (1959). *J. Physiol. (London)* **147**, 458.

Lewis, T. (1927). "The Blood Vessels of the Human Skin and Their Responses." Shaw, London.

Lewis, T., and Love, W. S. (1926). *Heart* **13**, 27.

Lindell, S. E., and Westling, H. (1966). *In* "Handbuch der experimentellen Pharmakologie" (O. Eichler and A. Farah, eds.), Vol. 18, Part 1, p. 734–788. Springer-Verlag, Berlin.

Logan, G., and Wilhelm, D. L. (1963). *Nature (London)* **198**, 968.

Logan, G., and Wilhelm, D. L. (1966a). *Brit. J. Exp. Pathol.* **47**, 286.

Logan, G., and Wilhelm, D. L. (1966b). *Brit. J. Exp. Pathol.* **47**, 300.

Logan, G., and Wilhelm, D. L. (1966c). *Brit. J. Exp. Pathol.* **47**, 324.

Lykke, A. W. J., and Cummings, R. (1969). *Brit. J. Exp. Pathol.* **50**, 309.

Lykke, A. W. J., and Cummings, R. (1970). *J. Pathol.* **101**, 319.

Lykke, A. W. J., Willoughby, D. A., and Kosche, E. R. (1967). *J. Pathol. Bacteriol.* **94**, 381.

McClugage, S. G. J., and McCluskey, R. T. (1971). *Microvac. Res.* **3**, 354.

Macfarlane, M. G. (1955). *Symp. Soc. Gen. Microbiol.* **5**, 57.

Macfarlane, M. G., and Knight, B. C. J. G. (1941). *Biochem. J.* **35**, 884.

Mackay, M. E., Miles, A. A., Schachter, M., and Wilhelm, D. L. (1953). *Nature (London)* **172**, 714.

Majno, G. (1964). *In* "Injury, Inflammation and Immunity" (L. Thomas, J. W. Uhr, and L. Grant, eds.), pp. 58–93. Williams & Wilkins Co., Baltimore, Maryland.

Majno, G. (1965). *In* "Handbook of Physiology" (Amer. Physiol. Soc., J. Field, ed), Vol. 3, Sect. 2, pp. 2293–2375. Williams & Wilkins, Baltimore, Maryland.

Majno, G., and Palade, G. E. (1961). *J. Biophys. Biochem. Cytol.* **11**, 571.

Majno, G., Palade, G. E., and Schoefl, G. (1961). *J. Biophys. Biochem. Cytol.* **11**, 607.

Majno, G., Shea, S. M., and Leventhal, M. (1969). *J. Cell Biol.* **42**, 647.

Marchesi, V. T., and Florey, H. W. (1960). *Quart. J. Exp. Physiol.* **45**, 343.

Margolis, J. (1957). *J. Physiol. (London)* **137**, 95.

Margolis, J. (1958). *J. Physiol. (London)* **144**, 1.

Margolis, J., and Bishop, E. A. (1963). *Aust. J. Exp. Biol. Med. Sci.* **41**, 293.

Massart, J., and Bordet, C. (1890). *J. Méd. Chir. Pharmacol., Bruxelles.* **90**, 169.

Massart, J., and Bordet C. (1891). *Ann. Inst. Pasteur, Paris* **5**, 417.

Melrose, G. J. H., Muller, H. K., and Vagg, W. J. (1970). *Nature (London)* **225**, 547.

Menkin, V. (1938). *J. Exp. Med.* **67**, 129.

Menkin, V. (1940). "Dynamics of Inflammation." Macmillan, New York.

Miles, A. A. (1958–1959). *Lect. Sci. Basis Med.* **8**, 198–225.

Miles, A. A. (1961). *Fed. Proc., Fed. Amer. Soc. Exp. Biol.* **20**, Suppl. 9, 141.

Miles, A. A. (1964). *Ann. N.Y. Acad. Sci.* **116**, 855.

Miles, A. A., and Miles, E. M. (1952). *J. Physiol. (London)* **118**, 228.

Miles, A. A., and Wilhelm, D. L. (1955). *Brit. J. Exp. Pathol.* **36**, 71.

Miles, A. A., and Wilhelm, D. L. (1958). *Nature (London)* **181**, 96.

Miles, A. A., and Wilhelm, D. L. (1960a). *In* "The Biochemical Response to Injury" (H. B. Stoner, ed.), pp. 51–79. Blackwell, Oxford.

Miles, A. A., and Wilhelm, D. L. (1960b). *In* "Polypeptides which Affect Smooth Muscles and Blood Vessels" (M. Schachter, ed.), pp. 309–316. Pergamon, Oxford.

Mongar, J. L., and Schild, H. O. (1962). *Physiol. Rev.* **42**, 226.

Moses, J. M., Ebert, R. H., Graham, R. C., and Brine, K. L. (1964). *J. Exp. Med.* **120**, 57.

Movat, H. Z., Poon, M. C., and Takeuchi. Y. (1971). *Int. Arch. Allergy Appl. Immunol.* **40**, 89.

Muller, H. K., Salasoo, I., and Wilhelm, D. L. (1968). *Aust. J. Exp. Biol. Med. Sci.* **46**, 165.

Mustard, J. F., Movat, H. Z., Macmorine, D. R. L., and Sényi, A. (1965). *Proc. Soc. Exp. Biol. Med.* **119**, 988.

Nicolaides, E. D., and DeWald, H. A. (1961). *J. Org. Chem.* **26**, 3872.

Northover, B. J. (1963). *J. Pathol. Bacteriol.* **85**, 361.

Northover, B. J. (1964). *J. Pathol. Bacteriol.* **87**, 395.

Ovary, Z. (1958). *Progr. Allergy* **5**, 459.

Oyvin, I. A., Gaponyuk, P. Ya., and Oyvin, V. J. (1967). *Experientia* **23**, 925.

Parizek, J. (1960). *J. Reprod. Fert.* **1**, 294.

Parizek, J., and Zahor, Z. (1956). *Nature (London)* **177**, 1036.

Parratt, J. R., and West, G. B. (1957). *J. Physiol. (London)* **137**, 169.

Paton, W. D. M. (1957). *Pharmacol. Rev.* **9**, 269.

Petri, G., Csipak, J., Kovacs, A., and Bentzik, M. (1952). *Acta Med. (Budapest)* **3**, 347.

Pierce, J. V. (1968). *Fed. Proc., Fed. Amer. Soc. Exp. Biol.* **27**, 52.

Pierce, J. V., and Webster, M. E. (1966). *In* "Hypotensive Peptides' (E. G. Erdös, N. Back, and F. Sicuteri, eds.), pp. 130–138. Springer-Verlag, Berlin and New York.

Pietra, G. G., Szidon, J. P., Callahan, E. J., and Fishman, A. P. (1971). *Fed. Proc., Fed. Amer. Soc. Exp. Biol.* **30**, 720.

Pisano, J. J., Tamura, Z., Furano, E., and Udenfriend, S. (1965). *Fed. Proc., Fed. Amer. Soc. Exp. Biol.* **24**, 488.

Ramsdell, S. G. (1928). *J. Immunol.* **15**, 305.

Rapport, M. M., Green, A. A., and Page, I. H. (1948a). *Science* **108**, 329.

Rapport, M. M., Green, A. A., and Page, I. H. (1948b). *J. Biol. Chem.* **176**, 1243.

Rawson, R. A. (1943). *Amer. J. Physiol.* **138**, 708.

Riley, J. F., and West, G. B. (1953). *J. Physiol. (London)* **120**, 528.

Rocha e Silva, M. (1964). *Ann. N. Y. Acad. Sci.* **116**, 899.

Rocha e Silva, M., Beraldo, W. T., and Rosenfeld, G. (1949). *Amer. J. Physiol.* **156**, 261.

Rowley, D. A., and Benditt, E. P. (1956). *J. Exp. Med.* **103**, 399.

Samuel, S. (1890). *Arch. Pathol. Anat. Physiol. Klin. Med.* **121**, 396.

Sano, I., Kakimoto, Y., and Taniguki, K. (1958). *J. Physiol. (London)* **195**, 495.

Schachter, M. (1966). *In* "Hypotensive Peptides" (E.G. Erdös, N. Back, and F. Sicuteri, eds.), pp. 275–278. Springer-Verlag, Berlin and New York.

Schachter, M. (1969). *Physiol. Rev.* **49**, 509.

Schayer, R. W. (1961). *Chemotherapia* **3**, 128.

Schayer, R. W. (1963). *Progr. Allergy* **7**, 187.

Schayer, M. (1966a). *In* "Handbuch der experimentellen Pharmakologie" (O. Eichler and A. Farah, eds.), Vol. 18, Part 1, pp. 672–683. Springer-Verlag, Berlin and New York.

Schayer, M. (1966b). *In* "Handbuch der experimentellen Pharmakologie" (O. Eichler and A. Farah, eds.), Vol. 18, Part 1, pp. 688–725. Springer-Verlag, Berlin and New York.

Schröder, E., and Hempel, R. (1964). *Experientia* **20**, 529.

Sevitt, S. (1957). "Burns: Pathology and Therapeutic Applications." Butterworth, London.

Sevitt, S. (1958). *J. Pathol. Bacteriol.* **75**, 27.

Sevitt, S. (1964). *In* "Injury, Inflammation and Immunity" (L. Thomas, J. Uhr, and L. Grant, eds.), pp. 183–210. Williams & Wilkins, Baltimore, Maryland.
Sevitt, S., Bull, J. P., Cruickshank, C. N. D., Jackson, D. M., and Lowbury, E. J. I. (1952). *Brit. Med. J.* **2**, 57.
Sim, M. F. (1965). *Int. Symp. Non-Steroidal Anti-Inflammatory Drugs, Proc., 1964 Int. Congr. Ser.* No. 82, pp. 207–213.
Simon, F. P., Polts, A. M., and Gerard, R. W. (1947). *Arch. Biochem.* **12**, 283.
Skinner, N. S., Jr., and Webster, M. E. (1968). *J. Physiol. (London)* **195**, 505.
Sollman, T., and Pilcher, J. D. (1917). *J. Pharmacol. Exp. Ther.* **9**, 309.
Soltay, M. J., Movat, H. Z., and Özge-Anwar, A. H. (1971). *Proc. Soc. Exp. Biol. Med.* **138**, 952.
Song, C. W., Anderson, R. S., and Tabachnick, J. (1966). *Radiat. Res.* **27**, 604.
Spalteholz, W. (1893). Cited by Majno (1964).
Sparrow, E. M., and Wilhelm, D. L. (1957). *J. Physiol. (London)* **137**, 51.
Spector, W. G. (1951). *J. Pathol. Bacteriol.* **63**, 93.
Spector, W. G. (1956). *J. Pathol. Bacteriol.* **72**, 367.
Spector, W. G. (1958). *Pharmacol. Rev.* **10**, 475.
Spector, W. G., and Willoughby, D. A. (1957). *J. Pathol. Bacteriol.* **73**, 133.
Spector, W. G., and Willoughby, D. A. (1959a). *J. Pathol. Bacteriol.* **77**, 1.
Spector, W. G., and Willoughby, D. A. (1959b). *J. Pathol. Bacteriol.* **78**, 121.
Spector, W. G., and Willoughby, D. A. (1960). *J. Pathol. Bacteriol.* **79**, 21.
Spector, W. G., and Willoughby, D. A. (1963). *Bacteriol. Rev.* **27**, 117.
Spragg, J., and Austen, K. F. (1971). *J. Immunol.* **107**, 1512.
Stacey, R. S. (1957). *Proc. Roy. Soc. Med.* **50**, 40.
Steele, R. H. (1969). Ph.D. Thesis, University of New South Wales.
Steele, R. H., and Wilhelm, D. L. (1966). *Brit. J. Exp. Pathol.* **47**, 612.
Steele, R. H., and Wilhelm, D. L. (1967). *Brit. J. Exp. Pathol.* **48**, 592.
Steele, R. H., and Wilhelm, D. L. (1970). *Brit. J. Exp. Pathol.* **51**, 265.
Stetson, C. A., and Good, R. A. (1951). *J. Exp. Med.* **93**, 49.
Stewart, J. M., and Wolley, D. W. (1967). *In* "Vaso-active Polypeptides: Bradykinin and Related Kinins" (M. Rocha e Silva and H. A. Rothschild, eds.), pp. 7–13. Edart Livraria Editora Ltda., Sao Paulo.
Stone, C. A., Wenger, H. C., Ludden, C. T., Stavorski, J. M., and Ross, C. A. (1961). *J. Pharmacol. Exp. Ther.* **131**, 73.
Thomson, J. (1813). "Lectures on Inflammation. Exhibiting a View of the General Doctrines, Pathological and Practical of Medical Surgery." William Blackwood, Edinburgh.
Treloar, N. P., and Movat, H. Z. (1970). *Fed. Proc., Fed. Amer. Soc. Exp. Biol.* **29**, 576.
Udenfriend, S. (1958). *In* "5-Hydroxytryptamine" (G. P. Lewis, ed.), pp. 43–49. Pergamon, Oxford.
Ungar, G. (1952). *Lancet* **2**, 742.
Ungar, G. (1956). Histamine, *Ciba Found. Synp., 1955* pp. 431–443.
Uvnäs, B. (1962). *Proc. Int. Congr. Inter. Union Physiol. Sci., 22nd, 1962* pp. 106–114.
Uvnäs, B. (1964). *Ann. N. Y. Acad. Sci.* **116**, 880.
Uvnäs, B. (1969). *In* "Inflammation Biochemistry and Drug Interaction" (A. Bertelli and J. C. Houck, eds.), pp. 221–227. Excerpta Med. Found., Amsterdam.
Vialli, M., and Erspamer, V. (1933). *Z. Zellforsch. Mikrosk. Anat.* **19**, 743.
Vogel, R., Trautschold, I., and Werle, E. (1969). "Naturliche Proteinasen–Inhibitoren." Thieme, Stuttgart.
Voisin, G. A., and Toullet, F. (1960). *Cell. Aspects Immunity, Ciba Found. Symp., 1959* pp. 373–405.

Voisin, G. A., and Toullet, F. (1963). *Ann. Inst. Pasteur, Paris* **104**, 169.

Waller, A. (1946). *Phil. Mag.* [4] **29**, 397.

Wasserman, K., Loeb, L., and Mayerson, H. S. (1955). *Circ. Res.* **3**, 594.

Webster, M. E. (1966a). *In* "Hypotensive Peptides" (E. G. Erdös, N. Back, and F. Sicuteri, eds.), pp. 648–653. Springer-Verlag, Berlin and New York.

Webster, M. E. (1966b). *In* "Hypotensive Peptides" (E. G. Erdös, N. Back, and F. Sicuteri, eds.), pp. 263–272. Springer-Verlag, Berlin and New York.

Webster, M. E. (1966c). *Arthritis Rheum.* **9**, 473.

Webster, M. E. (1968). *Fed. Proc., Fed. Amer. Soc. Exp. Biol.* **27**, 84.

Webster, M. E. (1969). *In* "Cellular and Humoral Mechanisms in Anaphylasis and Allergy" (H. Z. Movat, ed.), pp. 207–214. Karger, Basel.

Webster, M. E., and Pierce, J. V. (1963). *Ann. N. Y. Acad. Sci.* **104**, 91.

Webster, M. E., and Ratnoff, O. D. (1961). *Nature (London)* **192**, 180.

Webster, M. E., Jacobson, S., and Pierce, J. V. (1969). Cited by Webster (1969).

Weeks, R. E., and Gunnar, R. M. (1949). *AMA Arch. Pathol.* **48**, 178.

Wells, F. R., and Miles, A. A. (1963). *Nature (London)* **200**, 1015.

Werle, E., and Vogel, R. (1961). *Arch. Int. Pharmacodyn. Ther.* **131**, 257.

Werle, E., and von Roden, P. (1936). *Biochem. Z.* **286**, 213.

Werle, E., Gotze, W., and Keppler, A. (1937). *Biochem. Z.* **289**, 217.

Werle, E., Forell, M. M., and Maier, L. (1955). *Naunyn-Schmiedebergs Arch. Exp. Pathol. Pharmakol.* **225**, 269.

Werle, E., Vogel, R., and Kaliampetsos, G. (1963). *In* "Weltkongress fur Gastroenterologie" (E. Schmid, J. Tomenius, and G. Watkinson, eds.), Vol. 2, p 778. Karger, Basel.

Wharton Jones, T. (1851). *Guy's Hosp. Rep.* **14**, 1.

Wilhelm, D. L. (1962). *Pharmacol. Rev.* **14**, 215.

Wilhelm, D. L. (1971a). *Rev. Can. Biol.* **30**, 153.

Wilhelm, D. L. (1971b). *Annu. Rev. Med.* **22**, 63.

Wilhelm, D. L. (1971c). *In* "Pathology" (W. A. D. Anderson, ed.), pp. 14–67. Mosby, St. Louis, Missouri.

Wilhelm, D. L., and Mason, B. (1960). *Brit. J. Exp. Pathol.* **61**, 487.

Wilhelm, D. L., Miles, A. A., and Mackay, M. E. (1955). *Brit. J. Exp. Pathol.* **36**, 82.

Wilhelm, D. L., Mill, P. J., and Miles, A. A. (1957). *Brit. J. Exp. Pathol.* **38**, 446.

Wilhelm, D. L., Mill, P. J., Sparrow, E. M., Mackay, M. E., and Miles, A. A. (1958). *Brit. J. Exp. Pathol.* **39**, 228.

Wilhelm, G., and Domenjoz, R. (1951). *Arch. Int. Pharmacodyn. Ther.* **85**, 129.

Willms-Kretschmer, K., Flax, M., and Cotran, R. S. (1967). *Lab. Invest.* **17**, 334.

Willoughby, D. A. (1960). *Brit. J. Radiol.* **33**, 515.

Willoughby, D. A., and Giroud, J. P. (1969). *J. Pathol.* **98**, 53.

Windaus, A., and Vogt, W. (1907). *Chem. Ber.* **40**, 3691.

Winder, C. V., Wase, J., Burr, V., Been, M., and Rosiere, C. E. (1958). *Arch. Int. Pharmacodyn. Ther.* **116**, 261.

Wuepper, K. D., and Cochrane, C. G. (1972). *J. Exp. Med.* **135**, 1.

Wuepper, K. D., Tucker, E. S., and Cochrane, C. G. (1969). *Fed. Proc., Fed. Amer. Soc. Exp. Biol.* **28**, 363.

Wuepper, K. D., Tucker, E. S., and Cochrane, C. G. (1970). *J. Immunol.* **105**, 1307.

Yang, H. Y. T., and Erdös, E. G. (1967). *Nature (London)* **215**, 1402.

Chapter 9

MEDIATION OF INCREASED VASCULAR PERMEABILITY IN INFLAMMATION

D. A. WILLOUGHBY

I. Introduction

In considering the mediation of increased vascular permeability in inflammation, it is necessary to carefully define terms. In the first instance, this chapter will be devoted to those aspects of inflammatory response in which a dynamic state exists, and it will not concern itself with the physical destruction of blood vessels which can, of course, lead to extravasation of whole blood into the tissues. It will be concerned with the response of the blood vessels to injurious stimuli under conditions where it is reasonable to suppose that the changes in the vessel wall are brought about by endogenous vasoactive substances.

It is also necessary to carefully define the particular type of inflammation which is being discussed at any point in time. For purposes of simplicity it is proposed to divide inflammation into "immunological" and "nonimmunological." These two broad subdivisions are not clear, but for the purposes of this chapter immunological will be considered under the following categories: immediate hypersensitivity, or that brought about by humoral antibody, and delayed hypersensitivity, or cell-mediated immunity brought about by sensitized cells of lymphoid origin.

The nonimmunological inflammation will be divided into acute and chronic. Under acute, we will consider the inflammatory response to thermal injury, radiation, and simple chemicals, while, in the section dealing with chronic inflammation, we will discuss the more prolonged results arising from either chemicals or, e.g., cotton pellet implantation.

The impetus for the concept of chemical mediators of inflammation probably arose from the simple but elegant experiments of Lewis in 1929. In this work, he suggested that inflammation is brought about by "H" substance, the substance or substances resembling histamine which had been discovered a few years earlier by Barger and Dale (1910). It is worthwhile recording at this point that Dale in his third Dohme lecture stated,

> The discovery in artificial extract from an organ or tissue of a substance which on artificial injection provides a pharmaco-dynamic effect provides only a first item of presumptive evidence in support of a theory that the action of this substance plays a part in normal inflammation.

In the past, we and others have suggested that certain criteria must be fulfilled before accepting that a substance acts as a mediator of inflammation, and these are

1. The substance should be demonstrably present during an inflammatory reaction and absent when the reaction subsides.

2. The substance should possess properties which qualify it as a mediator of inflammation.

3. Inhibition of the substance by specific antagonists should lead to a diminution of that aspect of the inflammatory reaction for which the substance is assumed to be responsible.

4. Depletion of the tissues of the suspected mediator prior to the injurious stimulus should similarly suppress that part of the inflammatory reaction for which the substance is assumed to be responsible.

After Lewis, the interest waned until the 1940's when Menkin aroused enormous interest with his studies on chemical mediators of inflammation. He felt assured that there should be a series of mediators for each aspect of the inflammatory response, and he produced such exotic names as leukotaxine, exudin, necrosin, leukocytosis-promoting factor, etc. Unfortunately, much of his work did not stand the test of time, and pharmacologists, such as Roche e Silva, with their descriptions of bradykinin and its permeability-enhancing properties failed to confirm the findings of Menkin. Nevertheless, Menkin's contribution to this field was vast in that he stimulated other investigators to pursue the concept of chemical mediators of inflammation.

II. Acute Inflammation

In Chapter 8, Wilhelm describes the methods used for evaluating increased vascular permeability.

A. Site of Leakage of Plasma Protein

Thanks to the work of Majno et al. (1961), we now know that plasma protein usually leaves the inflamed vessel wall by passing between the endothelial cells. There is not a great deal of difference between the various permeability factors studied in this way. Usually, definite gaps appear between the cells permitting the egress of the plasma protein. The mechanism of the gap production is unknown, but gaps could be produced by rounding up of the cells or by cell contraction. Support for the latter concept has recently arisen from the findings of Majno who has shown a reduction in nuclear size associated with the formation of gaps, suggesting a positive contraction of the cell. Many of the permeability factors have in common the ability to cause a contraction of smooth muscle, but there are notable exceptions, e.g., RNA and the lymph node permeability factor (PF). It is possible that the permeability factors cause a leakage of small ions, e.g., potassium, which would result in a situation similar to that occurring in nerves, where there is depolarization and formation of an action potential. It must be restated at this point that the mechanism of gap formation is unknown.

The site of vascular permeability change during inflammation was the subject of great interest during the early 1960's, and it has been shown that most permeability factors do not act on all the vessels of the microcirculation in the same way. The main action has been shown to be on the venules with little or no effect on the capillaries. This has been studied by the use of the colloidal carbon method first described by Cotran and Majno (1964), Wells and Miles (1963), Hurley (1963), and Hurley and Spector (1965). In this method, colloidal carbon is injected IV into the animals, and, subsequently, either inflammation is introduced or a permeability factor is injected. At various times, the lesion is removed; the tissues are cleared and visualized using the light microscope. In permeable vessels, the carbon becomes trapped in the vessel walls and can, on occasion, accumulate outside the vessels.

On the basis of structure and size, it is easy to differentiate between venules and capillaries. The method, however, is fraught with danger; thus, sometimes vessels look blackened, but close examination show that they are constricted and occluded by carbon particles in the lumen. This has been well described by Bohm (1966) in his studies of vessels in the lung after various types of pulmonary edema. A further problem of the carbon particle method in demonstrating increased cytovascular permeability is the failure to correlate with local edema. It has been shown by Spector *et al.* (1965) that after thermal injury in the rat there is an accumulation of carbon in the venules which subsequently subsides; this is followed by an accumulation of carbon in the capillaries. When, however, the edema is indicated by the water content of burned skin, it is totally suppressed by massive doses of salicylate or by the use of monoamine oxidase inhibitors. Venular labelling with carbon was suppressed, but the capillary labeling was not modified. Such results caused the carbon to be regarded with suspicion. Nevertheless, it is usual to suggest that the initial increased vascular permeability is associated with leakage from venules and that the subsequent prolonged phase occurs more usually with leakage from capillaries. Furthermore, most pharmacological agents capable of increasing vascular permeability act on the venules and not on the capillaries. This has gained support not only from the colloidal carbon method, but also from direct observation of the interendothelial cell junction with the electron microscope. It is not proposed in this chapter to describe the phasic pattern of increased vascular permeability that occurs after injurious stimuli; see Chapter 8 for a detailed description.

B. *Potential Mediators*

1. WHY MEDIATORS?

The inflamed site is in a constant dynamic state of change, nad most of these changes are reversible. Thus, direct physical damage to the blood vessels alone would seem unlikely to be the whole answer to the pathogenesis of the permeability of blood vessels to plasma protein after an inflammatory stimulus. The early workers in the field of inflammation were impressed by the standard reply of the vasculature to a wide variety of insult; thus, heat, cold, and chemical injury all led to vasodilation and increased vascular permeability to plasma protein. This led Menkin, among others, to postulate the chemical theory of inflammation in which he suggested that inflammatory stimuli lead to the relaese of a series of endogenous substances endowed with the appropriate properties to bring about the typical picture of inflammation. Most of the work in this field has concentrated on so-called mediators of the acute inflammatory response. Many disciplines have been used to study this topic, but probably the most successful has been the use of autopharmacological methods. The ideal method demonstrates that a potential mediator has the appropriate properties to bring about that part of the inflammatory response for which it is deemed to be responsible. The mediator should then be demonstrably present for a phase of the inflammatory response. Finally, if it is possible to deplete the tissues of the mediator, this should also lead to a suppression of the inflammatory response. These are the ideal criteria for a mediator, but they are seldom fulfilled in all of these aspects. We will now consider some specific contenders for the role of mediator of the acute inflammatory process. The methods used for demonstrating that certain substances are capable of increasing vascular permeability will be discussed by Wilhelm (Chapter 8). It is necessary to briefly consider the models of acute inflammation.

a. THERMAL INJURY.   This method depends on the response of the animal to a standardized thermal injury. In our laboratory, we shave rat or guinea pig abdominal skin and then place the animal on a small cork platform through the center of which is a fine guage brass tube. The tube contains hot water supplied from a thermostatically controlled water bath which circulates at high speed. Immediately prior to the burn, the animal is injected with an azo dye, such as trypan or pontamine blue, which binds to the plasma albumin. From experience, we have found that a good response in rats can be obtained by using a temperature of 56°C for 27 seconds. This leads to a leakage of protein-bound dye from the vessels during the first hour, and, subsequently, by the fourth hour, there is up to a 300% increase in water content in the burned area. This particular model has the advantage of objective measurement (certainly during the later stages).

2. TURPENTINE PLEURISY

In this model, a small quantity of turpentine is injected (0.15 ml) into the pleural cavity of rats. Subsequently, the animals are killed by ether anesthesia and exsanguination from the carotid cartery, and the exudate is collected from the pleural cavity with a Pasteur pipette. This method has the advantage that the exudate may be harvested at various times and examined for the content of pharmacologically active mediators. Analysis of the exudate reveals that within 1 hour the exudate contains all the plasma protein in the same proportions as found in the serum. It is also convenient to follow migration of cells into the exudate, and it is easy matter carry out a total and differential white cell count. As in the case of the thermal injury, this method may be quantitated and objective measurements applied.

3. Various Hindpaw Edemas

It has long been practice for experimentalists to inject various noxious substances into the hindpaws of anaimals and to measure the subsequent edema by means of a foot paw edema machine possibly of the type produced by U. Basili (Milan). This allows a constant monitering of the development of the edema, but it is difficult to sample the edema. The advantage of the hindpaw edema method, however, is that it supplies quantitative results that can be easily obtained by relatively inexperienced workers. As we shall see later, the problems of rat paw edema arise from the type of noxious material injected into the foot. Thus, those inflammation-inducing agents that cause the release of only histamine or 5-hydroxytryptamine differ markedly from those agents that cause the release of other mediators. These differences become apparent during experiments with antagonists which attempt to define the various phases of the inflammatory response. Among the most commonly used irritants in this method are dextran, formalin, and carrageenan; the latter shows the best correlation between the ability of a potential anti-inflammatory agent to suppress edema and its subsequent clinical efficacy in human chronic inflammatory disease.

4. Ultraviolet Erythema

Until very recently, the use of ultraviolet rays to produce erythema on the skin of rats and mice as a model of inflammation has been made with little or no knowledge of its mechanism. However, as we shall see later, there have been attempts to define roles for certain mediators which have emerged only during the past year.

C. Substances Considered as Mediators

No mention will be made in this section of the host of early substances originally described by Menkin, as these have been referred to in an earlier edition of this treatise. Instead, the focus will be on those agents which have some substantive evidence in support of their role as mediators of the inflammatory response.

1. Histamine

The role of histamine in acute inflammation was reviewed in the previous edition of this treatise, however, histamine is widely distributed throughout the body in most tissues and also in many physiological fluids. Under normal circumstances, histamine is found in the tissues closely associated with the mast cells (Riley and West, 1953; West, 1955). Usually release of histamine is associated with mast cell degranulation. However,

Smith (1958a,b) showed that the mast cells were capable of actively releasing histamine without degranulation. The precise mechanism for the release of histamine from tissues by exogenous substances remains uncertain (see reviews by Paton, 1957; Uvnäs, 1958; Spector, 1958; Mongar and Schild, 1962). Histamine may be released by a wide variety of substances including proteolytic enzymes (Rocha e Silva, 1956), surface active compounds (Kranz et al., 1948), basic peptides and proteins (MacIntosh and Paton, 1949), and large molecular substances (Halpern, 1956; Paton, 1957). Probably the best known of a large group of basic substances is compound 48/80 (Paton, 1951).

Xanthisine was shown to release histamine in a certain proportion of the population with, apparently, a genetically linked specificity (Kalmus and Willoughby, 1960). On the other hand, nucleoside inosine released histamine in rats, but not in man (Moulton et al., 1957). It is now generally agreed that histamine can be released by at least four mechanisms as follows: splitting of a hypothetical bond linking histamine to a protein; leakage of histamine through a cellular or subcellular membrane rendered permeable or destroyed; an ion exchange reaction releasing histamine from combination with an acidic intracellular site; or rupture of a polar linkage with protein or lipoprotein (details of the controversy are given elsewhere, see Spector, 1958; Mongar and Schild, 1962).

EVIDENCE FOR THE PARTICIPATION OF HISTAMINE IN INFLAMMATION.   Evidence exists to support the hypothesis that histamine is released after burns, chemical injury, bacterial invasion, and X-ray injury (Spector and Willoughby, 1968). Unfortunately, many of these observations are difficult to interpret since they are based on either a rise or a fall in the histamine content of the tissues. Spector and Willoughby (1963a) found histamine to be present in pleural exudate from rats after the intrapleural injection of turpentine. Histamine concentration became maximal by 1 hour after injection of turpentine, after which the histamine content of the exudate fell rapidly.

In irradiation injury, histamine has long been the center of controversy, thus, Kawaguchi (1930) demonstrated an increase of histamine content in skin after irradiation—a finding that could not be confirmed by his contemporary Ellinger in 1928 and 1930, nor by the more recent work of Ungar and Damgaard (1954). Willoughby (1959a, 1960) found a loss of histamine from the intestine of rats during the first 24 hours after abdominal X irradiation. More consistent results have come from the assay of blood levels of this amine after irradiation, and there seems no doubt that irradiation is accompanied by a higher blood level of histamine. Indeed, a review by Ellinger supported the theory that histamine is the main contributing factor to the vascular changes after irradiation injury (Ellinger, 1930). More recently, Willoughby (1960) suggested that histamine is merely the first detectable pharmacologically active amine relased and that its role is as transitory in irradiation injury as in other types of inflammation. Thus, its release is merely the first in a sequence of events.

As stated earlier, the demonstration of the presence of histamine is by itself insufficient evidence of its role in inducing changes in vascular permeability. These observations would gain support if the inflammatory response could be diminished in some way by the action of antihistamine drugs. Ideally, the increased vascular permeability associated with inflammation should be suppressed by the antihistamine at the time when the release of histamine can be demonstrated. A necessary prerequisite is that the selected drug acts specifically and exclusively as an antagonist of histamine. Many antihistamines are not specific in their action in blocking histamine, e.g., promethazine, 1 mg/kg, has been shown to cause a 70% suppression of the permeability-inducing effect of the substance P (the vasoactive polypeptide) and, in doses of 5 mg/kg, 50% suppression of 5-HT (Spector and Willoughby, 1963b). Similar results showing this lack of specificity have been described by Halpern *et al.* (1963) in skin reactions in the mouse. These workers also found that chlorpromazine, a weak antihistamine, raised the threshold dose for histamine by a factor of 10. Even mepyramine maleate (anthisan neoantergan) administered in high doses can be shown to have a significant suppressive effect on permeability factors other than histamine. Antihistamines must be selected with some care. Mepyramine maleate is often favored for its high specificity when given in moderate systemic doses. This drug given in doses of 200–300 mg has long been established as a successful form of therapy for patients suffering from drug or food allergy; in these doses it sufficiently abolishes the urticarial weals. Evidencehas been found that after thermal injury in rats the earliest changes in vascular permeability may be suppressed by small doses of systmic antihistamine drug (Spector and Willoughby, 1959). However, after this initial suppression of increased vascular permeability, repeated administration of the antihistamine failed to affect edema formation suggesting that histamine is released only during the earliest phase of the inflammatory reaction. Similar results were obtained in rabbits and guinea pigs by Wilhelm and Mason (1960).

In turpentine-induced pleurisy, the volume of the exudate obtained 30 minutes after intrapleural injection of turpentine was reduced from 1 ml to a mean of 0.1 ml in those animals pretreated with the antihistamine mepyramine maleate (Spector and Willoughby, 1957). However, after 1 hour, i.e., the period during which histamine was demonstrable, the exudate volume rose rapidly and after 2–3 hours was not significantly different from that in control animals despite repeated administration of the antihistamine drug. Substantially similar results have been obtained after X irradiation of rats. Under these conditions, a marked loss of histamine from the intestine occurs during the first 24 hours after irradiation and is accompanied by an increase in vascular permeability. Pretreatment of rats with small doses of antihistamine drugs causes a striking suppression of this increase in vascular permeability. Pretreatment of rats with small doses of antihistamine drugs causes a striking suppression of this increase in vascular permeability. Once again, however, the effect of the antihistamine was short lived, and only the earliest permeability changes were abolished by this treatment (Willoughby, 1959b).

The role of histamine in injury induced by bacterial infection has been difficult to elucidate. Smith and Miles (1960) failed to modify the inflammatory response to experimental bacterial peritonitis in rats; nor did they find a significant release of histamine in the peritoneal fluid.

In addition to the demonstration of histamine in inflammatory exudates and the action of antihistamine drugs leading to the suppression of the inflammatory action, it has also been possible by means of histamine liberators to apply the injurious stimulus to animals depleted of histamine. Sheldon and Bauer (1960) found that after cutaneous inoculation of *Mucor myscitis* to the skin of rats there is a local increase in vascular permeability. If, however, the rats are depleted of tissue histamine by repeated daily injections of compound 48/80 before inoculation, the onset of the increased vascular permeability is delayed. Similar results were obtained in rats made diabetic by alloxan; here the onset of increased vascular permeability is again markedly delayed (Spector *et al.*, 1963). Alloxan apparently prevents granules from leaving the mast cells and thus inhibits histamine release. Compound 48/80, on the other hand, depletes the mast cells of their granules and histamine. Sheldon and Bauer also found that rats depleted of their tissue histamine heal more slowly than those with normal tissue levels of histamine, although the precise function of histamine in healing is not yet understood.

Thermal and chemical injury in histamine-depleted rats resulted in a delayed onset of increased vascular permeability comparable with that seen when the animals were treated with antihistamine drugs (Spector and Willoughby, 1959). It is important to bear in mind that certain "classic" histamine liberators release agents other than histamine. Compound 48/80 leads to a depletion of tissue 5-HT as well as tissue histamine. In turpentine-induced pleurisy, the effect of histamine and 5-HT depletion can be observed after 48/80 treatment. In this case, the suppression of increased vascular permeability persists slightly beyond the period of the inflamatory response believed to be due to histamine, and it probably has an effect on the part of the inflammatory reaction suspected to be mediated by 5-HT. Poly-mixin B appears to be a more specific liberator of histamine, as this agent tends to have little or no effect on the tissue 5-HT. When carrying out procedures after a course of injections with histamine liberator, it is impor-tant that the tissues be checked by assay of histamine to corroborate the actual existence of a low histamine content and that, furthermore, the vessels are not in a refractory state. Some confusion may have arisen in the past when workers, after treating rats with histamine liberator, assumed that the intestinal histamine was reduced: actually, histamine in the intestine is not depleted by 48/80.

One final aspect of histamine in acute inflammation which must be con-sidered is the role of histidine decarboxylase and intrinsic histamine. Schayer (1963) has carried out many experiments which show that after inury there is increased histidine decarboxylase activity. He assumes that this will be ac-companied by an increased histamine synthesis. Increased enzyme activity of this kind has been found after thermal injury, allergic reactions, injection of endotoxin, and systemic infection. Schayer is not impressed by the impor-tance of stored histamine released during the early phase of increased per-meability. He postulates that the newly formed or induced histamine is the candidate most likely to be responsible for the later changes as it is intrinsic. Sir Henry Dale (1948) coined the expression "intrinsic histamine" to refer to the histamine released during an antigen–antibody reaction which acts on the cells which release it and which is probably not susceptible to the action of antihistamine drugs. Schayer also postulates that such histamine would be rapidly destroyed orinactivated and, therefore, could not be detected in exudates or in the blood stream. Urinary assay for histamine breakdown products is also unsatisfactory due to the comparatively inaccurate methods of analysis. This is an extremely attractive hypothesis which defies criticism. Actually, the principal established fact is that histidine decarboxylase activ-ity is raised. No other positive evidence supports the view that newly formed histamine is responsible for the later stages of acute inflammation; indeed, an ever-increasing body of evidence suggests that the mediators of the late phase will prove to be of high molecular weight.

2.   5-Hydroxytryptamine (5-HT)

The role of this amine in acute inflammation was also previously discussed in the first edition of this treatise, and, in this chapter, only a brief survey will be made. Interest in 5-HT as a possible mediator of the inflammatory re-sponse was aroused by Rowley and Benditt's observation (1956) that on injec-tion in microgram amounts 5-HT causes immediate edema of rat paws. Spector and Willoughby (1957) found that 5-HT causes vasoconstriction of rat skin in doses above 50 μg/ml, but that it increases vascular permeability to plasma protein in lower doses. Parratt and West (1957a,b,c) confirmed the effect on rat paws and demonstrated the abolition of this edema by means of 2-bromo-d-lysergic acid diethylamide. Spector and Willoughby (1963a) reported that the development of turpentine-induced pleurisy is associated during the first hour after injection with a fairly high concentration of 5-HT. It was not possible to reduce the formation of the pleural exudate by the administration of 5-HT antagonists; on the other hand, rats depleted of their tissue histamine and 5-HT by means of the liberator 48/80 showed a more marked suppression of edema than did animals treated with an antihistamine drug. Although these observations do not permit an unequivocal conclusion to be drawn regarding the role of 5-HT as a mediator of permeability changes, it may be inferred in the rat that 5-HT exerts a short-lived effect which probably follows that of released histamine. This hypothesis gains support from the observations by Willoughby on the effects of irradiation on the rat intestine. In these experiments, rats were irradiated over the abdomen, and the permeability changes were followed by means of leakage of protein-bound trypan blue along the intestine. Permeability changes commenced at 1 day after irradiation and became maximal by 3–4 days. The gut was depleted of histamine by day 1 and of 5-HT by day 2. As with turpentine-induced pleurisy, these changes could not be modified by pretreatment with 5-HT antagonists. In addition, Moglinitsky and Brhumshstein (1949) found within 70 hours of irradiation a loss of staining ability in the argyrophil and argentaffin cells, which are believed to contain 5-HT (Jacobson, 1958).

Some types of edema in the rat are modified by the administration of 5-HT antagonists, particularly the type induced in the rat hindpaw by the injection of large molecular compounds such as egg white and dextran. These types of edema are probably of a specialized nature, and, in addition, the hindpaw of the rat is rich in 5-HT (see Spector and Willoughby, 1963a). The difficulty of using antagonists to confirm the role of 5-HT as a mediator is not surprising. Its action is probably of brief duration and in most instances is associated with some concomitant action of histamine. Also, it has been shown that 5-HT antagonists fail to modify the syndrome produced by the argentofinoma in man which seems to be due mainly to large amounts of circulating 5-HT. Very recently, it has been found in carrageenan-induced edema in the hindpaw of rats that the early stages of this edema are bought about by simultaneous release of histamine and 5-HT; thus, suppression of either histamine or 5-HT fails to influence the development of this early edema. However, simultaneous treatment with histamine and 5-HT antagonists leads to a total suppression of the early edema following such injections of carrageenan. Similarly, depletion of histamine and 5-HT from the tissues prior to the injection of carrageenan also leads to a similar suppression of the early edema.

3. EPINEPHRINE AND NOREPINEPHRINE

As far back as 1929, Krogh speculated on the possible release after injury of antipermeability hormone leading to the restoration of normal vascular permeability. These speculations received recent experimental confirmation, although not as envisaged by Krogh. Considerable evidence exists today that during inflammation vasoactive hormones are released and immediately destroyed and that these hormones in their active form restore vascular permeability to normal. The most likely substances to act as local anti-inflammatory hormones are epinephrine and norepinephrine. The activation of any sudden excess amounts of these amines is attributed to monoamine oxidase, whereas the normal regulation of levels is probably maintained by catechol O-methyltransferase. Monoamine oxidase inhibitors are effective in suppressing increased vascular permeability after thermal and chemical injury whereas paragalol has little or no effect on edema formation (Spector and Willoughby, 1960).

A number of monoamine oxidase inhibitors of varying chemical structure share this anti-inflammatory activity. If dibenamine, an adrenalytic drug, was given simultaneously with the monoamine oxidase inhibitor, no suppression of inflammatory edema occurred. Conversely, if bretyllium ptosalate was given simultaneously with the inhibitor of monoamine oxidase, the anti-inflammatory effect was potentiated. The significance of this observation is that bretyllium is a substance that potentiates circulating epinephrine and norepinephrine, but also prevents its release from nerve endings.

It was found that systemic administration of epinephrine suppresses the inflammatory response after thermal injury. A similar effect could be obtained after systemic administration of higher doses of norepinephrine. These results suggest that epinephrine or norepinephrine are released at the site of injury, and, when destruction of the amines is prevented, the inflammatory reaction is suppressed. Similar results were obtained by Setnikar *et al.* (1959) and Northover and Subramanian (1961). In addition to thermal injury, the vascular changes after other types of injury have also been suppressed, i.e., chemical injury (Willoughby and Spector, 1962) and X-ray injury to the intestine of rats (Willoughby, 1962). The increased vascular permeability that occurred in the intestine of rats after irradiation could be greatly diminished with a variety of monoamine oxidase inhibitors, the effect in every case being reversed by dibenamine. Simultaneous treatment with monoamine oxidase inhibitors and dibenamine failed to suppress the increased vascular permeability. At the time these experiments were being conducted, it was assumed that the anti-inflammatory hormone was probably eipinephrine, and work was carried out in an attempt to determine the source of this anti-inflammatory amine. Inasmuch as adrenalectomy failed to modify the inhibitory action of monoamine oxidase inhibitors, it did not appear that we were dealing with medullary epinephrine.

As previously stated, bretyllium ptosolate, which prevents the release of epinephrine and norepinephrine from nerve endings, failed to prevent the action of monoamine oxidase inhibitors. On the contrary, it potentiated their action. This would seem to eliminate epinephrine from the nervous system as a source of antipermeability hormone. At that time, we concluded that the epinephrine was probably released from platelets or vessel walls during inflammation. More recent work has taken into account the metabolic pathway for the formation of the epinephrines (Spector and Willoughby, 1964a; Willoughby and Spector, 1964b). Tyrosine is converted to dopa, the enzyme dopa decarboxylase converts dopa to dopamine, which is, in turn, converted to norepinephrine by the enzyme dopamine β-oxidase. Finally, epinephrine is formed from norepinephrine. The inactivation has already been discussed; suffice it to say that among the breakdown products we may expect to find adrenachrome, normetanephrine, and vanilyl mandelic acid (VMA). We found that prior administration of 4-bromo-3-hydroxybenzyloxiamine hydrogen phosphate, a compound that antagonizes the actions of both dopa and histidine decarboxylase and dopamine β-oxidase, led to a 50% suppression of edema after thermal injury. This inhibitory effect can be reversed completely by simultaneous treatment with the adrenalytic drug dibenamine. Compounds which block only dopa and histidine decarboxylase suppress the edema after thermal injury by 35%. In high doses (400 mg/kg) which were still nontoxic, this substance caused a total inhibition of inflammatory edema. Compounds thought to be specific antagonists of dopa β-oxidase reduced inflammatory edema by about 75%. It was concluded that the inflammatory reaction depends not only on the destruction of epinephrine and norepinephrine, but also possibly on the destruction of dopa by dopa decarboxylase and dopamine by dopamine β-oxidase.

On this basis, both dopa and dopamine should possess anti-inflammatory activity. Actually, dopamine given intraperitoneally in doses of 25–50 mg/kg reduced inflammatory edema after thermal injury by 80%. This effect could be prevented by concomitant treatment with dibenamine. Dopa also caused suppression of thermal edema, and the anti-inflammatory effects of these two amines were confirmed by their effects on turpentine-induced pleurisy when prior treatment led once again to a striking suppression of increased vascular permeability. The breakdown products of epinephrine, *viz.*, normetanephrine, adrenachrome, and vanilyl mandelic acid, had no effect on these two models of experimental inflammation. These results suggest that after injury monoamine oxidase, dopamine β-oxidase, and dopa decarboxylase are activated leading to the increased formation and inactivation of epinephrine, norepinephrine, dopa, and dopamine. Thus, the anti-inflammatory hormone would be inactivated, and the inflammatory reaction could proceed. Northover (1963) also found that inhibitors of monoamine oxidase suppress the permeability of the vessels of the peritoneum in the mouse. Other workers established increased monoamine oxidase activity in injured rat skin by histochemical methods (Raekallio, 1963). Finally, Molle (1962) described a fall in the catecholamine content in injured skin. In the first part of this chapter, the work of Schayer was referred to in which he described the increased histidine decarboxylase activity occurring after injury. Possibly, this is merely a reflection of general activation of those enzymes responsible for amine formation and breakdown. Augmented dopa decarboxylase and dopamine β-oxidase activities also serve to increase the formation of anti-inflammatory amine, especially epinephrine. Presumably, monoamine oxidase activity is adequate to deal with this process.

4. POLYPEPTIDES AND POLYPEPTIDE-FORMING SYSTEMS

This has recently been reviewed by Spector and Willoughby (1968). Of the six structures now known, three are mammalian plasma kinins, bradykinin, kallidin, and methionyl-lysyl-bradykinin. Two others are venom kinins from the wasp, *Polystes*, and the last is phyllokinin, which is a bradykinin-isoleucine-tyrosine-*O*-sulfate extracted from the skin of a South American amphibian. All these kinins are peptides of molecular weight 1000 or more. In this chapter, the remarks on polypeptides and polypeptide-forming systems will be restricted to the kinins mentioned above, since much has previously been written about the various polypeptides described at different times during the inflammatory response, and most of this is now merely of historical interest (see Spector and Willoughby, 1968).

Roche e Silva and his colleagues (1949) found that snake venom or trypsin caused the formation from blood serum of a substance which caused a slow contraction of plain muscle. The substance was soon characterized as a polypeptide named bradykinin by Rocha e Silva, and it is now known that such substances can be found in blood plasma or serum subjected to a variety of procedures. These substances are known collectively as plasma kinins and have the common property of producing a slow contraction of plain muscle of the isolated ileum or uterus, of dilating arterioles or increasing the permeability of venules to large molecules, of lowering the blood pressure, and of causing pain on application to a blister. Plasma kinins have an additional property: once formed, they are rapidly destroyed by further contact with plasma due to the action of endogenous peptidases. They are also rapidly inactivated by incubation with chymotrypsin. This makes their detection in demonstration during an inflammatory process an extremely difficult procedure. The substrate in plasma which yields kinins is present in all mammalian species and, in most species including man, consists of a globulin in the α_2 fraction.

Apart from snake venom protease and trypsin, other enzymes are known to produce kinins, notably kallikrein which is present in blood plasma and other body fluids. Using the α_2-globulin as substrate, kinin formed by the action of trypsin and kallikrein has been purified and subsequently synthesized. Bradykinin is a nonapeptide with the amine acid sequence arg-pro-pro-gly-phe-ser-pro-phe-arg. Kallidin is a decapeptide with the amino acid sequence lys-arg-pro-pro-gly-phe-ser-pro-phe-arg. Of the enzymes which form plasma kinins, the most important so far described is serum kallikrein. Kallikrein is a protein of rather small molecular size described by Werler and found in urine, pancreas, salivary glands, and serum. Kallikrein is present in serum in an inactive form and may be activated by a variety of simple procedures including dilution of the serum. Kallikrein increases vascular permeability upon intradermal injection. This effect is presumably due to formation of kinins *in vivo*, but it has been suggested that a portion of this action may result from other causes, e.g., a direct action on the vessel walls. Since it is far from certain that all kinin-forming activity inplasma is due to kallikrein, activity formerly attributed to serum kallikrein is now best described as plasma kininogenase.

In addition to kinin formation by the action of certain enzymes, similar peptides are formed when plasma from a number of species is diluted with saline and brought into contact with glass or highly charged surfaces. Plasma so treated causes a slow contraction of plain muscle, gives rise to pain on application to a blister base, and increases vascular permeability to plasma protein. With the exception of the vascular effects (see below), these actions are short lived due presumably to destruction of the kinins by the plasma peptidases. In surveying these results, it seemed likely that formation of kinins by dilution of plasma is due to activation of plasma kininogenases. In fact, a completely separate line of approach is also leading to this conclusion, although only after much uncertainty. The line of approach referred to concerns factors known as PF/dil and globulin permeability factor.

In 1955, Miles and Wilhelm reported that dilution of guinea pig plasma or serum gave the fluid the property of increasing vascular permeability. The active principles called PF/dil are traced to an activation of part of the α_2 globulin fraction, this latter fraction being called globulin PF. Further work revealed that globulin PF was present in all mammalian serum, including man. In some species, however, e.g., rabbit, dog, cat, horse, and ox, globulin PF is not activated by dilution, although this does occur in man, rat, mouse, guinea pig, and baboon. Serum was also found to contain a specific inhibitor of globulin PF present in guinea pig and rat plasma in the α_1

globulin fraction. Miles has suggested that PF/dil, which is formed or activated when plasma in contact with a glass surface is diluted with saline, is part of the pathway for the formation of kininogenase. It is now generally agreed that glass contact is an essential feature of activation and that dilution serves merely to decrease the concentration of inhibitor. Miles has also obtained some experimental evidence in support of this hypothesis and has shown that the *in vitro* activation of plasma leads to the formation of two distinct substances which increase vascular permeability. These permeability factors correspond to globulin PF and kininogenase and may be differentiated by their differing heat lability and their relative abilities to attack synthetic substrates or bovine globulin. Miles has shown also that these two substances bear certain similarities in that both are inactivated by soybean trypsin inhibitor and diisopropyl fluorophosphonate. Neither agent is formed in plasma deficient in Hageman factor.

Plasma kinins such as bradykinin are characterized by their rapid destruction in plasma; kinin may be formed by activated kininogenase within 2 or 3 minutes. Therefore, it cannot be expected that the experiments usually performed on inflammation will readily demonstrate their presence. In addition, there are no specific inhibitors of kinin or kininogenases, and, indeed, the problem of demonstrating the presence of kinin has been compared with attempts to demonstrate acetylcholine without the use of anticholinesterase. Nevertheless, five main methods have been used in attempts to determine the role of kinins in inflammation: (1) the appearance of kinins or kininogenases in tissues or draining lymph; (2) estimations of kininogenases or their precursors in plasma; (3) the detection of kinins or kininogenases in urine; (4) the estimation of kinins or kininogenase activity after perfusion of inflamed areas; (5) detection of kinins or kininogenases in inflammatory exudates or blister fluids.

In thermal injury, increased excretion of kinins has been demonstrated in patients suffering from burns. Attempts to demonstrate the formation of kinins at the site of thermal injury have also been made. In this experiment, saline was injected into an air pouch whose wall was formed by the in injured skin. It is open, therefore, to the objection that the kinins extracted by the saline may have owed their presence to the dilution of exuded plasma. In inflammation due to bacterial invasion, efforts to demonstrate kinins or kinin-forming enzymes in the affected tissue proved unsuccessful. Lewis in the past few years has used the method of careful drainage and collection of lymph from inflamed areas. Lymph has been collected and examined from the hindlimbs of anesthetized dogs which have been exposed to various forms of injury including thermal damage. When the kinin-forming activity, i.e., kininogenase content, of the lymph was assayed, it was increased about eightfold over the resting level. In some circumstances, the lymph flow itself showed a corresponding eight- or ninefold increase. Attempts to demonstrate the kinins themselves, however, was invariably unsuccessful. In addition, administration of antihistamine drugs, although they failed to suppress the increased lymph flow, nevertheless completely abolished the appearance of the augmented kininogenase activity. Antihistamine drugs also failed to significantly lessen the inflammatory changes themselves and notably did not suppress the increased vascular permeability for which the kinins might have been thought responsible. Where these results might be partially explained by postulating the release of histamine as a necessary step for activation of the kinin-forming system, it must be admitted that there is no unequivocal demonstration of a role for kinins as mediators of the inflammatory response. It is generally agreed that the antihistamine drugs suppress only the very early phase of the inflammatory response, and this makes it doubly difficult to reconcile the effect of the antihistamine drugs in suppressing kinin-forming activity and their failure to effect the later phase of increased fascular permeability. It may be, therefore, that the increased kininogenase activity found in the lymph draining injured areas is a consequence of the inflammatory reaction and not a cause.

Reference has already been made to estimation of kinins in plasma during anaphylactic shock. This technique has been extended to the estimation of the concentration of kininogenase precursors in the plasma of such animals. The basis of this approach is the demonstration of a depression of the circulating level of the precursor of the kinin-forming enzyme. The inference drawn from these results is that the precursor is depleted due to extensive conversion of the kinin-forming enzyme. Once again, however, such evidence cannot be regarded as conclusive.

Another approach, which, as plasma estimations, has been developed at Sao Paulo by Rocha e Silva and his colleagues, consists of coaxial perfusion of inflamed tissue. In this system, a piece of polythene tubing is placed in the area where the inflammatory edema is to develop. Through this is passed a second tube one-half the diameter through which tyrode solution can be passed. After injury, the resulting perfusate is collected from the large tube into vessels packed in ice. With this method, it was found that after mild thermal injury of 45°C the substance released was indistinguishable from bradykinin on pharmacological assay. This system has the merit that the temperature used is too low to result in the release of histamine and 5-HT. It could, however, be argued conversely that under these conditions the injury does not result in a true or typical inflammation. It is possible also that release of bradykinin is an artifact induced by the perfusion of the tissues, perhaps in conjunction with extensive vasodilation. We are once again seeing the results of dilution of tissue factors brought about by a perfusion technique. It will be appreciated from the foregoing that the demonstration of the role of kinins and kinin-forming enzymes as mediators of inflammation is fraught with many difficulties and uncertainties.

More recently, Di Rosa and Sorrentino (1970) used cellulose sulfate to deplete animals of their plasma kininogen. Animals depleted of their kininogens were unable to develop a normal inflammatory response to carrageenan injected into their hindpaws. This has recently been reevaluated by Di Rosa *et al.* (1971a) who found that in addition to depleting animals of kininogen the cellulose sulfate caused a dramatic lowering of total hemolytic complement levels; however, within 3 hours, the complement levels of the cellulose sulfate-treated animals returned to normal, while kininogen levels remained depressed for 18–24 hours. Thus it was possible to use animals with a normal complement level, yet depleted of kininogen. Under these circumstances, it was found that after the injection of carrageenan into the hindpaw of the rat there was a distinct phase that was affected by kininogen depletion. This was a phase which persisted from roughly $1\frac{1}{2}$ to $2\frac{1}{2}$ hours after the injection of carrageenan. If the animals were first depleted of histamine, of 5-HT by means of compound 48/80, and then of kininogen by cellulose sulfate, such animals, when carrageenan was injected into their feet, failed to develop any edema until $2\frac{1}{2}$–3 hours later. In other words, using this depletion method, these workers have established that the kinins probably occupy a very transitory role in the acute inflammatory response. On the other hand, Di Rosa and Willoughby (1971) have found that after injection of dextran or formalin into the hindpaws of rats depletion with 48/80 and cellulose sulfate of the tissue stores of histamine, of 5-HT, and of kininogen in the plasma results in total suppression of the edema, i.e., as in the carrageenan situation, the mediators involved appear to be histamine and 5-HT, closely followed by kinins and then another mediator, which, as we shall see later, is almost certainly one of the prostaglandins. However, with dextran and formalin, this later mediator is missing from the system.

In conclusion, it seems that the kinins will probably be responsible for merely a transient phase of the acute inflammatory response and will be of no greater importance than the initial histamine and 5-HT roles.

5. PROSTAGLANDINS

The term "prostaglandin" relates not to a single substance but to a group of chemically related long chain hydroxy fatty acids. The name prostaglandin was coined by von Euler in 1935 to a factor found in human seminal fluid which stimulated smooth muscle and lowered blood pressure. To date, thirteen different prostaglandins have been isolated from human semen (Bergstrom, 1968). They are present in many mammalian tissues and have a wide range of pharmacological actions. There seems little doubt that members of this family play an active role in mediation of the inflammatory response. Some confusion arises on occasion due to the conflicting modes of action of different members of this family. Wein has shown that both *in vitro* and *in vivo* anaphylactic shock can lead to the production of these substances, mostly of the E_1 type. The production of these substances may well be associated with cell death and, subsequently, are to be expected to be associated with the later stages of inflammation (Brocklehurst, 1971; Pickles, 1967). They are formed by the action of common lipid oxidase from polyunsaturated aliphatic acids such as arachidonic acid. Thus, the lysosomal enzymes may have a role to play in splitting suitable fatty acids from lecithin which is present in cell membranes. Similarly, lecithinase activated by complement could lead to the formation of these prostaglandins. It has been postulated by Brocklehurst that the prostaglandin system could be self-limiting in that formation of different types of prostaglandins with conflicting properties could lead to suppression of a particular reaction.

In more specific terms, Willis has shown that during carrageenan edema of the rat paw the prostaglandins are present in the edema during the later stage of the inflammatory response. Similarly, Greaves has suggested that prostaglandins may be responsible for the vasodilation caused by ultraviolet irradiation. Recently, Giroud and Willoughby (1970) have found an interrelationship between activity of prostaglandins *in vitro* and *in vivo* and the complement system. These authors have found that depression of total hemolytic complement titers leads to a reduction in the ability to form prostaglandins *in vitro* and also to a suppression of the delayed phase of the inflammatory response. These observations have been extended by Di Rosa *et al.* (1972a) who have shown that during carrageenan edema there is a distinct phase from $2\frac{1}{2}$ to 6 hours which appears to be mediated by prostaglandins. This prostaglandin phase is closely associated with migration of leukocytes into the inflamed area. Suppression of migration of leukocytes either by polymorphonuclear depletion or by methotrexate treatment leads to some depression, as does suppression of mononuclear cell migration by nonsteroidal anti-inflammatory drugs. If both polymorphonuclear and mononuclear cells are suppressed, this treatment results in total suppression of the later edema induced by carrageeenan.

Greaves (1972) has also implicated the prostaglandins in experimental ultraviolet erythema using a perfusion method after injury. Recent unpublished results from this laboratory have revealed basically similar mechanisms with the immunosuppressive agents. It is of interest that in situations where there is an edema of the hindpaw of rats with little or no cellular migration the phase of inflammation brought about by prostaglandins appears to be missing; thus, in dextran- or formalin-induced edema of the hindpaw of rats, depletion of histamine, of 5-HT with 48/80, and depletion of kininogen by cellulose sulfate result in complete suppression of the inflammatory exudate: thus, of course, being in marked contrast to the results obtained with carrageenan in which depletion of these phases results in a late-developing edema presumably being mediated by the prostaglandins. At this point, it is probably wise to suggest that the prostaglandins have a considerable amount of presumptive evidence to support their roles as mediators of the inflammatory response. This is not conclusive, and, as was the case with the kinins until fairly recently, much of the evidence comes from perfusing the inflamed tissues, and such evidence is not good since the procedure itself may lead to activation of the prostaglandins. Similarly, in the absence of specific antagonists, it is difficult to obtain the necessary evidence. (See note added in proof.)

6. Coagulation Factors

During the acute inflammatory process, it is almost inevitable that various aspects of the coagulation process be activated. Some of these factors will be briefly considered.

a. Platelets. Agglutination of platelets, which have been considered as mobile stores of vasoactive amines carrying histamine and particularly 5-HT, can lead to liberation of these amines during the early phase of the inflammatory response.

b. Factor XII or Hageman Factor. This has been clearly implicated as part of the possible pathway for the activation of kinins, and it is now thought that the contact factor responsible for the formation of the kinins is probably activated Hageman factor. Hageman factor seems to promote release of kinins by activating both kallikreinogen and plasminogen. Although the kinin-releasing effect of plasmin would be due to kallikreinogen activation, a direct effect of plasmin on kininogen has also been demonstrated. Similarly, plasmin becomes activated after tissue injury which potentially will also act on kininogen to form active kinins. The early mediators can also provide a feedback mechanism. Histamine released during the early phase of the inflammatory response enhances plasma fibrinolytic activity, possibly by speeding up the conversion of plasminogen to plasmin. A similar sequence of events has been postulated for the kinins.

c. Fibrinogen. Fibrinogen, which leaves vessels as a consequence of possibly a nonspecific response to injury, is converted to fibrin. Formed fibrin is a potent activator of the plasmin system (Astrup, 1966). Indeed, after injury, the tissues have been shown to release a variety of activators of plasminogen, and, as long ago as 1947, Astrup and Perunin named these activators "cytofibrinokinases." More recently in some elegant studies, Barnhart (1968) has shown that fibrin and related products may be of importance in acute inflammation due to their powerful chemotactic activity for polymorphonuclear leukocytes.

III. Trigger Mechanisms

What is responsible for launching the inflammatory response after an injurious stimulus? Recent studies from this laboratory have shown that the most likely sequence of events is based upon activation of complement. In the scheme proposed, it is suggested that inflammatory stimulus leads to production of some modified protein capable of activating the complement system. It has been found by Houck and his colleagues (1971) that a variety of simple dermal injuries can lead to the activation of collagenases. The action of these collagenases can produce breakdown products which are capable of causing leukocyte emigration in millimicrogram amounts *in vitro* and *in vivo*; this was shown with a modification of the Rebuck skin window technique. Probably more important is that such enzyme activation leading to modification of tissue protein serves as a stimulus for the activation of complement. That such a sequence of events may occur has been shown in experiments in which serum of known complement titer has been incubated with skin after thermal injury. This led to a rapid fall in the complement titer, suggesting an activation and exhaustion of the complement components. No such fall occurred when normal skin was incubated with serum.

Activation of the complement system leads to the formation of various vasoactive factors including histamine liberators, possibly kinins, and prostaglandinlike substances. This has recently been reviewed by Giroud and Willoughby (1970) and Di Rosa et al. (1972a,b). These workers found that activation of prostaglandinlike substances in inflammation depends upon the presence of an intact complement system and that suppression of total hemolytic complement titer results in a diminished ability to form these mediators. Similarly (Willoughby et al., 1969), it was found that suppression of total hemolytic complement led to a reduction in the acute inflammatory response to either thermal or chemical injury. Whereas the complement system was viewed merely as being associated with the immune reaction, it now seems necessary to consider its role as a trigger mechanism in acute, nonimmunological reactions.

IV. Leukocytes as Mediators

It has been suggested that the polymorphonuclear leukocytes may be involved in the acute inflammatory response as potential mediators of increased vascular permeability: the hypothesis being that the emigrated polymorphonuclear cell would discharge its contents of lysosomal enzymes and that these proteases would increase vascular permeability.

Recently, this concept has been disproved by Willoughby and Spector

(1968) and by Giroud and Willoughby (1969). These workers found that during the inflammatory response to either thermal injury or chemical injury in the rat animals rendered totally agranulocytic could still mount normal inflammatory responses. Furthermore, these animals depleted of their polymorphonuclear cells still responded normally to various irritants in terms of the numbers of mononuclear cells migrating to the site of injury. This would seem to indicate that both vascular and cellular sequelae proceed in a normal fashion in the absence of polymorphonuclear cells.

In contrast, during experiments with carrageenan injected into the hindpaw of rats, by measuring the subsequent edema, Di Rosa et al. (1972b) found that depletion of polymorphonuclear cells leads to a slight reduction in the edema normally associated with release of prostaglandins. Similarly, nonsteroidal anti-inflammatory drugs led to a reduction in the later edema which was associated with suppression of migration of mononuclear cells. Combining these two forms of treatment, i.e., depletion of polymorphonuclears and inhibition of mononuclear cell migration, resulted in almost total suppression of the prostaglandin-mediated phase of carrageenan edema. Furthermore, there was a highly significant correlation between inhibition of migration of mononuclear cells and inhibition of edema. It is of interest that in situations such as dextran- or formalin-induced edema that provoke a minimal cell migration the prostaglandin-mediated phase is virtually missing, thus providing negative evidence supporting the concept of the prostaglandin-mediated phase being associated with migration of cells.

Thus, it is of interest that apparently similar models of acute inflammation have different mediators present according to their ability to provide migrating leukocytes.

V. The Case Against Mediators

Probably, the best, most closely reasoned case against endogenous mediators is that put forward by Hurley et al. (1967). This is based on the carbon-labeling method applied to mild thermal injury, particularly during the delayed phase of increased vascular permeability. These workers point out that when using this model the delayed phase of increased permeability is via capillaries, whereas the known mediators have an action confined to venules (Majno, 1965). In addition, they feel it is necessary to postulate that if this change is brought about by an unknown mediator it must have different actions in skin and muscle, or, alternatively, that some noxious substance is released by these tissues under the influence of this unknown mediator. They felt that there was no evidence to support this concept.

In contrast, they suggested that all features of the delayed response are readily explicable if it is assumed that mild thermal injury causes direct damage to the wall of the vessels in the burned area. They supported this hypothesis by finding damage to both venules and capillaries which is detectable using the electron microscope (Ham and Hurley, 1968). Finally, an analogy is drawn to the toxic effects of certain agents in the liver. Thus, injected carbon tetrachloride reaches the liver within 2 hours (Dawkins, 1963). This results in minor and apparently nonspecific damage at this stage. Definite evidence of damage to liver cells appears during the next few hours with concomitant biochemical evidence of gross disturbance of cellular function. Clear evidence of necrosis in the more severely damaged areas is not seen until 10–12 hours after the injection of carbon tetrachloride (Judah et al., 1964; Rees, 1964).

From analogy, Hurley and his co-workers suggest that it is not surprising that the escape of plasma does not occur through vessel walls until some hours after the direct injury to the vessel walls.

If one bears in mind the possibility of the involvement of the complement system, it seems more likely that a system of mediators could be involved which appear later on in the acute inflammatory response. Possibly, the terminal components of complement are responsible for these changes in capillaries. Similarly, the activation of SH-dependent proteases postulated by Hayashi and his co-workers could produce changes in the capillaries. Certainly, proteases isolated from the skin (Lykke et al., 1967) have been shown to exert an effect upon both venules and capillaries.

VI. Delayed Hypersensitivity

Of all the mediators that have been considered above in nonimmunological inflammation and in immediate hypersensitivity, cell-mediated immunity alone seems to be unique in that none of these mediators appear to be involved. Thus, there is no evidence that histamine, 5-HT, kinins, or, thus far, prostaglandins is involved in this type of reaction.

The first mediator to be seriously considered for the role of mediator of these reactions was a membrane-free extract of lymph node cells named "lymph node permeability factor" (LNPF). This term was applied to the biologically active factors present within lymph node cells (Schild and Willoughby, 1967). Such extracts were potent in increasing vascular permeability (Willoughby et al., 1962), in causing leukocyte emigration (Willoughby and Spector, 1964b), and also in bringing about the deposition of something resembling connective tissue fibroid (Willoughby and Spector,

1964a). Thus, this material had many of the properties that one would wish to see in a potential mediator of a cell-mediated reaction.

It was subsequently found that bringing sensitized cells into contact with appropriate antigens caused the release of this material into the incubating fluid (Willoughby *et al.*, 1964). Later studies showed that the active principle rose in concentration at the site of various delayed hypersensitivity reactions: tuberculin (Willoughby *et al.*, 1964), DNCB (Willoughby *et al.*, 1965), thyroiditis (Willoughby and Coote, 1966), pertussis (Willoughby, 1966), and homograft reaction. In addition, antisera prepared against LNPF caused a suppression of the various cell-mediated reactions listed above. The final evidence for the role of LNPF, which is almost certainly a mixture of factors, is that neonatal treatment of rats with rat LNPF causes a diminished reactivity to this material in the adult rat, yet it still retains reactivity to other PF's. Such neonatally treated rats cannot develop normal delayed hypersensitivity reactions as adults. It has been shown that such unresponsive animals develop sensitized cells in response to antigenic stimulation, but that they fail to react to the released mediator, thereby demonstrating that neonatal treatment does not influence the basic immunological responsiveness, but only the response to the mediator and the subsequent inflammatory process.

Purification of the lymph node permeability factor has proved difficult, and it often appears to be bound to plasma protein fractions (Meacock and Willoughby, 1968). Removal of the active principle form the plasma protein fraction has resulted, so far, in loss of activity. Nevertheless, it would seem that this material is one of the most likely candidates for the role of mediator of delayed hypersensitivity or cell-mediated immune reactions.

More recently, Dumonde (1970) has coined the expression "lymphokines" to describe the biologically active factors released from sensitized lymph node cells after coming into contact with antigen. One of these factors bears a striking resemblance to the lymph node permeability factor described above. It was thought at one time (Pick *et al.*, 1969) that these were different factors based on the use of protein synthesis inhibitors. Thus, antigen in contact with sensitized cells in the presence of puromycin or actinomycin D failed to release the active lymphokine responsible for inflammation. However, subsequent work from this laboratory has shown that these inhibitors lead to an antagonism or destruction of the preformed lymphokine and also of lymph node permeability factor. Parish (1971) has also suggested a similar identity between these factors on the basis of chemical similarities between the phlogistic lymphokine released from sensitized lymphocytes and that found in nonsensitized cells (LNPF) (see Meacock and Willoughby, 1968).

Finally, Pick *et al.* (1970) have shown that normal guinea pig cells exposed to mitogens *in vitro* release an inflammatory substance similar to that liberated by sensitized lymphocytes incubated with specific antigen.

VII. Unifying Hypothesis of Inflammation

Recently, Willoughby and Di Rosa (1971) described the possible inter-relationships of these various factors and their roles in bringing about the complex picture of the inflammatory response. It has been suggested that the key factor is probably the production of "modified protein" such as can be produced by the collagenases described by Houck and his colleagues. Such modified proteins potentially may become antigenic and lead to the production of antibody. In acute inflammation, the more likely role of this modified protein would be to activate the complement system leading to release of histamine, leukocyte migration, and concomitant activation of prostaglandins. Simulataneoulsy, the coagulation system would become activated leading to formation of kinins, and these would be enhanced by the plasmin system. In such a scheme, it would be possible to activate relatively late phases of the complement system by virtue of the plasmin system.

It is of interest that in such a scheme there is provision for feedback mechanisms. Thus, the kinins can enhance the plasmin system as can histamine. Serum factors of the type described by Keller and Sorkin would be activated and would lead to migration of both polymorphonuclear and mononuclear cells.

It is this interaction of various factors that constitutes the challenge to workers of different disciplines to elucidate the precise mechanisms of both the acute inflammatory response and the transition to chronicity.

VIII. Conclusions

The relative importance of different endogenous mediators in inflammation would seem to vary considerably according to both the type of injury and also the intensity of the inflammatory response. It must be borne in mind that mediators effective in one species will be less important in other species. The relative importance of nonspecific injury to the endothelial cells and the contribution to the inflammatory response by this nonmediated injury again will depend on type and intensity and possibly site of injury. Once one postulates late leakage of plasma protein independent of mediators, the question becomes semantic. Thus, are lysosomal enzymes and other proteases truly mediators, or is this nonspecific response to injury a consequence of dying cells? Such questions often cause misunderstandings among groups of workers in this field.

It would appear that as postulated in 1957 by Spector and Willoughby histamine is at this present time the only mediator that fulfils all the criteria that one would demand. It is present at the site of injury at the appropriate time; its antagonism with low doses of antagonist causes suppression of that transient phase of inflammation for which it is deemed responsible. Histamine itself can reproduce the events which it is alleged to mediate. Depletion of the tissue stores of histamine similarly prevents that phase of the inflammatory response. However, it may well transpire that with the passing of time the antihistamines may exert a multiplicity of effects of which histamine antagonism is relatively unimportant. It has certainly been shown recently by J. P. Giroud (unpublished, 1971) that treatment with compound 48/80 decreases total hemolytic complement titers.

Nevertheless, it would seem safe to say that of all the mediators, the evidence for histamine seems most convincing. For the others, cases are being developed which at this point are not convincingly proved for any of them despite the welter of "substantial evidence."

Note Added in Proof

Since this chapter was written, enormous interest has been shown in prostaglandins. Papers on this subject are now appearing at the rate of 900 per year. Vane, Willis, and their colleagues at the Royal College of Surgeons of England have elaborated a theory of prostaglandin synthesis which occurs at the inflamed site. The PG-forming enzyme (PG synthetase) has been shown to be blocked by certain nonsteroidal anti-inflammatory drugs and has been proposed as the mode of action of these therapeutic agents. PGE, a member of this family of fatty acids, has, in turn, been shown to be present during anaphylactic reactions and in acute and chronic inflammatory exudates. It is capable of increasing vascular permeability and is chemotactic to leukocytes. On the other hand, it has also been shown to be anti-inflammatory under certain conditions, e.g., when tested on adjuvant-induced arthritis. It has been suggested by Weissman and his colleagues that this may be due to its ability to prevent the liberation of hydrolases from cells due to the buildup of intracellular cyclic AMP.

Space does not permit adequate description of the recent work on prostaglandins. The interested reader is referred to reviews by Kaley and Weiner (1971), Vane (1972), and Willoughby et al. (1973).

References

Astrup, T. (1966). *Fed. Proc., Fed. Amer. Soc. Exp. Biol.* **25**, 42.

Astrup, T., and Perinin, P. M. (1947). *Nature (London)* **159**, 681.

Barger, G., and Dale, H. H. (1910). *J. Physiol. (London)* **41**, 499.

Barnhart, M. I. (1968). *In* "Chemical Biology of Inflammation" (B. K. Forscher, ed.), p. 205. Pergamon, Oxford.

Bergstrom, S. (1967). *Science* **157**, 382.

Bergstrom, S., Carlson, L. A., and Weeks, J. R. (1968). *Pharmacol. Res.* **20**, 1.

Böhm, G. M. (1966). *J. Pathol. Bacteriol.* **92**, 151.

Brocklehurst, W. E. (1971). *Proc. Roy. Soc. Med.* **64**, 4.

Cotran, R. S., and Majno, G. (1964). *Amer. J. Pathol.* **46**, 589.

Dale, H. H. (1948). *Brit Med. J.* **2**, 281.

Dawkins, M. J. R. (1963). *J. Pathol. Bacteriol.* **85**, 189.

Di Rosa, M., and Sorrentino, L. (1970). *Brit. J. Pharmacol.* **38**, 214.

Di Rosa, M., and Willoughby, D. A. (1971). *J. Pharm. Pharmacol.* **23**, 297.

Di Rosa, M., and Willoughby, D. A. (1972). *J. Pathol.* (in press).

Di Rosa, M., Giroud, J. P., and Willoughby, D. A. (1971a). *J. Pathol.* **104**, 15

Di Rosa, M., Papadimitriou, J. M., and Willoughby, D. A. (1971b). *J. Pathol.* **105**, 239.

Dumonde, D. C. (1970). *Proc. Roy. Soc. Med.* **63**, 899.

Ellinger, F. (1928). *Naunyn-Schmiedeberss Arch. Exp. Pathol. Pharmakol.* **136**, 129.

Ellinger, F. (1930). *Naunyn-Schmiedeberss Arch. Exp. Pathol. Pharmakol.* **149**, 344.

Giroud, J. P., and Willoughby, D. A. (1969). *J. Pathol.* **98**, 53.

Giroud, J. P., and Willoughby, D. A. (1970). *J. Pathol.* **101**, 241.

Greaves, M. W. (1972). In press.

Halpern, B. N. (1956). *Histamine, Ciba Found. Symp., 1955* p. 140.

Halpern, B. N., Neven, T., and Spector, S. (1963). *Brit. J. Pharmacol. Chemather.* **20**, 389.

Ham, K. N., and Hurley, J. V. (1968). *J. Pathol. Bacteriol.* **95**, 175.

Hayashi, H. (1967). *Trans. Soc. Pathol. Jap.* **56**, 37.

Houck, J. C., Barnes, S. G., and Chang, C. (1971). *In* "Immunopathology of Inflammation," (B. K. Forscher and J. C. Houck, eds). Int. Congr. Ser. Excerpta M. Found., Amsterdam. No. 299, p. 39.

Hurley, J. V. (1963). *Aust. J. Exp. Biol. Med. Sci.* **41**, 171.

Hurley, J. V., and Spector, W. G. (1965). *J. Pathol. Bacteriol.* **89**, 245.

Hurley, J. V., Ham, K. N., and Ryan, G. B. (1967). *J. Pathol. Bacteriol.* **94**, 1.

Jacobson, W. (1958). *In* "5-Hydroxytryptamine" (G. P. Lewis, ed.), p. 38 Pergamon, Oxford.

Judah, J. D., Ahmed, K., and McLean, A. E. M. (1964). *Cell. Injury, Ciba Found. Symp., 1963* p. 187.

Kaley, G., and Weiner, R. (1971). *Ann N. Y. Acad. Sci.* **180**, 338.

Kalmus, H., and Willoughby, D. A. (1960). *Heredity* **14**, 227.

Kawaguchi, S. (1930). *Biochem. Z.* **221**, 232.

Kranz, J. C., Carr, C. J., Bird, J. G., and Cook, S. (1948). *J. Pharmacol. Exp. Ther.* **93**, 188.

Krogh, A. (1929). "The Anatomy and Physiology of Capillaries," 2nd ed. Yale Univ. Press, New Haven, Connecticut.

Lewis, G. P. (1960). *Physiol. Rev.* **40**, 647.

Lewis, T. (1929). "Blood Vessels of the Human Skin and Their Responses," Shaw, London.

Lykke, A. W. J., Willoughby, D. A., and Houch, J. C. (1967). *J. Invest. Dermatol.* **48**, 318.

Majno, G. (1965). *In* "Handbook of Physiology" (Amer. Physiol. Soc., J. Field, ed.), Vol. 3, Sect. 2, p. 2293. Williams & Wilkins, Baltimore, Maryland.

Majno, G., Palade, G. E., and Schoefl, G. I. (1961). *J. Biophys. Biochem. Cytol.* **11**, 607.

MacIntosh, F. C., and Paton, W. D. M. (1949). *J. Physiol. (London)* **190**, 199.

Meacock, S. C. R., and Willoughby, D. A. (1968). *Immunology* **15**, 101.

Miles, A. A., and Wilhelm, D. L. (1955). *Brit. J. Exp. Pathol.* **36**, 71.

Moglinitsky, B. N., and Brhumshstein, S. (1949). *Publ. Acad. Med. Sci. (Moscow)* **61**.

Molle, H. (1962). *Acta Dermato-Venereol.* **42**, 386.

Mongar, J. L., and Schild, H. O. (1962). *Physiol. Rev.* **42**, 226.

Moulton, R., Spector, W. G., and Willoughby, D. A. (1957). *Brit. J. Pharmacol. Chemother.* **12**, 365.

Northover, B. J. (1963). *J. Pathol. Bacteriol.* **85**, 361.

Northover, B. J., and Subramanian, G. (1961). *Brit. J. Pharmacol. Chemother.* **16**, 163.

Parratt, J. R., and West, G. B. (1957a). *J. Physiol. (London)* **137**, 169.

Parratt, J. R., and West, G. B. (1957b). *J. Physiol. (London)* **137**, 179.

Parratt, J. R., and West, G. B. (1957c). *J. Physiol. (London)* **139**, 27.

Parish, W. E. (1971). *In* "Immunology and the Skin" (W. Montagna and R. E. Billingham, eds.), p. 1. Appleton, New York.

Paton, W. D. M. (1951). *Brit. J. Pharmacol. Chemother.* **6** 499.

Paton, W. D. M. (1957). *Pharmacol. Rev.* **9**, 269.

Pick, E., Krejci, J., and Turk, J. L. (1970). *Nature (London)* **225**, 236.

Pick, E., Krejci, J., Cech, K., and Turk, J. L. (1969). *Immunology* **17**, 741.

Pickles, V. R. (1967). *Biol. Rev. Cambridge Phil. Soc.* **42**, 617.

Raekallio, J. (1963). *Nature (London)* **199**, 496.

Rees, K. R. (1964). *Cell Injury, Ciba Found. Symp., 1963* p. 53.

Riley, R. F., and West, G. B. (1953). "The Mast Cells." Livingstone, Edinburgh.

Rocha e Silva, M. (1956). *Histamine, Ciba Found. Symp., 1955* p. 178.

Rocha e Silva, M., Beraldo, W. T., and Rosenfeld, G. (1949). *Amer. J. Physiol* **156**, 261.

Rowley, D. A., and Benditt, E. P. (1956). *J. Exp. Med.* **103**, 399.

Schayer, R. W. (1963). *Progr. Allergy* **7**, 187.

Schild, H. O., and Willoughby, D. A. (1967). *Brit. Med. Bull.* **23**, 46.

Setnikar, I., Sulvaterra, M., and Temelcou, O. (1959). *Brit. J. Pharmacol. Chemother.* **14**, 484.

Sheldon, W. H., and Bauer, H. (1960). *J. Exp. Med.* **112**, 1069.

Smith, D. E. (1958a). *Amer. J. Physiol.* **193**, 573.

Smith, D. E. (1958b). *Science* **128**, 207.

Smith, D. E., and Miles, A. A. (1960). *Brit. J. Exp. Pathol.* **41**, 305.

Spector, W. G. (1958). *Pharmacol. Rev.* **10**, 475.

Spector, W. G., and Willoughby, D. A. (1957). *J. Pathol. Bacteriol.* **74**, 57.

Spector, W. G., and Willoughby, D. A. (1959). *J. Pathol. Bacteriol.* **78**, 121.

Spector, W. G., and Willoughby, D. A. (1960). *J. Pathol. Bacteriol.* **80**, 271.

Spector, W. G., and Willoughby, D. A. (1963a). *Bacteriol. Rev.* **27**, 117.

Spector, W. G., and Willoughby, D. A. (1963b). *J. Pathol. Bacteriol.* **78**, 121.

Spector, W. G., and Willoughby, D. A. (1964a). *Ann. N. Y. Acad. Sci.* **116**, 839.

Spector, W. G., and Willoughby, D. A. (1964b). *J. Pathol. Bacteriol.* **87**, 341.

Spector, W. G., and Willoughby, D. A. (1968). "The Pharmacology of Inflammation," English Univ. Press, London.

Spector, W. G., Willoughby, D. A., and Frears, J. (1963) *Nature (London)* **198**, 595.

Spector, W. G., Walters, M. N-I., and Willoughby, D. A. (1965). *J. Pathol. Bacteriol.* **90**, 635.

Ungar, G., and Damgaard, E. (1954). *Proc. Soc. Exp. Biol. Med.* **87**, 383.

Uvnäs, B. (1958). *J. Pharm. Pharmacol.* **10**, 1.

Vane, J. R. (1972). *Hosp. Pract.* **7**, 61.

Wells, F. R., and Miles, A. A. (1963). *Nature (London)* **200**, 1015.

Werle, E. (1955). *In* "Polypeptides which Stimulate Plain Muscle" (J. H. Gaddum, ed.), p. 20. Livingstone, Edinburgh.

West, G. B. (1955). *J. Pharm. Pharmacol.* **7**, 80.

Wilhelm, D. L., and Mason, B. (1960). *Brit. J. Exp. Pathol.* **41**, 487.

Willoughby, D. A. (1959a). *J. Physiol. (London)* **148**, 42.

Willoughby, D. A. (1959b). *Nature (London)* **184**, 1156.

Willoughby, D. A. (1960). *Brit. J. Radiol.* **33**, 515.

Willoughby, D. A. (1962). *J. Pathol. Bacteriol.* **83**, 389.

Willoughby, D. A. (1966). *J. Pathol. Bacteriol.* **92**, 139.

Willoughby, D. A., and Coote, E. (1966). *J. Pathol. Bacteriol.* **92**, 281.

Willoughby, D. A., and Di Rosa, M. (1971). *In* "Immunopathology of Inflammation," Int. Congr. Ser. No. 299, p. 28. Excerpta Med. Found., Amsterdam.

Willoughby, D. A., and Spector, W. G. (1962). *Int. J. Neuropharmacol.* **1**, 217.

Willoughby, D. A., and Spector, W. G. (1964a). *J. Pathol. Bacteriol.* **88**, 159.

Willoughby, D. A., and Spector, W. G. (1964b). *J. Pathol. Bacteriol.* **88**, 557.

Willoughby, D. A., and Spector, W. G. (1968). *Nature (London)* **219**, 1258.

Willoughby, D. A., Boughton, B., and Spector, W. G. (1964). *J. Pathol. Bacteriol.* **87**, 353.

Willoughby, D. A., Walters, M. N-I., and Spector, W. G. (1965). *Immunology* **8**, 578.

Willoughby, D. A., Coote, E., and Turk, J. L. (1969). *J. Pathol.* **97**, 295.

Willoughby, D. A., Boughten, B., Spector, W. G., and Schild, H. O. (1962). *Life Sci.* No. 7 p. 347.

Willoughby, D. A., Giroud, J. P., Di Rosa, M., and Velo, G. P. (1973). (In press).

Part II

HEMATOLOGICAL CONSIDERATIONS

Chapter 10

HEMOSTATIC MECHANISMS IN TISSUE INJURY

R. G. MACFARLANE

I. Introduction

A. Definition

In this chapter, the term "hemostasis" means the spontaneous arrest of bleeding by a physiological process based on the reactions of the blood and tissues to injury. It is not applied in its literal sense which would include the stasis of blood in mechanically intact blood vessels; nor does it include the therapeutic devices often used to control bleeding, such as clamps, cauteries, sutures, dressings, tourniquests, or the operation of "hemostatic" drugs.

B. Mechanical Factors in Hemostasis

It might be supposed that the process of hemostasis would be easy to analyze since it involves the sort of mechanical principles familiar to anyone who understands simple plumbing. A number of workers have, in fact, underestimated its complexity, including myself (Macfarlane, 1941), and it is salutory to refer to the view expressed by Jones in 1810: "We can no longer consider the suppression of haemorrhage as a simple or mechanical effect, but as a process performed by the concurrent and successive operations of many causes" [a statement which is quoted by Quick (1957)]. It requires extensive biological experience to realize that mechanical principles seldom operate either singly or simply in living systems and that behind every obvious change there lies a complex network, rather than a linear chain, of cause and effect. But at least an initial approach can be made by way of physical considerations. The first of these concerns the factors which determine bleeding. Bleeding means the loss of whole blood from the vascular system, and it can only occur if, in the wall of a blood vessel, there is a breach large enough to allow the passage of a substantial number of blood cells and if the blood pressure within the vessel exceeds the pressure outside it. In the case of an individual vessel, the rate of bleeding depends on the size of the hole and the pressure differential. In practice, the sort of vessel injured and the nature and extent of the injury are factors which determine the rate of blood loss, and they also invoke different hemostatic responses, varying widely in effectiveness. For example, incised wounds of large arteries are likely to cause bleeding beyond the control of natural hemostasis, and they may be fatal if artificial aids are not applied, whereas wounds to similar arteries involving crushing or laceration of the tissues may bleed surprisingly little. Injuries to large veins may bleed profusely, but the pressure within the vessel may be so low that elevation of the injured part, a fall in general blood pressure, or an accumulation of blood in the tissues will stop the bleeding. Blood loss from the small vessels depends initially on the number injured and the rate at which blood is supplied to them, that is, on the degree of hyperemia or ischemia of the tissues involved. In damage to this type of vessel, the hemostatic mechanism is highly effective; the bleeding ceases spontaneously within a few minutes, and its normal operation is only appreciated when its failure is observed in cases of hemophilia or purpura, in which hemorrhage from even slight injuries may be disastrously prolonged.

From the mechanical point of view, bleeding from an injured vessel will cease if the internal and external hydrostatic pressures become equalized or if the hole in the vessel wall, or the vessel itself, becomes blocked by solid material. Without too much analytical hairsplitting, it can be seen that these two eventualities can be brought about by a number of different factors, some of which are interrelated. Equalization of pressure may result from a rise in external pressure caused, for example, by accumulation of blood in the surrounding tissues, or it can result from a fall in the general blood pressure, from a local fall due to vascular constriction, or from diversion of the blood flow through shunt connections which bypass the area of damage.

Mechanical obliteration of an opening into a vessel may occur in two main ways: (1) by the formation of a solid plug derived from the blood and (2) by the active contraction of the vessel wall at or near the site of injury so that the lumen becomes obliterated. In some circumstances and in small vessels, mutual adhesion of intimal surfaces at the site of injury may cause sealing, perhaps independent of plug formation or contraction. Solid masses may form extravascularly in the wound orifice, thus impeding the escape of blood to the surface from vessels which have not yet been plugged or constricted by raising the hydrostatic pressure in the tissues. These events have been discussed in detail by Tocantins (1947), and some are well illustrated in the drawings made by Wharton Jones in 1851.

II. The Hemostatic Plug

The importance of coagulation of the blood as a hemostatic factor has been recognized for centuries. Petit (1731) applied the term *bouchon* to the adherent clot which forms in a damaged vessel, and Jones (1810) described "the formation of a coagulum at its mouth, the inflammation and consolidation of its extremity by an effusion of coagulable lymph within its canal, between its tunic and in the cellular substance surrounding it." The views applied mainly to large vessels and emphasized a coagulation which meant, to later workers, fibrin formation. Microscope studies of the hemostatic plug, particularly in small vessels, showed that fibrin was not the only and, perhaps, not the most important constituent. Wharton Jones (1851) described the formation of a "grey granulous substance" at the site of injury to frogs' web vessels, which might obstruct the flow of blood and which appeared to consist of colorless corpuscles as well as fibrin. Zahn (1872) found that bleeding from a cut vessel might be arrested by the formation of a white mass, not a blood clot. Hayem (1878, 1882) investigated the structure of the mass which forms at the site of an incision in a vein in dogs and which finally plugs the opening. He called this mass the *clou hemostatique*, and showed that it was mainly composed of "hemoblasts" (platelets), fibrin being apparently of secondary importance. He predicted that a deficiency of platelets would lead to persistent bleeding.

Subsequent work largely confirmed these early observations by Hayem. Bizzozero (1882) established the identity of platelets and their adhesive properties, and Schimmelbusch (1885) made further studies of their role in hemostasis. More recently, by microscope observations in living tissues and histological techniques. M. B. Zucker (1947), H. D. Zucker (1949), and Hugues (1953, 1959), among others, have shown that the aggregation of platelets is an early and, perhaps, essential part in the formation of the hemostatic plug. The subject is reviewed by Roskam (1960). Electron microscope studies have also been made by Kjaerheim and Hovig (1962) and by French *et al.* (1964a) which reveal the detailed structure of hemostatic plugs and of the platelets during aggregation.

In the early stages of the development of the hemostatic plug, platelet aggregation proceeds without visible fibrin formation. Later stages normally involve the laying down of fibrin strata. Later still, when bleeding has stopped, the wound area and some vessels opening into it may contain a typical blood clot derived from the massive coagulation of static blood, and consisting of a meshwork of fibrin entangling randomly distributed platelets, red cells, and leukocytes. It is probable that the early layering of fibrin and the later massive clotting may achieve a more permanent hemostasis than can be obtained by platelet aggregation alone. It has been observed that in vessels which have been injured but not disrupted platelet thrombi form rapidly, but also break down rapidly (Florey, 1925; Honour and Ross-Russell, 1962), and it is a feature of these "white bodies" that fibrin formation does not occur. By contrast, the hemostatic plug is relatively stable, and a renewal of bleeding is normally uncommon. It is, however, common in those conditions such as hemophilia in which fibrin formation is deficient, so that fibrin must be regarded as important hemostatically as the platelets. It would be useful at this point to consider in detail the factors concerned both in fibrin formation and in platelet aggregation.

A. Fibrin Formation and the Blood-Clotting Mechanism

1. THE THROMBIN–FIBRINOGEN REACTION

The formation of a network of fibrin which converts fluid blood into a solid is a complex process. Fibrin is produced by polymerization of a soluble plasma constituent, fibrinogen: a protein with the high molecular weight of about 340,000 (Caspary and Kekwick, 1954) and a normal concentration of 200–400 mg per 100 ml of plasma. The fibrinogen molecule is thought to be rod shaped with two terminal and one central nodule (Hall and Slayter, 1959). Although it is the least stable of the plasma proteins, being most readily precipitated by heat or salt, fibrinogen forms the typical strands of fibrin only as the result of the action of thrombin. Thrombin has been recognized as a clotting factor since the work of Schmidt (1895). The names "fibrin ferment" (Schmidt, 1895) and "thrombase" (Mellanby, 1933) applied to thrombin reflect the view that it was an enzyme which acted on fibrinogen, a supposition which was confirmed by the brilliant work of Laki (1953),

Lorand (1952, 1954), and Bettelheim and Bailey (1952). It is now known that thrombin is a highly specific proteolytic enzyme, capable of splitting the fibrinogen molecule into one major and several smaller fragments or peptides. The major fragments constitute the fibrin monomer, and, given the right physical conditions, they polymerize by end-to-end and side-to-side alignment to form fibers. The process of polymerization is thought to be assisted by the loss from the fibrinogen molecules of negatively charged peptides containing glutamic acid, thus reducing electrostatic repulsion.

Actual fiber formation is probably due to covalent bonding. Later, secondary linkages may be brought into play by another factor known as the "fibrin stabilizing factor" (Factor XIII). This makes the fibrin mechanically stronger and insoluble in substances such as urea or monochloroacetic acid which are solvents of unstabilized fibrin (Lorand and Jacobsen, 1958, 1964).

2. PROTHROMBIN AND ITS ACTIVATION

Thrombin is not present in detectable amounts in normal circulating blood, and the explanation of its appearance in shed blood was sought by many workers during the first half of this century. The so-called classic theory of Morawitz (1905) postulated an inert precursor, prothrombin, which was converted into thrombin by the action of calcium and a hypothetical factor, "thromboplastin," derived from damaged tissues. There were thus four factors required for clotting: fibrinogen, prothrombin, thromboplastin, and calcium. The existence of prothrombin as a chemical entity and the derivation of thrombin from its molecule seem to be established beyond doubt by the fundamental work of Seegers and his collaborators, which has extended over many years (for references, see Seegers, 1962). Purified prothrombin will give rise to smaller molecules with thrombin activity on incubation with citrate, although the reaction is slow. Extremely rapid activation occurs with various blood or tissue fractions, and there is evidence suggesting that this is due to enzymic splitting of the prothrombin molecule. Prothrombin has a molecular weight of about 68,000, and its amino acid composition has been determined. It is relatively stable and is absorbed by various inorganic precipitates. Its concentration in normal plasma is thought to be about 10 mg/100 ml, and 1 mg of the best preparations will yield about 2700 units of thrombin.

Although knowledge of prothrombin and thrombin has been put on a biochemical basis by this work, the natural process of prothrombin activation is still in doubt. Since the blood remains fluid in the normal circulatory system, it can be inferred that no significant amount of prothrombin activator is present. For many years, clotting was thought to be initiated, when blood was shed or vessels were damaged, by thromboplastin released from damaged tissues—a view based on the observation that tissue extracts when added to blood caused clotting within about 15 seconds. Many attempts were made to identify the active principle in these tissue extracts. Some workers thought that it was an enzyme (thrombokinase), and others thought that it was a phospholipid; attempts at purification have led, not to a gain, but to a loss of specific activity (Biggs and Bidwell, 1957).

Meanwhile, the activity of crude tissue extract was used to practical effect by Quick (1935, 1937) with the introduction of the prothrombin time test. This test consists of adding an excess of brain extract and an optimum amount of calcium to citrated blood and recording the clotting time. By the classic theory, this clotting time should be proportional to the prothrombin deficiency, which is a cause of bleeding in jaundice and liver disease. This test assisted in the discovery of vitamin K, paved the way for the discovery of the coumarin drugs, and is widely applied for controlling their use in treating thrombosis. Focus on the mechanism of prothrombin activation has led to the discovery of an unexpected complexity, the details of which are only now becoming appreciated.

The wide application of this test uncovered the fact that in some blood samples the prothrombin time might be abnormally long despite a normal

TABLE I

THE ROMAN NUMERAL SYSTEM OF CLOTTING FACTOR NOMENCLATURE AND SOME PREVIOUSLY USED SYNONYMS

Factor	Synonyms
I	Fibrinogen
II	Prothrombin
III	Thromboplastin (tissue extract)
IV	Calcium
V	Proaccelerin, labile factor, accelerator globulin
VI	Accelerin or some other intermediate product of pro-thrombin activator formation (not used now)
VII	Proconvertin, serum prothrombin conversion accelerator (SPCA), stable factor, autoprothrombin I
VIII	Antihemophilic factor (AHF), antihemophilic globulin (AHG), platelet cofactor I, antihemophilic factor A
IX	Plasma thromboplastin component (PTC), Christmas factor, platelet cofactor II, autoprothrombin II, antihemophilic factor B
X	Stuart-Prower factor
XI	Plasma thromboplastin antecedent (PTA)
XIII	Fibrin-stabilizing factor

prothrombin concentration as determined by other methods. Such discrepancies were clarified when it was shown independently by Quick (1943) and Owren (1947) that there was an additional (or fifth) clotting factor required for the activation of prothrombin, any deficiency of which would lengthen the prothrombin time. The newly recognized factor was named "Factor V" by Owren (1947) and was shown to be a labile β-globulin, differing from prothrombin in that it is not absorbed by inorganic precipitates and loses activity in stored blood.

Within the next few years, the existence of two other necessary factors was discovered. One of these was called Factor VII by Koller *et al.* (1951) as a continuation of Owren's numerical terminology, the term Factor VI having been already used in another context. The other became known as Factor X, a Roman numeral terminology having been recommended for new factors by an international committee (Koller, 1959). Previously used synonyms for these numbered factors are shown in Table I. Naturally occurring deficiencies of Factors VII and X have been observed, and, like prothrombin, both factors are dependent on vitamin K for their synthesis, probably in the liver; their blood levels are reduced by dicoumarin therapy. There is now evidence that tissue thromboplastin is itself a complex consisting of a labile, water-soluble component (tissue factor) and a stable, phospholipid component, as suggested 30 years ago by me (Macfarlane, 1942). In recent years, the system by which tissue factor activates prothrombin has been designated the "extrinsic system," and its components are shown on the left side of Fig. 1; all of these interact during the apparently simple prothrombin time test.

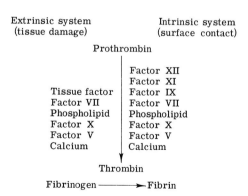

Fig. 1. The factors concerned in the extrinsic and intrinsic systems of prothrombin activation.

3. The Intrinsic Prothrombin Activation System.

Preoccupation with clotting produced by tissue thromboplastin distracted attention from the fact that normal blood clots effectively without the help of tissue factor when it comes into contact with a foreign surface.

This observation, which was emphasized by Lister as long ago as 1863, was not followed up with much enthusiasm for nearly 90 years. Study of the reactions of blood with tissue extract did not explain the clotting defect in hemophilia since the prothrombin time is normal in this condition; but the clotting time of the blood without added tissue extracts is usually prolonged. The observation that the addition of small amounts of normal plasma or its globulin fraction to hemophilic plasma corrected its clotting defect (Patek and Taylor, 1937) suggested that hemophilic blood must lack a normal factor previously unrecognized to which the term "antihemophilic globulin" was applied (Minot and Taylor, 1947). This factor is now known as Factor VIII, but its function could not then be defined, although Quick (1947) and Brinkhous (1947) showed independently that a reaction between the platelets and the normal plasma globulin was necessary for prothrombin conversion and that this did not occur with hemophilic plasma.

Subsequent work in Oxford showed that a powerful activator of prothrombin is, in fact, formed in normal plasma after contact by a process involving the platelets and Factors VIII and V (Biggs et al., 1953a,b,c). This led to the development of the "thromboplastin generation test" (Biggs and Douglas, 1953), the application of which has helped to reveal the existence of other factors concerned in what is now called the "intrinsic system" of prothrombin activation. The Christmas factor (now Factor IX) was so designated because investigation of the hemophilialike condition of a patient of this name revealed that the deficiency was not of Factor VIII, but of a stable, absorbable factor also required for the production of intrinsic prothrombin activator (Biggs et al., 1952). Factor XI (PTA; Rosenthal, 1954) and Factor XII (Hageman factor; Ratnoff and Colopy, 1955) have also been identified as factors concerned in the earliest stages of the contact activation process. The components of the intrinsic system are shown on the right side of Fig. 1, and it will be seen that Factors V and X are common to both systems. Moreover, there is evidence that the phospholipid component of the extrinsic system can substitute for the platelets in the intrinsic system (Bell and Alton, 1954). It is probable, therefore, that the clotting function of platelets lies in the provision of phospholipid. Much attention has been given to the problem of the identity of the phospholipids which cooperate in these systems, and it appears that purified preparations of phosphatidyl ethanolamine and phosphatidyl serine have activity, although mixtures may be more effective than their separated components (Marcus and Spaet, 1958; Troup *et al.*, 1960). Much confusion has resulted from the use of different methods for testing activity and from ignorance of their site of action in the clotting mechanism (Macfarlane, 1964a).

4. THE INTERACTION OF CLOTTING FACTORS.

It is most unlikely that all the components concerned with prothrombin activation operate simultaneously, and there is now convincing evidence that a sequential chain of reactions takes place between pairs of components, the product of each reaction becoming a participant in the next stage. The conversion of inert prothrombin to a proteolytic enzyme which reacts with fibrinogen seems to be the model for the preceding stages. The first definite evidence of this repetition came from observations on the activation of Factor X. It has been known for many years that Russell's viper venom is a powerful activator of the clotting mechanism (Macfarlane and Barnett, 1934), and it was found that the venom did not clot fibrinogen or activate

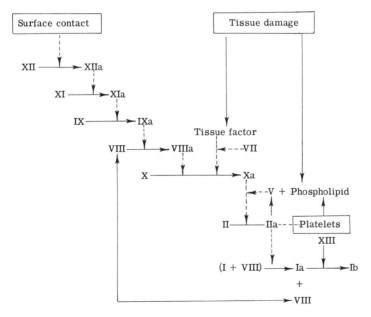

Fig. 2. A scheme for the coagulation mechanism based on the cascade principle. The extrinsic and intrinsic pathways both act on Factor X. Factors VII and V are shown as accelerators. The effects of thrombin (IIa) on fibrinogen, Factor V, and the platelets are indicated, as well as a possible explanation of its effect in mobilizing Factor VIII. Ia, fibrin; Ib, stabilized fibrin; solid line, transformation; dashed line, action. (From Macfarlane, 1965.)

prothrombin directly, but, in addition, required phospholipid (Macfarlane *et al.*, 1941), Factor V (Rapaport *et al.*, 1954), and Factor X (Hougie, 1956). By using a specific antivenom, it is possible to show that the venom reacts specifically and probably enzymically with Factor X and that it is the product of this reaction which activates prothrombin in the presence of phospholipid and Factor V (Macfarlane, 1961). The enzymic nature of the venom–Factor X reaction has been confirmed by Esnouf and Williams (1962), the Factor X molecule being split and the product itself having esterase activity. There is evidence that tissue factor and Factor VII interact to form a Factor X activator (Straub and Duckert, 1961). It has been shown that Factor X is probably activated enzymically during the clotting of plasma after contact with glass (Macfarlane and Ash, 1964). Margolis (1963) has shown that surface contact activates Factor XII, probably by causing an unfolding of the molecule. Activated Factor XII then reacts with Factor XI (Ratnoff *et al.*, 1961), and evidence has been presented by Biggs and Macfarlane (1962) to suggest that the product of such a reaction activates Factor IX; it has been shown that activated Factor IX probably reacts with Factor VIII to form the activator of Factor X (Macfarlane *et al.*, 1964).

Factor X can therefore be activated by different systems: by the intrinsic (contact-activated) system of the plasma; by the extrinsic (tissue-damage) system, and by such agents as Russell's viper venom. The product in each case seems to be the same, an enzyme known as "Xa" (Esnouf and Macfarlane, 1968), "autoprothrombin C" (Marciniak and Seegers, 1966), and "thrombokinase" (Milstone *et al.*, 1965). Its activity as an activator of prothrombin depends on the presence of a suitable phospholipid and of Factor V. It now seems likely that Factor V acts as a cofactor, and the phospholipid acts as a surface-active catalyst for the reaction between Xa and prothrombin. The probable sequential reactions of the intrinsic and extrinsic clotting systems are shown in Fig. 2, which also shows the autocatalytic action of thrombin in potentiating the activity of Factors V and VIII and of the platelets as a source of phospholipid. The details of the reactions are reviewed by Esnouf and Macfarlane (1968).

In this long chain of reactions, the different stages overlap considerably in time. During the process of activation of any particular factor, the first appearance of the product initiates the next stage, so that activation proceeds concurrently in several stages and with only a short time lag between them. This situation is most apparent in the final stage, since the first appearance of thrombin leads rapidly to the conversion of fibrinogen, but thrombin continues to be generated for 10–15 minutes after fibrin formation is complete. A further complication is that all activated factors are rapidly destroyed or inactivated in whole blood, plasma, or serum. At each stage, the concentration of active product at any one time is the result of the opposing rates of production and destruction, and only if the former outstrips the latter can the next stage be activated. It is these complications which have made the analysis of the clotting mechanism so difficult.

Recognition of a repetitive sequence of proenzyme–enzyme transformations as the probable basis of the clotting mechanism provides a rational explanation for its apparently fortuitous complexity. The hemostatic efficiency of clotting seems to depend upon the sudden conversion of fibrinogen to fibrin, which takes place after a latent period of 3 or 4 minutes from the time of contact activation. A more gradual conversion of fibrinogen, such as that which occurs in hemophilia, is hemostatically ineffective, even though the latent period may be not prolonged. The normally sudden appearance of fibrin is related to almost explosive generation of thrombin, and the function of the clotting mechanism is to link the minute physical stimulus of surface contact with a final outburst of enzymic activity. During the clotting of 100 ml of plasma, about 250 mg of fibrinogen are clotted within a few seconds, and available data suggest that this is brought about by the activation of not more than 15 mg of prothrombin, 1.8 mg of Factor X, 0.17 mg of Factor VIII, and an even smaller amount of Factor IX is involved. The whole sequence appears to function as a sort of biochemical amplifier, each enzyme being analogous to a valve or transistor stage in an electronic amplifier. If, for example, each enzyme activates ten times its own weight of substrate during its time of action, the "gain" in the cascade of enzymes in the clotting sequence would be 1×10^6. It might be further suggested that as the demands on hemostatic efficiency have increased during the evolution of the higher animals so additional stages have become "plugged in" between the existing stages of the simpler clotting mechanisms of lower animals if this would increase the chances of survival. There is reason to believe that a primitive prothrombin and fibrinogen may have become modified to produce these additional proenzymes, because Factors V and VIII are similar to fibrinogen, and Factors VII, IX, and X are similar to prothrombin in ways suggesting a common origin. A model illustrating how an additional stage might become inserted is provided by the action of trypsin. This enzyme, which might resemble the proteases derived from damaged tissues, is capable of activating both prothrombin and Factor X (Ferguson and Ennis, 1963). In a clotting system in which trypsin acts directly on prothrombin, the clotting time was 144 seconds; if in a similar system, it was allowed to activate Factor X as well as prothrombin, the clotting time was 19 seconds, suggesting that Factor X acted as a competitive substrate and produced more effective prothrombin activation than the trypsin itself (R. G. Macfarlane, 1963, unpublished). Thus, a tissue enzyme which might activate prothrombin directly in a primitive system would be more effective if an alternative stage could be provided during the process of evolutionary adaptation.

B. Platelet Aggregation

Among the studies that carry the problem closer to the inflammatory mechanism as defined are those dealing with platelet aggregation. Platelet aggregates form an important, possibly essential part of the hemostatic plug. Perhaps the simplest illustration of platelet adhesion *in vivo* is the formation of white bodies, or microthrombi, after slight trauma to small vessels. These bodies have been observed in the cerebral vessels of the rabbit and cat by Florey (1925), have been studied by Honour and Ross-Russell (1962) in the rabbit cerebral and guinea pig mesenteric circulation, and have been seen in the hamster cheek pouch by French *et al.* (1964a). All these workers agree that after minor injury to the vessel wall a white body begins to form at the injured site, increasing in size until it almost fills the lumen. Part or all of this body may then become detached and be swept away in the bloodstream, but rapid reformation usually occurs, breakdown and rebuilding being repeated many times. French *et al.* (1964a,b) used a microelectrode and a 1-second period of electrical stimulation to the vessel wall to produce the injury—a technique similar to that of Fulton *et al.* (1953). At the appropriate time, the cheek pouch area was fixed, dissected out, and sectioned for electron microscopy of the injury site. Figures 3–5 show three sections through an arteriole

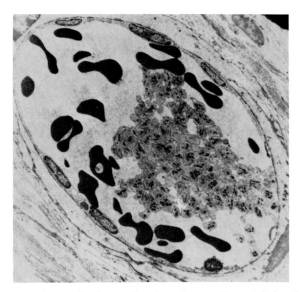

Fig. 3. Electron micrograph of a section through a small arteriole in a hamster cheek pouch just proximal to a point of (electrical) injury showing platelets adherent to an area denuded of endothelium. (× 3182.5.) (From French *et al.*, 1964a.)

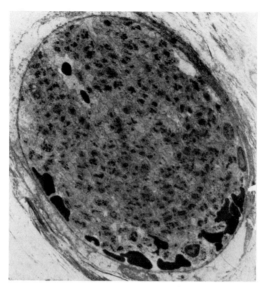

Fig. 4.   Section through the same vessel as in Fig. 3 at the point of injury showing aggregated platelets almost filling the lumen. (× 2960.) (From French *et al.*, 1964b).

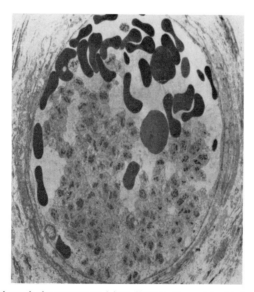

Fig. 5. Section through the same vessel just distal to the point of injury showing the tail end of the platelet mass. In all cases the platelet are distinct. (× 2960.) (From French *et al.*, 1964b.)

from one such experiment. In Fig. 3, the platelets can be seen adhering to an area of the vessel denuded of endothelium by the injury and cohering to form the beginning of a platelet mass. Figure 4 is a section further downstream showing the platelet mass almost filling the vessel, and Fig. 5 shows a section toward the tail of the white body. It will be seen that the outline of the individual platelets is distinct, that most of them contain granules, and that there is no visible fibrin formation or leukocyte adhesion.

A greater degree of trauma producing mechanical disruption of the vessel wall or actual transection is followed by platelet aggregation which procedes beyond the stage seen in the case of the white body. Electron micrographs of sections through the hemostatic plug which formed at the site of transection of a small arteriole in the hamster cheek pouch are shown in Figs. 6–9. Figure 6 is a section through the mass slightly beyond the tip of the severed vessel, and the higher power view (Fig. 7) shows massed platelets, many having lost their granules, and the clarity of their membrane outlines. In certain areas, fibrin formation has occurred (Fig. 8), and the platelets can be seen to be closely applied to the damaged tissues, particularly to collagen fibers (Fig. 9). In contrast to the white body, the hemostatic plug seldom breaks down once it has formed.

The Mechanism of Platelet Aggregation

In an attempt to analyze the process of platelet aggregation, it is tempting to define a series of separate events and the possible mechanisms responsible for them. Such a separation seems to be justified by the fact that some stages in the aggregation process can operate more or less independently of each other.

a. Platelet Adhesion.   The earliest observable event in the formation of a white body or hemostatic plug is the adhesion of platelets to the surface of the damaged vessel or tissues. This implies a difference between these surfaces and those presented to the platelets in the normal circulation, since platelets do not usually stick to other blood cells or normal vascular endothelium. It also implies a special quality in the platelets, since other blood cells do not adhere to the surface which forms the base of the hemostatic plug. It may be inferred, therefore, that under certain conditions platelets have or acquire the property of adhering to certain surfaces. These surfaces include glass (Hellem, 1960), metals, certain tissue cells (O'Brien, 1961), and connective tissue fibers, particularly collagen (Bounameaux, 1959; Zucker and Borrelli, 1962; Hugues, 1962). The physical or chemical properties which distinguish such surfaces from others to which platelets do not adhere have not yet been defined. Wetability by plasma is probably not the significant property, since Copley et al. (1964) have shown that in normal and intact vessels in the hamster the endothelium is wetted by the circulating

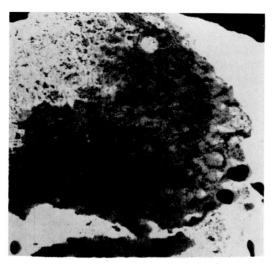

Fig. 6. Electron micrograph showing a section through a hemostatic plug which formed after transection of a small arteriole in a hamster cheek pouch. (× 3200.) (From French *et al.*, 1964a.)

blood. Some of the possible factors concerned with the reaction of blood with foreign surfaces are discussed by Margolis (1963). Platelet adhesion can take place within 1 or 2 seconds of contact, and will occur readily at 0°C (O'Brien, 1964), suggesting that the process must be independent of the enzymic and time-consuming reactions of the clotting mechanism.

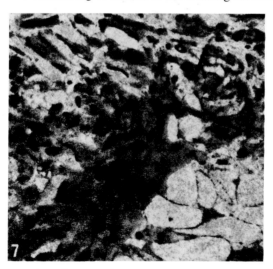

Fig. 7. High power view of an area of the hemostatic plug showing the loss of platelet outline granules (× 13,360.) (From French *et al.*, 1964a.)

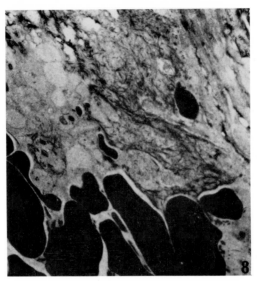

Fig. 8. Part of a hemostatic plug showing fibrin formation. (× 12,000.) (From French *et al.*, 1964b.)

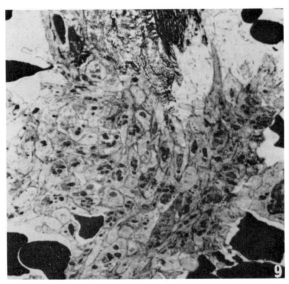

Fig. 9. Part of a hemostatic plug showing the close association of platelets to collagen at the wound edge. (× 5200.) (From French *et al.*, 1964b.)

There is still very little knowledge of the forces involved and of their possible relationships to the activation of the clotting mechanism which is also brought about by surfaces to which platelets adhere. Electrostatic attraction has been suggested as a cause of adhesion of the negatively charged platelets *in vivo* (Sawyer *et al.*, 1953) as a result of the positive charge developed by damaged tissues, but such potential differences between platelets and other adhesive surfaces have not been demonstrated.

If there is no electrostatic attraction, then adhesion may be due to impact, which overcomes the repulsion of a similarly charged surface by bringing the platelet close enough for short range forces of attraction to operate. Impact may result from the velocity with which the platelets are thrown against a surface in an area of turbulent flow or against a projection in a laminar stream. These conditions may occur at injury sites, and they are certainly produced in experimental studies of platelet adhesion in which mechanical stirring is used. In regard to the actual process of adhesion, perhaps the forces which cause the absorption and possibly unfolding of Factor XII on a fixed surface may also bind the platelet, and calcium may act as a cationic binding molecule, as suggested by Bangham and Pethica (1959). Much work remains for the elucidation of a phenomenon which is fundamental to the problems of hemostasis and thrombosis.

b. PLATELET COHESION. The second stage might be called "platelet cohesion," that is, the adhesion of platelet to platelet so that clumping takes place. Cohesion can occur without adhesion to a fixed surface, as in the case of platelets in a suspension, but the formation of hemostatic plugs or thrombi involves both processes, and platelet clumps, unlike agglutinated blood cells, are usually adhesive as well as cohesive. For many years it was supposed that platelet cohesion was related to the clotting process. Osler (1874), Hayem (1878), and Bizzozero (1882) noted that the two phenomena usually occurred together, and Burker (1904) showed that inhibition of clotting was associated with inhibition of platelet changes. A simple explanation would be the adhesion of platelets to fibrin, which can be seen to occur if clotting is studied microscopically. But, even though it seems to be induced by the clotting mechanism, platelet clumping often precedes visible fibrin formation (Sharp, 1958).

Wright and Minot (1917) concluded that it was dependent on a plasma factor which they identified as a labile globulin, and Roskam (1922) suggested that the platelets absorbed an adhesive protein film, which Apitz (1939) believed was profibrin. The observations of Fonio (1940), Desforges and Bigelow (1954), Zucker and Borrelli (1959), and Bounameaux (1957) that thrombin seems to promote platelet cohesion have led to the obvious conclusion that fibrinogen, absorbed to the platelet surface or contained within it, reacts with thrombin to form a cohesive polymer (Grette, 1962). There are objections to this view also: platelet cohesion occurs with normal activity in the blood of patients with a constitutional and complete lack of fibrinogen (Pinniger and Prunty, 1946; Alexander et al., 1954; Sharp, 1961), and it would be expected that if platelet fibrinogen normally exists it would be reduced or absent in such cases. It has also been observed that platelet aggregation takes place in the presence of sufficient heparin to prevent thrombin formation (Zucker, 1947; Hugues, 1953), so that even if thrombin does act as a cohesive agent it is probably not an essential one. Factors in the clotting mechanism other than thrombin have been shown to be active in producing cohesion, such as the "Product I" of Bergsagel (1956) and a product derived from Factors XI and XII (Sharp, 1958; Biggs et al., 1958). Moreover, it has been pointed out by Bettex-Galland et al. (1963) that the platelet changes induced by heparinoids, endotoxin, and antibody–antigen complexes are probably the cause and not the result of the fibrin formation which may accompany them.

Within the last few years, a new line of approach to the mechanism of platelet aggregation has opened up. In 1960, Hellem reported that adhesion of platelets to glass was promoted by the presence of red cells, and further investigation showed that this and cohesion were also brought about by red cell extracts. The active agent was soon identified as adenosine diphosphate (ADP) by Gaarder et al. (1961), an observation which links with Born's discovery of the carriage of adenosine triphosphate (ATP) by the platelets (Born, 1956a,b) and its breakdown to ADP and adenosine monophosphate (AMP) during clotting. Confirmation has come from a number of workers (Born and Cross, 1963; O'Brien, 1962a; Mitchell and Sharp, 1964), and it has been shown that ADP applied locally greatly enhances the formation of white bodies in vivo (Honour and Mitchell, 1963). Work on a number of other pharmacological cohesive agents and their inhibitors has been assisted by the development of quantitative methods (Born, 1962; O'Brien, 1962b), and it has now been found that, beside ADP, 5-hydroxytryptamine (Grette, 1962), adrenaline, and noradrenaline (Mitchell and Sharp, 1964) are active, whereas adenosine, antiadrenalines, and antiserotonins inhibit these actions (O'Brien, 1964; Born and Cross, 1963). It is, perhaps significant that collagen, to which platelets adhere directly, yields an extract which causes them to release ADP and to undergo clumping in about 1 minute (Hovig, 1963), and that thrombin also causes a release of ADP and 5-hydroxytryptamine (Grette, 1962; Holmsen et al., 1969). Platelet cohesion may therefore be brought about by these agents released first by tissue contact and later by the action of thrombin. How these substances actually cause cohesion is not known, but, as previously suggested, they may operate with calcium to form a binding molecule between the platelet surfaces, since calcium is necessary for their effect (O'Brien, 1964). It should be noted that Garvin (1961) suggests on the basis of *in vitro* studies that the adhesion of platelets requires either calcium or magnesium ions. Wide species differences in these reactions have been emphasized by Mills (1970).

    c. PLATELET FUSION. The last stage in aggregation has been called "fusion" (Sharp, 1961). In the general description of the platelet changes which take place during clotting, the term "viscous metamorphosis" was used by Wright and Minot (1917), and, besides aggregation, this includes the protrusion of pseudopodia, the discharge of granules, and the eventual loss of the individual outlines of the compacted platelets which thus become fused into an amorphous mass. Some of these appearances may be misleading. For example, platelets seemingly fused when observed by light microscopy can be shown to have intact boundaries when studied with the electron microscope (French and Poole, 1963). But electron microscopy does show that within 0.5–1.0 hour of formation of the hemostatic plug *in vivo* platelet outlines begin to merge, and loss of granules is clearly taking place (French *et al.*, 1964a). These changes seem to be concurrent with the appearance of fibrin, and it has been suggested that this later stage is due to the action of thrombin which produces an irreversible aggregation, in contrast to the reversible cohesion brought about by ADP (Roskam, 1963; Sokal, 1963). It is more probable that any coagulation of platelet fibrinogen, as postulated by Grette (1962), would occur during this final stage, rather than causing the initial platelet clumping, as proposed by earlier workers. It may be relevant also that although platelet plugs are formed at the site of an injury in the presence of heparin (which inhibits thrombin formation) they remain permeable, fragile, and hemostatically ineffective (Zucker, 1947; Hugues, 1959).

C. The Platelets and the Clotting Mechanism

    Having discussed intimate aspects of the reaction of platelets in tissue injury, we can now return to the relationship of the platelets to the clotting mechanism.

    In blood which has been deprived of platelets, the coagulation time in glass tubes is prolonged, the activation of prothrombin is incomplete, and the clots formed do not retract. The presence of platelets is therefore important to the intrinsic clotting mechanism. One of their components is "platelet Factor 3," probably phospholipid in nature, which, as described in an earlier section, participates in the conversion of prothrombin by Factors X and V (Hardisty and Hutton, 1966). It seems likely that the release of this substance during the clotting process accounts for the action of platelets, since phospholipid preparations free from protein can be used as adequate platelet substitutes in the activation of prothrombin. French and Poole (1963) have obtained electron micrographs of platelets during the formation of artificial thrombi which show vesicles apparently opening at the platelet surface and discharging their contents. Perhaps it is by this mechanism that platelet Factor 3 is made available, and it is not inconceivable that hydrolytic enzymes originating in lysosomal granules may also be involved in the process (see Volume I, Chapter 4).

The platelets also have an effect on the fibrin network after its formation. When the platelets are normal in function and number, clots formed by whole blood retract spontaneously so that serum is squeezed out of them until the mass of retained red cells is tightly compacted. Clot retraction has been much studied, particularly by Budtz-Olsen (1951), and many theories have been propounded. The most convincing of these ascribes retraction to a shortening of the fibrin fibers produced by active contraction of attached platelet pseudopodia. Budtz-Olsen has recorded the changes in shape of platelet clumps attached to fibrin, which certainly suggest active contraction. The theory is supported by the discovery of a contractile protein resembling actomyosin in the platelets by Bettex-Galland and Luscher (1959) and the demonstration of the breakdown of platelet ATP during clotting by Born (1956b). A source of motive power has thus been revealed (Bettex-Galland and Luscher, 1960), and it is significant that agents which poison or inhibit cell metabolism or enzyme activity also inhibit clot retraction (Budtz-Olsen, 1951). The physiological importance of retraction is not established, although it might be supposed that the clot when compacted is likely to be more effective as a hemostatic plug.

III. Vascular and Tissue Factors in Hemostasis

A. Vascular Constriction

Up to this point, we have discussed the clotting mechanism and some aspects of platelet physiology, and then we have attempted to link these two areas, admitting that much of this may be speculative. The participation of tissue and vascular factors will now be examined.

The most obvious hemostatic vascular reaction is constriction after injury. In smaller vessels, active constriction may be observed microscopically in various preparations such as the cerebral cortex of the rabbit and cat (Florey, 1925), frog's web, the mesentery in various animals, and the hamster cheek pouch. Damage to or transection of these vessels usually, but not always, results in constriction, although this seldom completely obstructs the blood flow. French *et al.* (1964b) observed that the local constriction which often followed the electrical injury was sufficient to cause white body formation, but this was short lived, and, though the white body might grow to a size that expanded the lumen, blood continued to flow past the obstruction, suggesting that there was little constrictive tone. When a vessel was transected, however, constriction was often maintained in the vicinity of the hemostatic plug, thus appearing to assist its impedence of the blood flow.

The mechanism of vascular constriction as a response to injury depends on factors which are discussed in Chapter 1. The reactions of vascular smooth muscle have been extensively studied and are the subject of a recent symposium. The chain of events linking the traumatic stimulus with the response of contraction is by no means understood, and it is probable that the pattern varies, not only from species to species, but from one anatomical site to another in the same animal. Florey (1925), for example, found that the small cerebral vessels in the cat and rabbit were nonreactive to adrenaline, but responded by marked contraction to stroking with a glass needle.

Apart from any direct effect of trauma on the constrictor motor elements and their possible innervation, there is evidence that the blood itself contributes to their stimulation. The fact that clotted blood contains constrictor substances has been known since the observations of Stevens and Lee (1884) and O'Connor (1911). Janeway and Park (1912) showed that they acted directly on smooth muscle, and Stewart and Zucker (1913) found that constrictor activity seemed to arise as a result of the clotting process and that agents which preserved the platelets prevented its appearance. They suggested the possible importance of this phenomenon in hemostasis. Zucker (1947) recorded the association of vascular constriction with the formation of platelet masses in living preparations, suggesting that they were releasing a diffusible and active substance. Shortly afterward, Rapport (1949) identified the serum constrictor substance as 5-hydroxytryptamine (serotonin), and Zucker and Borrelli (1955) showed that this was released from platelets during clotting, apparently by the action of thrombin. But it is now known that besides 5-HT the platelets carry histamine, adrenaline, noradrenaline, lysosomal enzymes, and ATP and that the effect of these substances on the vascular reactions to injury is likely to be complex and important. The situation is further complicated by the fact that the clotting mechanism is involved not only with the platelet changes leading to the release of these active amines, but also with the release of the vasoactive peptides of the kinin group (Margolis, 1963).

The response to injury of vessels, such as the true capillaries, has been a matter of dispute for many years. A number of workers have reported observations suggesting the active contraction of capillaries after a variety of stimuli, including direct trauma, but the majority view seems to be that these vessels are simply passive endothelial tubes, the diameter of which is determined only by the pressure of the blood they happen to receive. It is not appropriate here to cite the considerable evidence for these two opposing views, but it might be mentioned that the absence of any discernible motor elements which could cause capillary contraction has been advanced as an argument in favor of passivity. But, 15 years ago, few would have suspected the existence of a contractile protein in the platelets, and the recently demonstrated filamentous structures in vascular endothelial cells (Rhodin, 1962) may well have some type of contractile function [see Majno *et al.* (1969)]. Again, it is necessary to bear in mind the species and anatomical differences in the experimental preparations which have served as the basis for sweeping generalizations. Inasmuch as capillary contraction after injury has not been reported to occur, a hemostatic mechanism, as it applies to these vessels, is difficult to comprehend. Zucker (1949), in a careful histological examination of needle puncture wounds in human subjects, could find no platelet plugs sealing damaged capillaries, though there might be some fibrin; yet clinical experience shows that capillary bleeding is arrested with normal efficiency in cases of severe clotting defects in which fibrin formation does not occur.

B. Endothelial Adhesion

It is often found that after the clean transection of a small vessel in an experimental preparation no bleeding occurs despite the visible patency of the vessel on each side of the injury. Further mechanical disturbance, such as stretching the tissue or touching the cut area with a needle, may than cause immediate bleeding. The explanation of this phenomenon is probably that the pressure of the knife edge forces the vascular walls together before cutting them so that the endothelial surfaces adhere and seal the cut ends of the vessel. Chen and Tsai (1948) studied this adhesive sealing produced by mechanical pressure in the vessels of the toad, and have shown that it will withstand a pressure of 200 mm Hg. Earlier, it was suggested by Stegemann (1922) that intimal adhesion might occur after vascular constriction, and Roskam (1922) believed that it resulted from the deposition of an adhesive protein. This may happen within minutes, or even seconds, of an injury, but it can hardly explain the instantaneous adhesion of endothelial cells brought into contact by the knife in the moment of transection. One must infer that under these conditions the endothelium is inherently and mutually adhesive, and it is clear that the same factors may operate in the cohesion of endothelial cells as in platelet cohesion or adhesion, but little experimental work has been done in this field. (See Chapter 2 for a further discussion of endothelial "stickiness.")

C. Vascular Permeability and Shunt Mechanisms

A seldom-considered factor in hemostasis is the loss of plasma through the hemostatic plug while it is still porous and, also, probably through the intact but permeable walls of vessels in the injured area (see Chapter 1). Wounds which have ceased to lose whole blood still continue to ooze plasma or serum for a considerable time, as can be demonstrated by observing the flow of blood from the severed tip of a mouse's tail immersed in saline (Copley and Lalich, 1941). A thin stream of blood falls through the saline for a few minutes, and then ceases after one or two intermissions, but a stream of clear fluid can be seen to continue for several minutes afterward. In the hamster cheek pouch, transected vessels often become filled with tightly packed red cell masses similar to those characteristic of inflammatory "stasis." Occasionally, these viscous cell masses appear to obstruct the flow of blood despite the absence of a visible hemostatic plug or marked constriction. The aggregation of red cells as the result of plasma loss may be an important ancillary mechanism for curtailing hemorrhage.

Another factor, the importance of which is realized when the microcirculation is observed after experimental injury, is the opening up of vascular shunts. These have the effect of reducing the blood pressure in the damaged vessel in which the flow is also reduced by constriction and increased viscosity. In such cases, the bloodstream avoids the injured area by passing through dilated but previously invisible side channels, as illustrated by Wharton Jones (1851), and it is not unusual for the direction of flow to be reversed in parts of the injured area. The mechanism of these changes probably involves the vasoactive amines and peptides released by the blood and damaged tissues already mentioned, and the latter are discussed in detail in Chapters 1 and 7.

IV. Hemostasis as a Whole

Even from this brief account of some of the recognizable factors concerned with hemostasis, it will be appreciated that no simple or single picture can be given of the mechanism in operation. The order in which these factors come into play and their relative importance will vary with the nature and extent of the vascular injuries. Some insight into the integrated functions of these separate components can be gained from observation of the effects of their deficiencies. In platelet deficiency, the typical abnormality is the prolonged bleeding from even the slightest injury to the skin or mucous membranes; in clotting defects, it is the more severe damage to deeper structure that leads to serious hemorrhage. It is likely that a deficiency in any one component may be compensated to some extent by the normal working of the others; relatively mild defects in two components may have consequences far more severe than would be expected with either alone. Further complication is added by the feedback mechanisms which have already been described; activation of the clotting mechanism promotes platelet aggregation which, in turn, promotes clotting. Platelet adhesion releases active

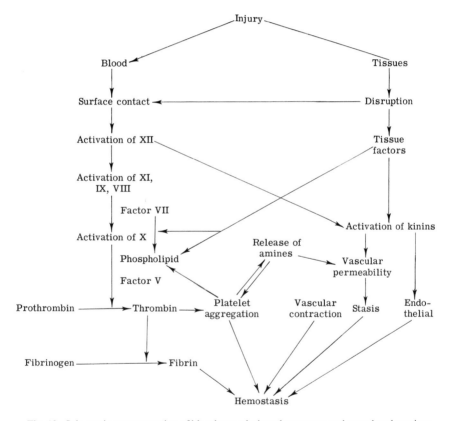

Fig. 10. Schematic representation of blood coagulation phenomena and vascular alterations after injury. Note that surface contact may cause platelet aggregation, and disruption may cause vascular contraction directly in each case, but these reactions are not indicated in the diagram in the interest of simplicity.

amines which cause further platelet adhesion and also vascular reactions. Vascular stasis allows time for the activation of the plasma–kinin system, leading to increased permeability, increased adhesion, and thus further stasis. Some of these tentative interrelationships are illustrated in Fig. 10.

These complexities are no doubt the result of the long history of adaptations required to combat the growing danger of exsanguination imposed by the increasing blood pressures and activities of the higher species during their evolution, and which have been discussed by Hawkey (1970). Platelet aggregation is probably the descendant of an almost exclusively cellular sort of "clotting" as seen in Crustacea and some insects today. Fibrin formation may be an adaptation of an even older intracellular precipitation reaction to injury (Heilbrunn, 1961), and coordinated vascular contractions are, of course, a feature of the circulatory mechanism of many lower animals. These three basic elements have been developed and combined to respond as an integrated mechanism to injury in the mammalian kingdom. The trigger in this response is the surface contact activation of the blood and platelets which follows disruption of the vessels. The sensitivity of the blood to this contact effect is indeed remarkable, but not more so than its lifetime of peaceful coexistence with a vast surface area of the normal vascular endothelium.

References

Alexander, B., Goldstein, R., Rich, L., Le Bolloc'h, A. G., Diamond, L. K., and Borges, W. (1954). *Blood* **9**, 843.

Apitz, K. (1939). *Z. Gesamte Exp. Med.* **105**, 89.

Bangham, A. D., and Pethica, B. A. (1959). *Proc. Roy. Phys. Soc. Edinburgh* **28**, 43.

Bell, W. N., and Alton, H. G. (1954). *Nature (London)* **174**, 880.

Bergsagel, D. E. (1956). *Brit. J. Haematol.* **2**, 130.

Bettelheim, F. R., and Bailey, K. (1952). *Biochim. Biophys. Acta* **9**, 578.

Bettex-Galland, M., and Luscher, E. F. (1959). *Nature (London)* **184**, 276.

Bettex-Galland, M., and Luscher, E. F. (1960). *Thromb. Diath. Haemorrh.* **4**, 178.

Bettex-Galland, M., Luscher, E. F., Simon, G., and Vassalli, P. (1963). *Nature (London)* **200**, 1109.

Biggs, R., and Bidwell, E. (1957). *Brit. J. Haematol.* **3**, 387.

Biggs, R., and Douglas, A. S. (1953). *J. Clin. Pathol.* **6**, 23.

Biggs, R., and Macfarlane, R. G. (1962). "Human Blood Coagulation and Its Disorders," 3rd ed. Blackwell, Oxford.

Biggs, R., Douglas, A. S., Macfarlane, R. G., Dacie, J. V., Pitney, W. R., Merskey, C., and O'Brien, J. R. (1952). *Brit. Med. J.* **2**, 1378.

Biggs, R., Douglas, A. S., and Macfarlane, R. G. (1953a). *J. Physiol. (London)* **119**, 89.

Biggs, R., Douglas, A. S., and Macfarlane, R. G. (1953b). *J. Physiol. (London)* **122**, 538.

Biggs, R., Douglas, A. S., and Macfarlane, R. G. (1953c). *J. Physiol. (London)* **122**, 554.

Biggs, R., Sharp, A. A., Margolis, J., Hardisty, R. M., Stewart, J., and Davidson, W. M. (1958). *Brit. J. Haematol.* **4**, 177.

Bizzozero, J. (1882). *Arch. Pathol. Anat. Physiol. Klin. Med.* **90**, 261.

Born, G. V. R. (1956a). *Biochem. J.* **62**, 33P.

Born, G. V. R. (1956b). *J. Physiol. (London)* **133**, 61P.

Born, G. V. R. (1962). *J. Physiol. (London)* **162**, 67P.

Born, G. V. R., and Cross, M. J. (1963). *J. Physiol. (London)* **168**, 178.

Bounameaux, Y. (1957). *Rev. Hematol.* **12**, 16.

Bounameaux, Y. (1959). *C. R. Soc. Biol.* **153**, 865.

Brinkhous, K. M. (1947). *Proc. Soc. Exp. Biol. Med.* **66**, 117.

Budtz-Olsen, O. E. (1951). "Clot Retraction." Blackwell, Oxford.

Burker, K. (1904). *Pfluegers Arch. Gesamte Physiol. Menschem Tiere* **102**, 36.

Caspary, E. A., and Kekwick, R. A. (1954). *Biochem. J.* **56**, XXXV.

Chen, T. I., and Tsai, C. (1948). *J. Physiol. (London)* **107**, 280.

Copley, A. L., and Lalich, J. J. (1941). *Amer. J. Physiol.* **135**, 547.

Copley, A. L., Glover, F. A., and Scott-Blair, G. W. (1964). *Biorheology* **2**, 29.

Desforges, J. F., and Bigelow, F. S. (1954). *Blood* **9**, 153.

Esnouf, M. P., and Macfarlane, R. G. (1968). *Advan. Enzymol.* **30**, 255.

Esnouf, M. P., and Williams, W. J. (1962). *Biochem. J.* **84**, 62.

Ferguson, J. H., and Ennis, E. G. W. (1963). *Thromb. Diath. Haemorrh.* **9**, 62.

Florey, H. (1925). *Brain* **48**, 43.

Fonio, A. (1940). *Schweiz Med. Wochenschr.* **21**, 510.

French, J. E., and Poole, J. C. F. (1963). *Proc. Roy. Soc., Ser. B* **157**, 170.

French, J. E., Macfarlane, R. G., and Sanders, A. G. (1964a). *Thromb. Diath. Haemorrh., Suppl.* **13**, 341.

French, J. E., Macfarlane, R. G., and Sanders A. G. (1964b), unpublished.

Fulton, G. P., Akers, R. P., and Lutz, B. R. (1953). *Blood* **8**, 140.

Gaarder, A., Jonsen, J., and Owren, P. A. (1961). *Nature (London)* **192**, 531.

Garvin, J. E. (1961). *J. Exp. Med.* **114**, 51.

Giacomelli, F., Wiener, J., and Spiro, D. (1970). *J. Cell. Biol.* **45**, 188.

Grette, K. (1962). *Acta Physiol. Scand.* **56**, Suppl., 195.

Hall, C. E., and Slayter, H. S. (1959). *J. Biophys. Biochem. Cytol.* **5**, 11.

Hardisty, R. M., and Hutton, R. A. (1966). *Brit. J. Haematol.* **12**, 764.

Hawkey, C. M. (1970). *Symp. Zool. Soc. Lond.* No. 27, 217.

Hayem, G. (1878). *Arch. Physiol. Norm. Pathol.* **2**, 692.

Hayem, G. (1882). *C. R. Acad. Sci.* **95**, 18.

Heilbrunn, L. V. (1961). In "Functions of the Blood" (R. G. Macfarlane and A. H. T. Robb-Smith, eds.), pp. 283–301. Academic Press, New York.

Hellem, A. J. (1960). *Scand. J. Clin. Lab. Invest.* **12**, Suppl., 51.

Holmsen, H., Day, H. J., and Stormorken, H. (1969). *Scand. J. Haematol., Suppl.* **8**, 1–26.

Honour, A. J., and Mitchell, J. R. A. (1963). *Nature (London)* **197**, 1019.

Honour, A. J., and Ross- Russell, R. W. (1962). *Brit. J. Exp. Pathol.* **43**, 350.

Hougie, C. (1956). *Proc. Soc. Exp. Biol. Bed.* **93**, 570.

Hovig, T. (1963). *Thromb. Diath. Haemorrh.* **9**, 264.

Hugues, J. (1953). *Arch. Int. Physiol.* **61**, 565.

Hugues, J. (1959). *Thromb. Diath. Haemorrh.* **3**, 177.

Hugues, J. (1962). *Thromb. Diath. Haemorrh.* **8**, 241.

Janeway, T. C., and Park, E. A. (1912). *J. Exp. Med.* **16**, 541.

Jones, A. F. D. (1810). "A Treatise on the Process Employed by Nature in Suppressing its Haemorrhage of Divided and Punctured Arteries and the Use of the Ligature." Longman, Hurst, Rees, Orine & Brown, London.

Kjaerheim, A., and Hovig, T. (1962). *Thromb. Diath. Haemorrh.* **7**, 1.
Koller, F. (1959). *Thromb. Diath. Haemorrh.* **4**, Suppl., 58.
Koller, F., Loeliger, A., and Duckert, F. (1951). *Acta Haematol.* **6**, 1.
Laki, K. (1953). *Blood* **8**, 845.
Lister, J. (1863). *Proc. Roy. Soc.* **12**, 580.
Lorand, L. (1952). *Biochem. J.* **52**, 200.
Lorand, L. (1954). *Physiol. Rev.* **34**, 742.
Lorand, L., and Jacobsen, A. (1958). *J. Biol. Chem.* **230**, 420.
Lorand, L., and Jacobsen, A. (1964). *Biochem. J.* **3**, 1939.
Macfarlane, R. G. (1941). *Quart. J. Med.* **10**, 1.
Macfarlane, R. G. (1942). *Proc. Roy. Soc. Med.* **35**, 410.
Macfarlane, R. G. (1961). *Brit. J. Haematol.* **7**, 496.
Macfarlane, R. G. (1964a) *In* "Metabolism and Physiological Significance of Lipids" (R. M. C. Dawson and D. N. Rhodes, eds.), p. 325, Wiley, New York.
Macfarlane, R. G. (1964b). *Nature (London)* **202**, 498.
Macfarlane, R. G. (1965) *Thromb. Diath. Haemorrh., Suppl.* **17**, 45.
Macfarlane, R. G., and Ash, B. J. (1964). *Brit. J. Haematol.* **10**, 217.
Macfarlane, R. G., and Barnett, B. (1934). *Lancet* **2**, 985.
Macfarlane, R. G., Trevan, J. W., and Attwood, A. M. P. (1941). *J. Physiol. (London)* **99**, 7P.
Macfarlane, R. G., Biggs, R., Denson, K. W., and Ash, B. J. (1964). *Brit. J. Haematol.* **10**, 530.
Majno, G., Shea, S. M., and Leventhal, M. (1969). *J. Cell Biol.* **42**, 647.
Marciniak, E., and Seegers, W. H. (1966). *Nature (London)* **209**, 621.
Marcus, A. J., and Spaet, T. H. (1958). *J. Clin. Invest.* **37**, 1836.
Margolis, J. (1963). *Ann. N. Y. Acad. Sci.* **104**, 133.
Mellanby, J. (1933). *Proc. Roy. Soc., Ser. B.* **113**, 93.
Mills, D. C. B., (1970). *Symp. Zool. Soc. Lond.* No. 27, 99.
Milstone, J. H., Qulianott, N., and Milstone, V. K. (1965). *Proc. Soc. Exp. Biol. Med.* **119**, 804.
Minot, G. R., and Taylor, F. H. L. (1947). *Ann. Intern. Med.* **26**, 363.
Mitchell, J. R. A., and Sharp, A. A. (1964). *Brit. J. Haematol.* **10**, 78.
Morawitz, P. (1905). *Ergeb. Physiol. Biol. Chem. Exp. Pharmakol.* **4**, 307.
O'Brien, J. R. (1961). *J. Clin. Pathol.* **14**, 140.
O'Brien, J. R. (1962a). *J. Clin. Pathol.* **15**, 446.
O'Brien, J. R. (1962b). *J. Clin. Pathol.* **15**, 452.
O'Brien, J. R. (1964). *Blood* **24**, 309.
O'Connor, J. M. (1911). *Muenchen. Med. Wochenschr.* **58**, 1439.
Osler, W. (1874). *Proc. Roy. Soc.* **22**, 391.
Owren, P. A. (1947). *Acta Med. Scand.* **128**, Suppl. 194.
Patek, A. J., and Taylor, F. H. L. (1937). *J. Clin. Invest.* **16**, 113.
Petit, J. E. (1731). *Mem. Acad. Roy. Sci.* p. 90 (quoted by Quick, 1957).
Pinniger, J. L., and Prunty, F. T. G. (1946). *Brit. J. Exp. Pathol.* **27**, 200.
Quick, A. J. (1935). *J. Biol. Chem.* **109**, lxxiii.
Quick, A. J. (1937). *Amer. J. Physiol.* **118**, 260.
Quick, A. J. (1943). *Amer. J. Physiol.* **140**, 212.
Quick, A. J. (1947). *Amer. J. Med. Sci.* **214**, 272.
Quick, A. J. (1957). "Hemorrhagic Diseases." Kimpton, London.
Rapaport, S. I., Aas, K., and Owren, P. A. (1954). *Blood* **9**, 1185.
Rapport, M. M. (1949). *J. Biol. Chem.* **180**, 961.
Ratnoff, O. D., and Colopy, J. E. (1955). *J. Clin. Invest.* **35**, 602.
Ratnoff, O. D., Davie, E. W., and Mallett, D. L. (1961). *J. Clin. Invest.* **40**, 803.
Rhodin, J. A. G. (1962). *Phys. Rev.* **42**, Suppl. 5, 48.

Rosenthal, R. L. (1954). *J. Clin. Invest.* **33**, 961.

Roskam. J. (1922). *C. R. Soc. Biol.* **86**, 733.

Roskam, J. (1960). *Schweiz. Med. Wochenschr.* **90**, 947.

Roskam, J. (1963). *Thromb. Diath. Haemorrh.* **10**, 253.

Sawyer, P. N., Pate, J. W., and Wildon, C. S. (1953). *Amer. J. Physiol.* **175**, 108.

Scheraga, H. A. (1958). *Ann. N. Y. Acad. Sci.* **75**, 189.

Schimmelbusch, C. (1885). *Arch. Pathol. Anat. Physiol. Klin. Med.* **101**, 201.

Schmidt, A. (1895). "Weitere Beitrage zur Blutlehre." Bergmann, Weisbaden.

Seegers, W. H. (1962). "Prothrombin." Harvard Univ. Press, Cambridge, Massachusetts.

Sharp, A. A. (1958). *Brit. J. Haematol.* **4**, 28.

Sharp, A. A. (1961). *In* "Blood Platelets" (S. A. Johnson *et al.*, eds.), pp. 67–88. Little, Brown, Boston, Massachusetts.

Sokal, G. (1963). *Thromb. Diath. Haemorrh.* **10**, 235.

Stegemann, H. (1922). *Bruns' Beitr. Klin. Chir.* **127**, 657.

Stevens, L. T., and Lee, F. S. (1884). *Johns Hopkins Hosp. Biol. Stud.* **3**, 99.

Stewart, G. N., and Zucker, T. F. (1913). *J. Exp. Med.* **17**, 152.

Straub, W., and Duckert, F. (1961). *Thromb. Diath. Haemorrh.* **5**, 402.

Tocantins, L. M. (1947). *Ann. Surg.* **125**, 292.

Troup, S. B., Reed, C. F., Marinetti, G. V., and Swischer, S. N. (1960). *J. Clin. Invest.* **39**, 342.

Wharton Jones, T. (1851). *Guy's Hosp. Rep.* **7**, 1.

Wright, J. H., and Minot, G. R. (1917). *J. Exp. Med.* **26**, 395.

Zahn, F. W. (1872). *Zentralbl. Med. Wiss.* **10** , 129.

Zucker, H. D. (1949). *Blood* **4**, 631.

Zucker, M. B. (1947). *Amer. J. Physiol.* **148**, 275.

Zucker, M. B., and Borelli, J. (1955). *J. Appl. Physiol.* **7**, 432.

Zucker, M. B., and Borelli, J. (1959). *J. Appl. Physiol.* **14**, 575.

Zucker, M. B., and Borelli, J. (1962). *Proc. Soc. Exp. Biol. Med.* **109**, 779.

Chapter 11

THROMBOSIS

NATHANIEL F. RODMAN

It is well known that thrombosis may either complicate or precede inflammation. This general knowledge stems from a wealth of experience by many observers of the pathology of inflammation. Thrombosis is prone to occur in inflammatory focuses, particularly those in which necrosis is prominent. Conversely, inflammation is frequently prominent in processes resulting from thrombosis. Classic among these is the zone of inflammatory infiltrate about an ischemic infarct.

I. Thrombosis as an Initiator of Inflammation

In addition to the classic example already mentioned, it has recently been demonstrated that platelet thrombi which impinge on a vessel wall may damage the wall with resultant inflammation (Jørgensen *et al.*, 1970). Adenosine diphosphate (ADP) infused intra-arterially or intravenously into swine induced platelet aggregation, and aggregates persisted as thrombi or emboli which became lodged in small arteries or veins. Endothelial cells underlying these thrombi degenerated, and at 6 hours there was accumulation of polymorphonuclear leukocytes.

A. *Thrombosis Due to Changes in the Blood Vessel Wall*

Thrombosis may also complicate any of several abnormalities in blood vessel walls. It is generally accepted that these include entities with vascular wall deformity such as atherosclerosis or aneurysm. Only recently has it become evident that minimal damage to the vascular wall may result in thrombosis. The spectrum of minimal damage might extend from limited endothelial cell damage alone to loss of endothelial cells with exposure of basement membrane or other subendothelial structures.

1. ENDOTHELIAL CELL DAMAGE

The least conceivable form of injury to the blood vessel wall is mild damage to the endothelial cells. Two groups of workers have reported formation of platelet thrombi upon damaged endothelial cells at least partially covering subendothelial structures (Johnson, 1968; McGrath and Stewart, 1969). Clear demonstration of platelets adhering to damaged endothelial cells without exposure of subendothelial structures has not been reported.

2. EXPOSURE OF SUBENDOTHELIAL STRUCTURES

Evidence of platelet adhesion to subendothelial structures, sometimes with subsequent thrombus formation, has appeared recently and is well documented. Tranzer and Baumgartner (1967) reported single platelets adherent to subendothelial basement membrane which was exposed during vascular dilation. Platelet degranulation was not observed, and other platelets did not attach to single adhering platelets. It was concluded that on termination of dilation the endothelial cells displace and release the adherent platelet. In contrast, on injured vessel walls with divided endothelial cells and exposed basement membrane, platelets are reported to adhere and to aggregate (French *et al.*, 1964; Baumgartner *et al.*, 1967; Ashford and Freiman, 1967; Branemark and Ekholm, 1968; Honour *et al.*, 1971; Stemerman *et al.*, 1971). It is well established that collagen fibrils in the basement membrane layer induce platelet adhesion and aggregation, and there is recent evidence that a basement membrane component other than collagen may act similarly (Hugues and Mahieu, 1970; Stemerman *et al.*, 1971). The latter group concluded that elastin may induce adhesion and aggregation of platelets.

3. PLATELET ADHESION TO VESSEL WALL FOLLOWED BY AGGREGATION AND THROMBOSIS

As noted above, platelets adhere to denuded subendothelial basement membrane in a variety of circumstances. Only where the vessel wall is damaged, as by electrical stimulation, transection, or by other physico-chemical trauma, do additional platelets attach to the initially adhering platelet. These additional platelets attach by the process known as agglutination or aggregation, and thereby form a thrombus. The mechanism by which other platelets are stimulated to aggregate with and about the initial adherent platelet and thus form the thrombus has been the subject of much study. ADP, itself a powerful aggregating agent, is released from platelets after exposure to any of several aggregating agents, including collagen fibrils (Hovig, 1963). This release of platelet constituents is also stimulated by thrombin (Davey and Lüscher, 1968; Holmsen and Day, 1970), epinephrine (Mills et al., 1968), and ADP itself (Mustard et al., 1964; Mills et al., 1968). In addition to ADP, other compounds released include ATP (Grette, 1962; Ireland, 1967; Thomas et al., 1970), 5-hydroxytryptamine (5-HT, serotonin) (Grette, 1962), K^+ (Buckingham and Maynert, 1964), β-glucuronidase (Dohrmann and Klesper, 1960; Holmsen and Day, 1968), β-N-acetylglucosaminidase, β-galactosidase, arylsulfatase, cathepsin (Holmsen and Day, 1970), fibrinogen (Grette, 1962), Platelet Factor 3 (Spaet and Cintron, 1965), and Platelet Factor 4 (Niewiarowski et al., 1968). Release of these multiple substances from the platelet has become commonly known as the "release reaction."

From a physiological and pathological standpoint, the released ADP is perhaps the most significant, since it seems most likely that endogenous, released ADP is the messenger by which additional platelets are stimulated to aggregate with those already present. Obviously other messengers, notably thrombin or catecholamines, may also stimulate platelet aggregation and thrombus formation. In addition, it has further been shown that some aggregating agents, at concentrations below the minimum required to induce platelet aggregation, will potentiate the action of other aggregating agents. For example, low concentrations of epinephrine potentiate the aggregating effect of ADP (Born et al., 1967; Mills and Roberts, 1967) and of thrombin (Thomas et al., 1968). Similarly, 5-HT potentiates the aggregating effect of epinephrine and of ADP (Baumgartner and Born, 1967, 1968). Thus, the presence of any such messenger or combination of messengers in sufficiently high concentration to produce platelet aggregation would constitute changes within the blood which might lead to thrombus formation.

B. Thrombosis Related to Changes within the Blood

Thrombus formation and evolution as well as the process usually termed "clotting" or "coagulation" require participation of the cellular and non-cellular components of the mechanism. Once any component of the thrombus-forming or clotting mechanism is activated, thrombosis may result.

Activation of either platelets or plasmatic clotting factors may thus stimulate thrombus formation.

1. PLATELET AGGREGATION

It is well established that platelets aggregate in response to any of several agents. The intensity or degree of the platelet aggregation response varies with concentration of the aggregating agent. The platelet response to each agent requires divalent cations such as Ca^{2+} or Mg^{2+}. With each aggregating agent, platelets follow an orderly sequence of events unique to that aggregating agent. Platelet responses to each of several well known agents which may, under appropriate circumstances, be physiologically or pathologically significant are presented below.

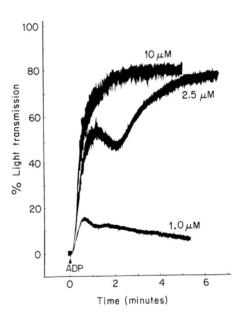

Fig. 1. Aggregometer tracings of responses of normal human platelets in citrated plasma to adenosine diphosphate (ADP). In each instance, ADP was added at the time marked by the arrow. The intermediate tracing, a response to 2.5 μM ADP, has distinct primary and secondary aggregation waves, separated by a pause or plateau. At the first peak, small aggregates form a loose mosaic (see Fig. 2). At the height of the second peak, aggregates are large, compact and complex (see Fig. 3). The upper tracing is a response to 10 μM ADP, in which virtually all of the platelets aggregate very rapidly with absence of a pause. At the height of this curve, aggregates are morphologically identical with those at the second peak of the intermediate tracing (Fig. 3). The lower tracing illustrates the platelet response to 1 μM ADP, with minimal aggregation (see Fig. 4) followed by deaggregation (see Fig. 5).

a. ADENOSINE DIPHOSPHATE. ADP has been widely recognized as a platelet-aggregating agent since the reports of Hellem *et al.* (1961) and Gaarder and associates (1961), and its effect on platelets has been extensively studied. It is now generally known that platelets in citrated platelet-rich plasma (PRP) of a donor known to have "normal" platelet responses to aggregating agents, normal prothrombin time (Quick, 1940) and partial thromboplastin time (Langdell *et al.*, 1953; Rodman *et al.*, 1958) and who have ingested no drugs within the previous 7 days have characteristic responses to ADP. Initial changes seen after addition of ADP to citrated PRP consist of pseudopod formation and organelle movement from random distribution to close apposition in the central part of the platelet (Rodman and Mason, 1967). This alteration was defined as Stage I in a spectrum of aggregation responses (Rodman *et al.*, 1963b). In addition, microtubules form a tight web or envelope about the centrally apposed organelles (Rodman, 1967; White, 1968). These initial morphological changes are followed by aggregation, the Stage II change (Rodman *et al.*, 1963a). At intermediate

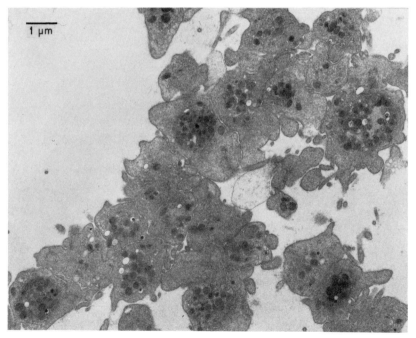

Fig. 2. A typical aggregate seen at the first peak of aggregation, induced by 2.5 μM ADP and sampled 55 seconds after addition of ADP. Platelets form a mosaic, and each platelet is easily identified as an individual cell. Organelles are intact and are in close apposition in the center of each platelet, while pseudopods extend outward.

plasma ADP concentrations, platelets aggregate in separate and distinct primary and secondary waves (Fig. 1). Although there is variation from one donor to another, this intermediate concentration range is usually from about 0.8 μM to 2.5 μM ADP. In the primary wave, a limited number of platelets, usually 60–70%, aggregate promptly but loosely (Fig. 2). After a pause of 1–2 minutes, seen as a plateau in aggregometer tracings, virtually all of the platelets aggregate and form large, very compact and complex aggregates (Fig. 3). In these aggregates, platelets are very closely apposed, and platelet bodies are in the central portion of the aggregate, while platelet pseudopods present to the periphery. These pseudopods are usually devoid of organelles, and their cytoplasm is continuous with that of the main body of the platelet in the central part of the aggregate. It is in association with the second wave of aggregation that the release reaction occurs. Although some of the released substances have been localized within platelet granules (Holmsen et al., 1969), there is no specific evidence that degranulation occurs during this release (Hardisty et al., 1970). Aggregates formed in this

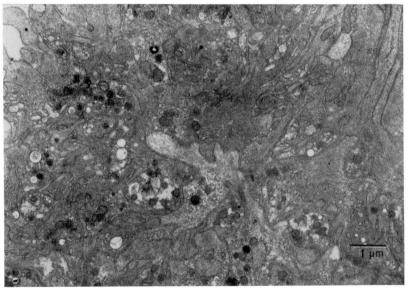

Fig. 3. A small portion of a large, compact, and complex aggregate from the peak of the intermediate curve in Fig. 1. The margin of the aggregate is in the upper left and upper right, where several elongated pseudopods extend outward from the aggregate center. Cytoplasm of several pseudopods on the far right is seen to be continuous with platelet cytoplasm in the aggregate center. In the aggregate center, occupying the middle and lower portions of the micrograph, there is a highly intricate mosaic pattern. Even in this area, organelles and plasma membranes are intact.

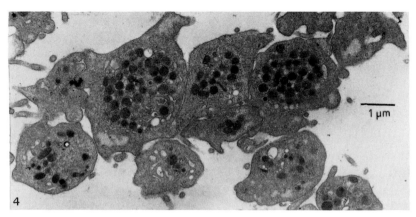

Fig. 4. A typical small aggregate from the peak of the lower tracing (see Fig. 1) in response to 1 μM ADP. A few platelets, all intact, form very small aggregates. Plasma membranes and organelles are intact.

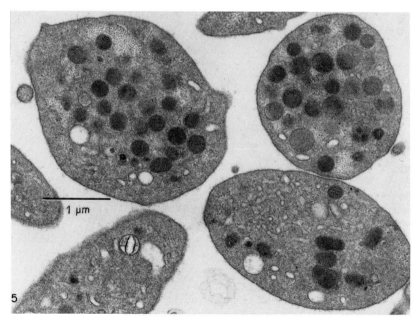

Fig. 5. A sampling of unaggregated platelets at the end of the lower tracing in Fig. 1 after deaggregation had occurred. These platelets have rounded contours, randomly dispersed organelles, and microtubules arranged in marginal bundles. These bundles are especially well noted in the platelet at the lower right.

second wave are stable, at least for 1 hour or more. In response to lower ADP concentrations, usually about 1 μM or lower, platelets aggregate and then rapidly deaggregate (Figs. 1, 4, and 5). At concentrations greater than 2.5 μM ADP, virtually all of the platelets aggregate rapidly, with the primary and secondary waves merging and with elimination of the plateau or pause. These aggregates are similar in size, compactness, and complexity to those seen at the peak of the secondary wave obtained with intermediate ADP concentrations (see Fig. 3).

b. CATECHOLAMINES.   Epinephrine and norepinephrine stimulate plate-lets to aggregate in a stepwise fashion similar to that observed with inter-mediate concentrations of ADP (O'Brien, 1963) (Fig. 6). The initial aggre-gation wave, at least in the response to ephinephrine, is thought to result from a direct effect of epinephrine on the platelets. The secondary wave is associated with release of ADP and other substances (Grette, 1962; Mills *et al.*, 1968), and the secondary wave has been thought to be mediated by the released, endogenous ADP. These aggregates are also stable for consider-able periods of time. As noted above, epinephrine at concentrations less

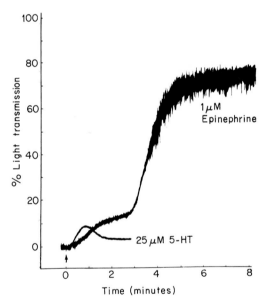

Fig. 6. Aggregometer tracing illustrating responses of normal human platelets in citrated plasma to epinephrine and to 5-HT. In the upper tracing, the epinephrine response occurs in two waves separated by a plateau. This resembles the tracing obtained with intermediate concen-trations of ADP (see Fig. 1). Aggregates at the peak of the secondary wave are similar to those at the secondary wave peak in the response to intermediate ADP concentrations. The lower tracing shows minimal aggregation in response to 5-HT, followed rapidly by deaggregation.

than those required to initiate aggregation potentiates the platelet aggregation response to ADP (Born *et al.*, 1967; Mills and Roberts, 1967) and to thrombin (Thomas *et al.*, 1968).

c. 5-HYDROXYTRYPTAMINE (5-HT).   5-HT is released from platelets after exposure to other aggregating agents and also induces platelet aggregation to a limited degree (Baumgartner, 1969). At concentrations of 0.1 μM and above, 5-HT added to citrated PRP causes aggregation of a small percentage of platelets, and most of these deaggregate within 2 or 3 minutes (see Fig. 6).

d. THROMBIN.   Thrombin is the time-honored proteolytic agent which induces the conversion of fibrinogen to the insoluble fibrillar protein fibrin,

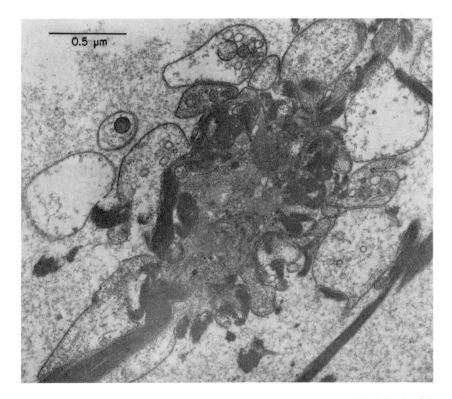

Fig. 7. A small mass of aggregated platelets recovered from citrated recalcified platelet-rich plasma, fixed just after a solid clot formed, and showing the Stage III change, thrombocytorrhexis. In the aggregate center, there are finely granular material and an occasional, poorly defined, short membrane segment. This is characteristic of organelle disintegration and plasma membrane disruption. Specific granules are not identified. Note the fibrin fibrils in both longitudinal and cross section toward the periphery of the aggregate and the very long fibrils in the lower left and right.

and is thus responsible for formation of the familiar fibrin clot. Thrombin is also a potent aggregator of platelets (Shermer *et al.*, 1961), and requires for its action divalent cations, preferentially Ca^{2+} or Mg^{2+}. The exact mechanism by which thrombin induces platelet aggregation is not entirely clear, although Haslam (1964) has presented evidence suggesting that its action is mediated through ADP which is released from the platelet by thrombin. Thrombin, however, induces extremely profound ultrastructural changes in platelets which far exceed those induced by ADP. The orderly sequence of events which constitutes the platelet response to thrombin has been described in detail (Rodman *et al.*, 1962, 1963a,b, 1966; Rodman and Mason, 1967). The response was divided into four stages (Rodman *et al.*, 1963b) as follows: Stage I, formation of pseudopods and central apposition of cytoplasmic organelles; Stage II, aggregation of altered platelets; Stage III, termed thrombocytorrhexis, consists of organelle disintegration and disruption of plasma membranes in the centers of aggregates (Fig. 7); Stage IV, thrombocytolysis, is the slow, progressive disintegration of platelet organelles and membranes. This occurs during the period of clot retraction when thrombin evolves and a clot forms in PRP or whole blood.

e. COLLAGEN. Platelet responses to collagen are certainly of utmost importance in thrombus formation. Kjaerheim and Hovig (1962) first described the formation of a hemostatic plug using ultrastructural techniques. They observed platelets first adhering to collagen fibrils adjacent to the site of blood vessel transection in a rabbit mesentery. Several other workers have studied the platelet response to collagen by adding finely divided collagen fibrils to citrated PRP. The morphological sequence of platelets exposed to collagen suspensions is similar to that of platelets exposed to thrombin. Within platelet aggregates, morphological sequences lead to thrombocytorrhexis and, ultimately, thrombocytolysis (Rodman and Mason, 1967) (Fig. 8). Evidence regarding the mechanism of the platelet–collagen reaction has included the observation that young platelets adhere to collagen more readily than older platelets (Hirsch *et al.*, 1968) and data which suggest that initiation of platelet aggregation requires a molecule of sufficient size containing rigidly spaced polar groups (Wilner *et al.*, 1971). Still more recently, Jamieson and associates (1971) have suggested that platelet to collagen adhesion is dependent upon a collagen:glucose transferase which is present in the platelet plasma membrane. They further suggest that platelet to collagen adhesion may be a specific case of a general cell adhesion mechanism which involves mutual interaction of glycosyl transferases and incomplete glycoproteins (Roseman, 1970). It seems likely that such a general cell adhesion mechanism may well be the initial event in the platelet collagen reaction. Perhaps this stimulates other reactions which lead to the

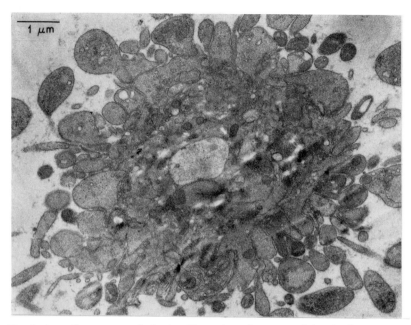

Fig. 8. A small aggregate of platelets illustrating a late stage of the platelet response to collagen. In the aggregate center, organelles have disintegrated; plasma membranes have undergone disruption; and the cytoplasmic remnants are in an advanced stage of lysis (Stage IV). Cytoplasm of pseudopods at the periphery frequently is seen to be continuous with cytoplasm of the aggregate center.

profound response by platelets to collagen, progressing through aggregation to thrombocytorrhexis and lysis.

f. FATTY ACIDS. Aggregation of platelets by fatty acids has been reported by Warner and associates (1967) and Hoak and associates (1966, 1967). Platelets in these aggregates retained their plasma membranes, and cytoplasmic organelles were intact. Evidence reported by Haslam (1964) suggests that the effect of fatty acids is mediated through endogenous ADP released by the fatty acids.

g. BACTERIA. Platelet aggregation responses to each of several bacteria have been reported by Clawson and White (1971). Bacteria in a 1:1 ratio with platelets induced marked platelet aggregation, while reduced numbers of bacteria induced a proportionately lesser aggregation response. Heat-killed *Staphylococcus aureus* was as effective as the living organism. The aggregation response, but not the change in platelet shape, was ablated by the potato ADPase, apyrase, suggesting that the aggregation response is dependent upon released, endogenous ADP. These data may be significant in the pathogenesis of some cases of disseminated intravascular coagulation.

h. BACTERIAL ENDOTOXIN. In addition to intact bacteria, it has been demonstrated that *Escherichia coli* endotoxin induces platelet aggregation and release of 5-HT (Des Prez *et al.*, 1961). Subsequently, it was shown that Factor V is a necessary cofactor in the aggregation response (Ream *et al.*, 1965) and that granule disintegration and plasma membrane disruption occurs in the aggregate centers (Davis, 1966). In other experiments, platelet aggregates were observed in vessels of a rabbit ear chamber after injection of lipopolysaccharides derived from *E. coli* or *Salmonella typhosa* (Silver and Stehbens, 1965).

i. RELATION TO CLINICAL STATES OF SHOCK. Hardaway (1962) has studied the occurence and mechanism of intravascular coagulation associated with experimental shock due to severe blood loss, incompatible transfusion, amniotic fluid infusion, *E. coli* endotoxin, or thrombin infusion. Preheparinization partially prevented shock except after severe hemorrhage. Later, Hardaway (1965) concluded that intravascular coagulation associated with shock resulted from capillary stasis. This depended in turn on decreased blood volume and arteriolar constriction. It could be relieved by expansion of blood volume and relief of arteriolar constriction with correction of microcirculatory stasis. More recently, Meagher and associates (1971) observed the late appearance of platelet aggregates in blood obtained from exsanguinating pigs. This may reflect intravascular activation of the clotting mechanism and the response by platelets to thrombin.

2. DISSEMINATED INTRAVASCULAR COAGULATION (DIC)

DIC is a variable and complex syndrome which should be viewed from each of several distinct perspectives. These must include consideration of the underlying disease, the triggering event which sets off the initial clotting episode, pathogenesis or evolution of the syndrome, and characteristics of the fully developed syndrome. Therapy should also be considered, at least insofar as its success or failure may provide information regarding mechanisms of the syndrome.

a. PREEXISTING DISEASE OR UNDERLYING CAUSES. Diseases known to precede the onset of DIC and therefore considered underlying causes are many and varied. They include abruptio placentae (Schneider, 1951; Coopland *et al.*, 1968; Sutton *et al.*, 1971), massive pulmonary embolism (McKay *et al.*, 1967), neoplasm (Rapaport and Chapman, 1959), severe trauma or burns (Eeles and Sevitt, 1967), severe infection (Conley *et al.*,

1951; Trigg, 1964; Verstraete *et al.*, 1965; Mason *et al.*, 1970), virus diseases (McKay and Margaretten, 1967), intravascular hemolysis or the intravascular presence of tissue thromboplastin, bacterial endotoxin or proteolytic enzymes (McKay, 1969a,b), long bone fracture with fat embolism (Keith *et al.*, 1971), and cirrhosis (Johansson, 1964).

b. TRIGGERING EVENT INITIATING INTRAVASCULAR COAGULATION. Any event which might stimulate either the extrinsic or intrinsic clotting system could initiate the DIC syndrome. The extrinsic system may be activated by release of tissue thromboplastin or tissue factor from any tissue undergoing necrosis, as in a case of severe trauma or sepsis with tissue necrosis. The intrinsic system may be activated by exposure of plasma or platelets to a denuded surface such as basement membrane or collagen with activation of Factor XII. *Neisseria meningitidis* septicemia with the Waterhouse-Friderichson syndrome would be an example of this, although tissue necrosis with release of tissue factor might also play a part in this instance.

c. EVOLUTION OF THE SYNDROME. The pathogenesis of the syndrome has been described and reviewed by numerous workers, including McKay (1965, 1969a,b), Verstrate and associates (1965), Merskey and associates (1967), Bachmann (1969), Deykin (1970), and Yoshikawa and associates (1971). Evolution of the DIC syndrome, as it is usually seen, first requires formation of thrombin. Frequently, but not necessarily always, the fibrinolytic system is also activated, with formation of fibrin split products. It seems likely that the syndrome arises as a response to a preexisting illness which provokes widespread activation of either the intrinsic plasmatic or extrinsic clotting mechanism or both. It further seems likely that the later occurrence of fibrinolysis, the appearance of fibrin split products with hypofibrinogenemia, decreased coagulability, and hemorrhagic phenomena all reflect the initial event and underlying disease state and could be viewed as an attempted protective mechanism gone awry.

When activation of the intrinsic clotting mechanism occurs, the sequence of events would probably begin with activation of Factor XII. This would lead through the now well-known cascade sequence to the consecutive activation of Factors XI, IX, and VIII. This complex of activated clotting factors, in the presence of lipid, would activate Factor X. Factor X may then induce the conversion of prothrombin to thrombin slowly by itself or more rapidly in the presence of Factor V and platelet phospholipid (Platelet Factor 3). The alternate extrinsic or tissue pathway requires formation of a complex of tissue factor with Factor VII in the presence of phospholipid. This complex then activates Factor X, which again stimulates the conversion of prothrombin to thrombin.

Thrombin formed by either of the above sequences then converts fibrinogen into the soluble fibrin monomer by cleaving the alpha (α) and beta (β) chains to remove, respectively, fibrinopeptides A and B. This fibrin monomer rapidly polymerizes, again under the influence of thrombin, to form the familiar insoluble protein macromolecule, fibrin. Finally, in order to become stable, the fibrin clot requires the action of Factor XIII, an enzyme activated by thrombin, which converts to covalent linkages those hydrogen bonds which initially bind the monomers.

As a balance to the above series of reactions, each of several varied actions tends to hold the clotting mechanism at least partly in check. For example, the liver removes from the circulation the particulate tissue thromboplastin (Spaet and Kropatkin, 1958) and activated Factors XI, IX, and X (Deykin, 1966; Deykin et al., 1968). Thrombin is readily adsorbed onto fibrin fibrils, and antithrombin III alone slowly neutralizes unadsorbed thrombin. Antithrombin III also is identical with heparin cofactor (Abildgaard, 1968). The combination of heparin and heparin cofactor is a powerful anticoagulant, perhaps through rapid inactivation of activated Factor X (Yin and Wessler, 1970), as well as through direct and rapid inactivation of thrombin (Abildgaard et al., 1970).

Plasminogen may be activated by any of several mechanisms. There is evidence that plasminogen levels increase with inadequate liver perfusion or blood pressure changes in either direction (von Kaulla, 1966). This suggests that plasminogen is continually being activated to its active form, plasmin; that the liver ordinarily controls the plasma plasmin level; and that poor liver perfusion, as in shock, would increase the plasmin level. Additionally, there is evidence that plasmin may be activated by catecholamines (Holemans, 1963), by histamine (Holemans and Langdell, 1964), or by the action of tissue factor itself (Astrup, 1966).

Activation of plasminogen to plasmin has profound effects on the fibrinogen molecule and its polymerization, thus markedly affecting coagulability of the blood. The degradation of fibrinogen to smaller fragments known as fibrin split products or fibrinogen degradation products and their effect on coagulation have been extensively studied by several groups of workers (Kowalski, 1960, 1968; Kowalski et al., 1964, 1965; Marder et al., 1967; Marder and Shulman, 1969). Plasmin degrades fibrinogen stepwise into several smaller fragments, some with alphabetical designations. Initially, several small fragments are cleaved, leaving a large fragment, designated X. This is then further cleaved into a large fragment, Y, and a small fragment, D. Fragment Y is further cleaved into another D and a different fragment called E. Fragments X and Y are slowly clottable by thrombin and compete with the intact fibrinogen molecule for thrombin action. They therefore have potent anticoagulant activity, while fragments D and E have less effective anticoagulant action.

d. CHARACTERISTICS OF THE FULLY DEVELOPED SYNDROME. The balancing effect of the thrombin-evolving mechanism and the antithrombin actions noted above plus the anticoagulant effects of fibrin split products produce a complex syndrome in which two basically opposing and highly potent systems are active. Furthermore, the stimuli, consisting of the underlying disease and its complications (such as sepsis with tissue necrosis), may persist. The situation is variable in that one system may temporarily outdistance the other. If the thrombin forming mechanism predominates, widespread thrombosis may be evident. If procoagulants are depleted or if fibrinolysis predominates, or both, then widespread hemorrhage may result as well. Such events may be clinically manifested as petechial or ecchymotic hemorrhages of the skin and mucous membranes, massive gastrointestinal bleeding, hematuria, or other similar events.

The effect on blood-clotting factor levels and platelet counts are variable and frequently profound. Merskey and associates (1967) found that in more than 50% of seven patients with DIC complicating abruptio placentae there was moderate to severe reduction of Factors XI, VIII, X, V, and prothrombin and fibrinogen. Factors VII and IX were mildly to moderately decreased in all patients. Of nine similar patients in whom platelet counts were done, all had platelet counts less than 200,000/mm³, six had less than 150,000 platelets/mm³, and, of these, three had less than 100,000/mm³. In most of a group of nonobstetrical patients with DIC, all clotting factors were moderately to severely reduced except Factors VII and IX. These factors were only mildly reduced in 50% of the patients and moderately to severely reduced in the remaining 50%. It is to be emphasized that clotting factor levels as well as levels of plasminogen and firbin split products will vary with the duration and severity of the disease.

e. EFFECTS OF THERAPY. Specific therapy, of course, would always be directed at the underlying disease and would include general supportive measures. However, disseminated intravascular coagulation is a complication which may overshadow the underlying disease to the extent that if it is not dealt with rapidly and effectively it may prove fatal. Several approaches have been proposed, including blood replacement therapy, anticoagulants such as heparin and dicoumarol, and activators and inhibitors of the fibrinolytic system (see McKay and Muller-Berghaus, 1967 and the several reviews of DIC cited above). Blood replacement, mandatory in hemorrhagic shock, could be expected to decrease stasis and help correct acidosis, each reported to be capable of triggering DIC (Hardaway, 1967). Vasopressors should perhaps be used with caution, since α-adrenergic stimulation via intravenous epinephrine infusions has been demonstrated experimentally to induce DIC by activation of Factor XII (McKay et al., 1970). Heparin, enhancing the action of antithrombin III, is well known to prevent the generation and action of thrombin and is widely though cautiously advocated in the treatment of DIC. It has been used frequently and has sometimes been successful in terminating the DIC episode. While heparin would be expected to halt thrombin formation and its action on both fibrinogen and platelets, it would not be expected to prevent platelet aggregation induced by other agents such as ADP, catecholamines, or exposed basement membrane and collagen fibrils. It has been suggested that short periods of heparinization would be highly effective, particularly if administered early, even in anticipation of a DIC episode (McKay and Muller-Berghaus, 1967). Drugs which affect the fibrinolytic system are advocated with considerably more caution. Current knowledge and experience offer no particularly illuminating understanding of mechanisms of the DIC syndrome.

3. Hypercoagulability States

There are a number of clinical states characterized by repeated thrombotic episodes which are thought to result from persistent increase in blood coagulability. These hypercoagulable states have been associated with an increased level of activity of one or more plasmatic clotting factors, decreased fibrinolytic activity, or increased platelet reactivity. Presumably, the hypercoagulable state also requires a triggering event or mechanism for the production of intravascular coagulation. The intravascular coagulation may be severe and widespread and therefore may resemble, at least to a limited degree, the DIC syndrome. Hypercoagulable states are to be distinguished, however, by the persistent high level of activity of one or more factors in the thrombus-forming mechanism.

a. Increased Factor VIII Levels.   Penick and associates (1966) first described a group of patients with multiple episodes of thrombosis and very high levels of Factor VIII. One patient who succumbed to complications of her illness had thrombi in vessels of the myocardium, cerebrum, mesentery, adrenal glands, and pelvic region and on the mitral valve. She had previously suffered abruptio placentae complicated by bilateral renal cortical necrosis. Her Factor VIII level was persistently in the range of 850% of normal during her 6 months of hospitalization. Other procoagulants were normal or only slightly elevated.

Additional patients were studied, including three families with a high incidence of recurrent thrombophlebitis and cerebral thrombosis. Each patient who had a history of thrombosis also had an elevated plasma Factor VIII level.

High levels of Factor VIII have also been reported to occur postoperatively (Ygge, 1970), and, in one such patient, Factor VIII activity was increased still further during a period of thrombosis.

b. INCREASED FACTOR V LEVELS. High levels of Factor V have been associated with sporadic thromboembolic disease (Olwin and Fahey, 1950) and also in several members of a family, one of whom had a thrombotic episode at age 6 (Gaston, 1966). The Factor V of one of these subjects, the father of the child with thrombosis, was chromatographically indistinguishable from normal Factor V.

c. TRANSIENT INCREASES IN FACTOR XI LEVELS. Egeberg (1966) demonstrated that ingestion of a meal high in certain fats produced a rise in Factor XI activity, as measured 5 hours after ingestion of the meal. He concluded that high titers of activated Factor XI increase the likelihood of thrombosis.

d. IMPAIRED FIBRINOLYTIC SYSTEM. A group of four patients with thrombotic episodes were studied by Brakman and associates (1966). In each of these patients, there was decreased spontaneous fibrinolytic activity. Each patient also had increased inhibition of tissue plasminogen activator.

e. INCREASED PLATELET ACTIVITY. Increased platelet reactivity has been reported in physiological and pathological situations, sometimes with associated thrombosis. Ikkala and associates (1966) demonstrated that each of several healthy subjects had an elevated platelet count, increased platelet adhesiveness to glass, and increased aggregability in response to ADP during and after brief, heavy muscular exercise. Additionally, they found elevated levels of Factors VIII and XII. Increased platelet adhesiveness and a hastened aggregation response to ADP in late pregnancy has been reported by Farbiszewski and Skrzydlewski (1970). Increased platelet adhesiveness to glass has also been reported in patients with hypertensive cardiovascular disease (Poplawski and associates 1968). Dawson and Ogston (1970) reported that patients with polycythemia vera who have thrombocytosis also have more thrombotic and hemorrhagic complications than those in whom the platelet count is normal. This last finding may represent an increase in the total Platelet Factor 3 available to the thrombus-forming mechanism.

O'Brien et al. (1966) studied platelet responsiveness in patients who had had myocardial infarcts. Platelets of those patients with recent infarcts gave greater responses to ADP and 5-HT, and these increased responses were unaffected by anticoagulant therapy. In another series, patients with nonacute ischemic heart disease had increased Platelet Factor 3 activity as estimated by the stypven time test (Nordøy and Rødset, 1970).

It seems likely, in our current state of knowledge, that adhesion and aggregation are two separate and distinct platelet functions. Nevertheless, it also seems probable that increased aggregability, increased adhesiveness, and increased availability of Platelet Factor 3 all reflect an elevation of general platelet reactivity or responsiveness and therefore an increased propensity to initiate thrombosis.

f. EFFECTS OF PROGESTATIONAL AGENTS.   The possible thrombotic effect
of oral contraceptive agents has been the subject of extensive study. Earlier
retrospective studies were generally not conclusive (Eastman and Winter,
1966). More recently, in a clinical study Vessey and Doll (1968) reported that
45% of 58 women between the ages of 16 and 40 with thromboembolic
disease and without evident predisposing cause had been taking oral contraceptives. In contrast, only 9% of 116 matched controls had been taking
oral contraceptives.

A few groups have studied specific parameters of the thrombus-forming
mechanism. Rutherford and associates (1964) found that patients taking
norethindrone with mestranol had increased levels of prothrombin and
Factors VII, IX, and X, while Factor VIII levels were normal. Hougie and
associates (1965) obtained similar results, but did not determine Factor IX
levels. Beller and Porges (1967) studied coagulation factors in groups of
women taking norethynodrel with mestranol or medroxyprogesterone
acetate, either cyclically for three cycles or continuously and in increasing
doses for several months. They found no significant variations from normal
levels except in patients taking high doses of the progestational agent. In
these patients, there was elevation of Factor VIII, fibrinogen, and plasminogen. In contrast, Ambrus and associates (1969) found that in patients on
combined norethindrone acetate and ethinyl estradiol therapy prothrombin,
fibrinogen, and Factor X were initially elevated, as was plasminogen. They
also found that levels of these factors had returned to normal after 24 months
of therapy.

More recently, other workers have studied still other parameters. Von
Kaulla and associates (1971) studied levels of antithrombin III in 21 women
during a single cycle consisting of twenty daily doses of 1 mg of progestogen
plus 0.08 mg of estrogen. At the end of 20 days, antithrombin III levels had
decreased so that their frequency distribution was similar to that of 45
patients with thromboembolic disease. This loss of antithrombin III activity,
taken together with the elevated levels of procoagulants discussed above,
was interpreted as a hypercoagulable state. In addition, Poller and associates
(1971) found that contraception with progestogen alone was associated with
shortened platelet aggregation times.

C. Rheologic Factors

The differences between the white thrombi formed in arteries and the red
thrombi formed in veins have long been thought to be related to rates of
blood flow and, perhaps, to disturbances in flow. However, specific mechanisms which determine the character of the thrombus have been poorly

understood. Only in the last decade have reports appeared which begin to identify and define the rheologic factors which may induce or affect composition of the thrombus.

1. DISTURBANCES IN FLOW PATTERNS

Murphy and associates (1962) reported the formation of platelet thrombi in an extracorporeal circulation device. In a curved tube, platelets were deposited on the lesser curvature. At a bifurcation, platelets were deposited laterally across the hips of the bifurcation, with most of the deposit being on the lateral walls of the secondary vessels and with nearly complete sparing of the primary or parent vessel wall. In an aneurysmal dilation, there were heavy deposits laterally, while the central channel was relatively free of deposit. In each vessel configuration, the platelet deposit was in the area where there was decreased or disturbed flow. Elsewhere, it has been shown that platelet aggregates may form in areas of vortices associated with change

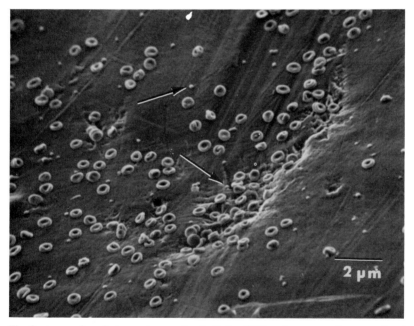

Fig. 9. A scanning electron micrograph of a Teflon TFE surface exposed to normal native human blood moving irregularly for 4 minutes. Erythrocytes and platelets (arrows) are collected densely in and about the deep crevice to the right of center and are scattered much more sparsely in smoother areas. Fibrin was not demonstrated. (From Rodman and Mason, 1970. Reprinted with permission of *Thromb. Diath. Haemorrh.*)

in direction of flow (Kwaan *et al.*, 1967). Using erythrocytes in a flowing system, Goldsmith (1970) showed that vortices occur just distal to sites of obstruction. It seems likely that the disturbed flow resulting from surface irregularities may be at least partly responsible for platelet aggregation and thrombus formation. In a study of blood compatibility with foreign surfaces, Rodman and Mason (1970) found that platelets adhere to a Teflon surface in areas of extreme irregularity earlier than they do in smooth areas (Fig. 9).

2. RATES OF FLOW

A series of studies has been undertaken to define the effects of high and low rates of shear on the character of the thrombus (Rozenberg and Dintenfass, 1964; Dintenfass and Rozenberg, 1965, 1967). Using a cone-in-cone viscometer, they demonstrated that at low rates of shear a red thrombus is formed, with cellular components randomly dispersed. With increasing rates of shear, there was progressively more platelet aggregation, with formation of a white thrombus at high shear rates. These white thrombi were composed of large masses of aggregated platelets with fibrin and peripheral leukocytes. This is consistent with the thesis that white thrombi form in arteries, where the flow is rapid, and that red thrombi form in veins, where the rate of flow is much slower.

3. STASIS

Stasis has been one of the time honored and generally well accepted causes of venous thrombosis. Penick and associates (1966) established that the clotting time of normal dog blood in an isolated segment of vein varied from 340 to 380 minutes. This clotting time was shortened to 195 minutes by the prior injection of Factor VIII concentrate or to 74 minutes by the prior injection of serum thrombotic accelerator (STA, prepared from aged serum). The clotting time was shortened even further by prior injection of both Factor VIII and STA. These data suggest that extremely prolonged stasis is required for the occurrence of venous thrombosis unless some other stimulus is also introduced. In this context, Wessler and associates (1967) concluded, from an experimental study, that stasis may trigger thrombosis in the presence of activated Factor IX or XI.

II. Thrombosis as a Complication of Inflammation

Up to this point, thrombosis has been viewed as an initiator of inflammation. The demonstration that thrombi regardless of their genesis may induce an inflammatory response (Jørgensen *et al.*, 1970) impels a full discussion of thrombogenesis. That discussion has required consideration of mechanisms stimulated by infections which also induce the inflammatory process. In this section, thrombosis will be viewed from the other perspective, that is, thrombosis resulting from or being an integral part of the inflammatory process itself. Where possible, reference will be made to subjects already discussed, especially disseminated intravascular coagulation (DIC).

A. Severe Infection

Severe infection of any etiology may produce marked local signs only, or it may overwhelm or nearly overwhelm the host. In any event, regardless of the identity of the specific etiologic agent, stimuli may activate the thrombus-forming mechanism. Tissue factor released from necrotic tissue in the infected, inflammatory focus may combine with Factor VII to activate Factor X and then prothrombin so that platelets aggregate, fibrin polymerizes, and thrombosis results. This could occur locally so that thrombosis occurs only in the area of inflammation. Alternately, release of tissue factor might be more generalized, or there may be activation of Factor XII or XI. Activation of procoagulants, release of tissue factor, depressed antithrombin levels, or some combination of these might act to induce the DIC syndrome. As already presented, this may produce a varied picture with widespread thrombosis and/or hemorrhagic manifestations.

1. SEPTICEMIA

Classic examples of severe infections would include the spectrum of septicemia caused by any organism. The induction of platelet aggregation due to the presence of any of several bacteria and the aggregation response to endotoxin or lipopolysaccharide derived from gram-negative bacteria have been noted above. This would suggest that at least in the case of infection with a gram-negative organism the presence of bacteria in the blood stream is not necessary for stimulation of the thrombus-forming mechanism. Merely a persistent focus of infection such as an abscess, with endotoxin release, could induce intravascular coagulation.

2. INFECTIVE ENDOCARDITIS

Thrombosis must have at least a local role in infective endocarditis, with thrombi or vegetations in one or more locations on heart valves or on parietal endocardium. Historically, bacterial endocarditis was classified into acute and subacute varieties, but, with the changing pattern resulting from successful use of antibiotics, these are now best considered as infective endocarditis, and are classified as active or healed. The active form may involve a previously normal valve, but more commonly attacks a valve previously distorted. The distortion may be of congenital origin or it may be acquired, as in rheumatic heart disease or from a previous bout of active infective endocarditis. The active form has frequently been associated with bacteremia or septicemia caused by pyogenic organisms such as *Neisseria gonorrhoeae*, *Neisseria meningitidis*, the more virulent staphylococci or streptococci, occasionally *E. coli*, and even fungi (Korns, 1965). Vegetations are large and friable and frequently contain organisms in sufficient numbers that embolizing fragments may induce septic infarcts. The well-known clinical phenomenon of changing heart sounds and murmurs may reflect valve destruction or a change in the character of vegetations. Changes in the vegetations, in turn, must reflect active intravascular coagulation and perhaps opposing mechanisms such as fibrinolysis.

In healed endocarditis with distortion or partial destruction of a valve, disturbances in flow are to be expected about the area of distortion. These flow disturbances may well explain the high incidence of recurrent episodes of active infective endocarditis after the initial episode. The frequent location of vegetations at lines of closure suggests that endothelial cell damage with, perhaps, exposure of subendothelial structures may play a role in initial platelet adhesion, followed by aggregation and formation of the vegetation. For more extensive discussion, the reader is referred to Spain (1968), Hudson (1970), or to any standard clinical or pathology text.

3. GENERALIZED SHWARTZMAN REACTION

This syndrome has been extensively studied in the human and in other animals. Produced experimentally in the rabbit by two intravenous injections of *E. coli* endotoxin approximately 24 hours apart, the syndrome progresses to bilateral renal cortical necrosis in a majority of animals. After a single injection of endotoxin, platelet aggregation is observed, as already noted (Silver and Stehbens, 1965). In a few hours, platelet thrombi have partially disappeared, while fibrin thrombi have appeared (McKay, 1965), suggesting persistent intravascular coagulation. Thrombin evolution has also been confirmed in the dog, since the respiratory symptoms which ordinarily follow a single injection of endotoxin can be prevented by prior heparinization (Stein and Thomas, 1967). In the fully developed generalized Shwartzman reaction, seen in the rabbit several hours after the second injection, there are multiple fibrin thrombi in numerous locations, including liver, lungs, and spleen. Their predominant location, however, is in the kidney, where fibrin thrombi fill almost every glomerular capillary, producing cortical necrosis. The basic mechanism is almost certainly one of persistent or repeated intravascular coagulation.

4. RICKETTSIAL DISEASE

The primary lesion of rickettsial disease has been generally considered to be vascular, consisting of endothelial cell proliferation and thrombosis (Ashburn, 1960). An extensive study of the pathogenesis of Rocky Mountain spotted fever in rhesus monkeys clarified many uncertainties (Wolf *et al.*, 1967). Six hours after the monkeys were infected by inhalation, endothelial cells of alveolar septal capillaries contained organisms and were swollen to the extent of producing capillary occlusion. On the eleventh day, there was widespread vasculitis involving capillaries plus arteries and veins of various sizes. In the involved vessels, there was endothelial degeneration and sloughing with thrombosis and necrosis of vascular walls. Organisms were observed in thrombi in the nasal septum of one animal. Also at this time, the whole blood clotting time was longer than 60 minutes. This syndrome of widespread thrombosis with tissue necrosis strongly suggests extensive intravascular coagulation through the mechanism of Factor VII activation by tissue factor. The delayed blood coagulation also suggests that procoagulants were depressed or that the fibrinolytic system was active, or both. A recent report of several cases in humans described a marked though transient thrombocytopenia (Hand *et al.*, 1970), suggesting DIC.

5. PYLEPHLEBITIS

Inflammation and thrombosis of the portal vein is now seen much less frequently than several decades ago. This is probably largely because antibiotic therapy and earlier, more specifically definitive medical care have all but eliminated full development of severe inflammatory disease in that area which drains to the liver. Unimpeded infection and inflammation of the appendix, for example, may well lead to abscess formation. An abscess, particularly if not well delimited, may be expected to release tissue factor thromboplastin to react with Factor VII, leading, in turn, to subsequent activation of Factor X. Since this activation would occur in a location proximal to the hepatic site of inactivation of tissue thromboplastin (Spaet and Kropatkin, 1958) and Factor X (Deykin *et al.*, 1968) and since the flow of blood is somewhat sluggish, these influences might tend toward thrombosis. In fact, such cases are seldom seen, or at least they do not often progress to a point of recognition. It should be emphasized, however, that since passage of blood through the liver should result in inactivation of both the tissue thromboplastin and activated Factor X, this mechanism could operate locally and still not stimulate the disseminated syndrome.

In addition to pyogenic infections of this region, infestations with parasites such as *Schistosoma japonicum* may induce localized phlebitis with thrombosis in radicles of the portal vein (Hsü *et al.*, 1969). Adult worms of *S. japonicum* frequently elicited, late in the reaction in the rhesus monkey, a segmental thrombophlebitis and periphlebitis.

B. *Specific Noninfectious Inflammatory Processes with Associated Thrombosis*

Several inflammatory diseases which are not fully understood are nevertheless complicated by or associated with thrombosis. In these situations, thrombosis is, in all likelihood, secondary to the inflammatory process. Several of these will be presented.

1. POLYARTERITIS NODOSA

This disease may be acute, chronic, or recurring, and segmentally involves small arteries and arterioles in many locations. It may therefore have varied manifestations. Etiology is obscure, and the disease may represent a response to any of several stimuli. The mechanism may be that of delayed autoimmune hypersensitivity. Nevertheless, histological progression of the specific, localized arterial lesion is well delineated. After endothelial cell loss and necrosis of arterial intima, there is intense neutrophilic infiltration and thrombosis. This lesion progresses through destruction of vessel wall structures to resolution by organization. Characteristically, thrombosis involves only the localized, specific inflammatory lesion. There have been, however, three reports of polyarteritis nodosa with associated renal vein thrombosis (Miller *et al.*, 1954; Mandelbaum *et al.*, 1965; Beard and Taylor, 1969). In addition, there is a report of polyarteritis nodosa with disseminated platelet thrombosis (Benitez *et al.*, 1964).

2. HYPERSENSITIVITY REACTIONS

These reactions are varied as to mechanism and pathogenesis, and therefore have somewhat dissimilar histological patterns. One aspect which they have in common is thrombosis.

a. ARTHUS REACTION.   This local lesion results from an antigen–antibody (Ag–Ab) reaction of the precipitin type. These lesions have been produced experimentally by two approaches and with different patterns of thrombosis. In the direct active Arthus reaction, antigen is injected locally with antibody in the circulation. Large masses of Ag–Ab precipitate in the vessel lumina at the site of antigen injection; leukocytes gather; and platelet thrombi form rapidly (Uriuhara and Movat, 1964; Venkatachalam and Cotran, 1970). Endothelial changes were also observed early, and later there was vessel wall necrosis. The relationship of thrombosis to basement membrane exposure is not clear in this instance.

In contrast, the reversed Arthus reaction results from antigen in the circulation with antibody injected locally. In this situation, Ag–Ab precipitates are within the vessel wall, in the endothelial cell layer, or beneath the basement membrane. Necrosis of the vessel wall was occasionally seen early and commonly seen at later stages. Platelet aggregation was observed only occasionally and then late in the reaction (Uriuhara and Movat, 1966).

b. LOCAL SHWARTZMAN REACTION. In contrast to the Arthus reaction, the local Shwartzman reaction is produced by a local preparatory injection of *E. coli* endotoxin followed, in 18–24 hours, by a provocative parenteral injection of identical material. In rabbits or hamsters, the local reaction after the provocative injection included occlusive thrombi consisting of leukocytes, aggregated platelets, and fibrin. Ag–Ab precipitates were not observed, and endothelial cell damage was not demonstrated (Taichman *et al.*, 1965). The thrombotic part of this lesion appears to be minor.

III. Prevention of Thrombosis

It is apparent that thrombosis plays a significant role in the pathogenesis of many inflammatory diseases. Avoidance of thrombus formation may well alter beneficially the course of some of these diseases. The ideal objective in avoidance or prevention of thrombosis should be to reduce the reactivity of the thrombus-forming mechanism to a point at which harmful thrombi would not generate and, at the same time, the hemostatic mechanism would retain adequate function.

A. Traditional Approach

Inhibition of the plasmatic blood-clotting mechanism has been the avenue of traditional attack on the problem of thrombosis prevention. Most extensively, bishydroxycoumarin or other coumarin deriviates have been used, largely as preventive therapy after an initial episode of thrombosis. That initial episode has most frequently been a complication of atherosclerotic vascular disease, thrombosis of deep leg veins, or thrombophlebitis. The coumarin drugs reduce the plasma levels of prothrombin and Factors VII,

IX, and X, and effectively delay clotting as measured by the prothrombin time. Similarly, heparin, used in many acute situations including thrombotic episodes and in the DIC syndrome, prevents formation of thrombin. None of these drugs, however, would be expected to decrease or inhibit platelet function, and success with them has been less than desirable.

B. Newer Approaches: Inhibition of Platelet Function

The realization that inhibitors of the plasmatic clotting system alone were only marginally effective in preventing thrombosis has stimulated interest in compounds which limit platelet function. Many commonly known and widely used compounds now known to inhibit platelet function have been studied. These include acetylsalicylic acid (Weiss and Aledort, 1967; Zucker and Peterson, 1968; O'Brien, 1968), diphenylhydantoin (Rodman et al., 1971a), dipyrridamole (Cucuianu et al., 1971), and others. Perhaps it is even more important that an extensive search has been initiated for new compounds which may be used as antiaggregating agents. There have been reports on aggregation inhibition (Mills et al., 1970), adhesion inhibition (Bicher, 1970), and studies of ultrastructural alteration correlated with inhibition of several platelet functions and change in enzyme activity (Rodman et al., 1971b). .

An overview of the subject with a look at some of the various agents currently available has been published by Hampton (1971). He suggests that it is reasonable to begin clinical investigation of agents which affect platelet behavior. It seems most likely that overall effective prevention of damaging thrombosis will require judicious use of agents which inhibit thrombin evolution combined with those which limit platelet reactivity.

Acknowledgments

This work was supported, in part, by a grant from the National Heart and Lung Institute, No. HL-14230 and by a grant from the Veterans Administration.

References

Abildgaard, U. (1968). Scand. J. Clin. Lab. Invest. 21, 89.
Abildgaard, U., Fagerhol, M. K., and Egeberg, O. (1970). Scand. J. Clin. Lab. Invest. 26, 349.
Ambrus, J. L., Niswander, K. R., Courey, N. G., Wamsteker, E. F., and Mink, I. B. (1969). Amer. J. Obstet. Gynecol. 103, 994.

Ashburn, L. L. (1960). *In* "Symposium on the Spotted Fever Group of Rickettsiae" (C. L. Wisseman, ed.), Publ. No. 7, WRAIR, pp. 19–21. US Gov. Printing Office, Washington, D.C.
Ashford, T. P., and Freiman, D. G. (1967). *Amer. J. Pathol.* **50**, 257.
Astrup, T. (1966). *Fed. Proc., Fed. Amer. Soc. Exp. Biol.* **25**, 42.
Bachmann, F. (1969). *In* "Disease-a-Month" (H. F. Dowling, ed.), pp. 3–44. Yearbook Publ., Chicago, Illinois.
Baumgartner, H. R. (1969). *J. Physiol. (London)* **201**, 409.
Baumgartner, H. R., and Born, G. V. R. (1967). *J. Physiol. (London)* **194**, 92P.
Baumgartner, H. R., and Born, G. V. R. (1968). *Nature (London)* **218**, 137.
Baumgartner, H. R., Tranzer, J. P., and Studer, A. (1967). *Thromb. Diath. Haemorrh.* **18**, 592.
Beard, M. E. J., and Taylor, D. J. E. (1969). *J. Clin. Pathol.* **22**, 396.
Beller, F. K., and Porges, R. F. (1967). *Amer. J. Obstet. Gynecol.* **97**, 448.
Benitez, L., Mathews, M., and Mallory, G. K. (1964). *Arch. Pathol.* **77**, 116.
Bicher, H. I. (1970). *Thromb. Diath. Haemorrh., Suppl.* **42**, 197.
Born, G. V. R., Mills, D. C. B., and Roberts, G. C. K. (1967). *J. Physiol. (London)* **191**, 43P.
Brakman, P., Mohler, E. R., and Astrup, T. (1966). *Scand. J. Haematol.* **3**, 389.
Brånemark, P.-I., and Ekholm, R. (1968). *Blut* **16**, 274.
Buckingham, S., and Maynert, E. W. (1964). *J. Pharmacol. Exp. Ther.* **143**, 332.
Clawson, C. C., and White, J. G. (1971). *Amer. J. Pathol.* **65**, 367.
Conley, C. L., Ratnoff, O. D., and Hartmann, R. C. (1951). *Bull. Johns Hopkins Hosp.* **88**, 402.
Coopland, A. T., Israels, E. D., Zipursky, A., and Israels, L. G. (1968). *Amer. J. Obstet. Gynecol.* **100**, 311.
Cucuianu, M. P., Nishizawa, E. E., and Mustard, J. F. (1971). *J. Lab. Clin. Med.* **77**, 958.
Davey, M. G., and Lüscher, E. F. (1968). *Biochim. Biophys. Acta* **165**, 490.
Davis, R. B. (1966). *Exp. Mol. Pathol.* **5**, 559.
Dawson, A. A., and Ogston, D. (1970). *Postgrad. Med. J.* **46**, 76.
Des Prez, R. M., Horowitz, H. I., and Hook, E. W. (1961). *J. Exp. Med.* **114**, 857.
Deykin, D. (1966). *J. Clin. Invest.* **45**, 256.
Deykin, D. (1970). *N. Engl. J. Med.* **283**, 636.
Deykin, D., Cochios, F., DeCamp, G., and Lopez, A. (1968). *Amer. J. Physiol.* **214**, 414.
Dintenfass, L., and Rozenberg, M. C. (1965). *J. Atheroscler. Res.* **5**, 276.
Dintenfass, L., and Rozenberg, M. C. (1967). *Thromb. Diath. Haemorrh.* **17**, 112.
Dohrmann, R., and Klesper, R. (1960). *Klin. Wochenschr.* **38**, 595.
Eastman, N. J., and Winter, I. C. (1966). *In* "F. D. A. Report on the Oral Contraceptives," p. 17.. US Gov. Printing Office, Washington, D.C.
Eeles, G. H., and Sevitt, S. (1967). *J. Pathol. Bacteriol.* **93**, 275.
Egeberg, O. (1966). *Thromb. Diath. Haemorrh.* **15**, 390.
Farbiszewski, R., and Skrzydlewski, Z. (1970). *Haematologia* **4**, 187.
French, J. E., Macfarlane, R. G., and Sanders, A. G. (1964). *Brit. J. Exp. Pathol.* **45**, 467.
Gaarder, A., Jonsen, J., Laland, S., Hellem, A., and Owren, P. A. (1961). *Nature (London)* **192**, 531.
Gaston, L. W. (1966). *J. Pediat.* **68**, 367.
Goldsmith, H. J. (1970). *Thromb. Diath. Haemorrh., Suppl.* **40**, 91.
Grette, K. (1962). *Acta Physiol. Scand., Suppl.* **195**.
Hampton, J. C. (1971). *Amer. J. Cardiol.* **27**, 559.
Hand, W. L., Miller, J. B., Reinarz, J. A., and Sanford, J. P. (1970). *Arch. Intern. Med.* **125**, 879.
Hardaway, R. M. (1962). *Ann. Surg.* **155**, 325.
Hardaway, R. M. (1965). *Amer. J. Surg.* **110**, 298.

Hardaway, R. M. (1967). *Amer. J. Cardiol.* **20**, 161.

Hardisty, R. M., Hutton, R. A., Montgomery, D., Rickard, S., and Trebilcock, H. (1970). *Brit. J. Haematol.* **19**, 307.

Haslam, R. J. (1964). *Nature (London)* **202**, 765.

Hellem, A. J., Borchgrevink, C. F., and Ames, S. B. (1961). *Brit. J. Haematol.* **7**, 42.

Hirsh, J., Glynn, M. F., and Mustard, J. F. (1968). *J. Clin. Invest.* **47**, 466.

Hoak, J. C., Connor, W. E., and Warner, E. D. (1966). *Arch. Pathol.* **81**, 136.

Hoak, J. C., Warner, E. D., and Connor, W. E. (1967). *Circ. Res.* **20**, 11.

Holemans, R. (1963). *Med. Exp.* **9**, 5.

Holemans, R., and Langdell, R. D. (1964). *Proc. Soc. Exp. Biol. Med.* **115**, 584.

Holmsen, H., and Day, H. J. (1968). *Nature (London)* **219**, 760.

Holmsen, H., and Day, H. J. (1970). *J. Lab. Clin. Med.* **75**, 840.

Holmsen, H., Day, H. J., and Stormorken, H. (1969). *Scand. J. Haematol., Suppl.* **8**, 3.

Honour, A. J., Pickering, G. W., and Sheppard, B. L. (1971). *Brit. J. Exp. Pathol.* **52**, 482.

Hougie, C., Rutherford, R. N., Banks, A. L., and Coburn, W. A. (1965). *Metabo., Clin. Exp.* **14**, 411.

Hovig, T. (1963). *Thromb. Diath. Haemorrh.* **9**, 264.

Hsü, H. F., Davis, J. R., and Hsü, S. Y. Li. (1969). *Z. Tropenmed. Parasitol.* **20**, 184.

Hudson, R. E. B. (1970). *In* "Cardiovascular Pathology," pp. 683–720. Williams & Wilkins, Baltimore, Maryland.

Hugues, J., and Mahieu, P. (1970). *Thromb. Diath. Haemorrh.* **24**, 395.

Ikkala, E., Myllylä, G., and Sarajas, H. S. S. (1966). *Ann. Med. Exp. Biol. Fenn.* **44**, 88.

Ireland, D. M. (1967). *Biochem. J.* **105**, 857.

Jamieson, G. A., Urban, C. L., and Barber, A. J. (1971). *Nature (London), New Biol.* **234**, 5.

Johansson, S.-A. (1964). *Acta. Med. Scand.* **175**, 177.

Johnson, S. A. (1968). *Thromb. Diath. Haemorrh., Suppl.* **28**, 65.

Jørgensen, L., Hovig, T., Rowsell, H. C., and Mustard, J. F. (1970). *Amer. J. Pathol.* **61**, 161.

Keith, R. G., Mahoney, L. J., and Garvey, M. B. (1971). *Can. Med. Ass. J.* **105**, 74.

Kjaerheim, A., and Hovig, T. (1962). *Thromb. Diath. Haemorrh.* **7**, 1.

Korns, M. E. (1965). *Circulation* **32**, 589.

Kowalski, E. (1960). *Thromb. Diath. Haemorrh., Suppl.* **4**, 211.

Kowalski, E. (1968). *Semin. Hematol.* **5**, 45.

Kowalski, E., Kopec, M., and Wegrzynowicz, Z. (1964). *Thromb. Diath. Haemorrh.* **10**, 406.

Kowalski, E., Budzynski, A. Z., Kopec, M., Latallo, Z. S., Lipinski, B., and Wegrzynowicz, Z. (1965). *Thromb. Diath. Haemorrh.* **13**, 12.

Kwaan, H. C., Harding, F., and Astrup, T. (1967). *Thromb. Diath. Haemorrh., Suppl.* **26**, 207.

Langdell, R. D., Wagner, R. H., and Brinkhous, K. M. (1953). *J. Lab. Clin. Med.* **41**, 637.

McGrath, J. M., and Stewart, G. J. (1969). *J. Exp. Med.* **129**, 833.

McKay, D. G. (1965). "Disseminated Intravascular Coagulation." Harper, New York.

McKay, D. G. (1969a). *Calif. Med.* **111**, 186.

McKay, D. G. (1969b). *Calif. Med.* **111**, 279.

McKay, D. G., and Margaretten, W. (1967). *Arch. Intern. Med.* **120**, 129.

McKay, D. G., and Muller-Berghaus, G. (1967). *Amer. J. Cardiol.* **20**, 392.

McKay, D. G., Franciosi, R., and Zeller, J. (1967). *Amer. J. Cardiol.* **20**, 374.

McKay, D. G., Latour, J.-G., and Parrish, M. H. (1970). *Thromb. Diath. Haemorrh.* **23**, 417.

Mandelbaum, J., Aftalion, B., Brody, C. P., and Hoffman, I. (1965). *N. Y. State J. Med.* **65**, 1790.

Marder, V. J., and Shulman, N. R. (1969). *J. Biol. Chem.* **244**, 2120.

Marder, V. J., Shulman, N. R., and Carroll, W. R. (1967). *Trans. Ass. Amer. Physicians* **80**, 156.

Mason, J. W., Kleeberg, U., Dolan, P., and Colman, R. W. (1970). *Ann. Intern. Med.* **73**, 545.

Meagher, D. M., Piermattei, D. L., and Swan, H. (1971). *J. Thorac. Cardiov. Surg.* **62**, 822.

Merskey, C., Johnson, A. J., Kleiner, G. J., and Wohl, H. (1967). *Brit. J. Haematol.* **13**, 528.

Miller, G., Hoyt, J. C., and Pollock, B. E. (1954). *Amer. J, Med.* **17**, 856.

Mills, D. C. B., and Roberts, G. C. K. (1967). *J. Physiol. (London)* **193**, 443.

Mills, D. C. B., Robb, I. A., and Roberts, G. C. K. (1968). *J. Physiol. (London)* **195**, 715.

Mills, D. C. B., Smith, J. B., and Born, G. V. R. (1970). *Thromb. Diath. Haemorrh., Suppl.* **42**, 175.

Murphy, E. A., Rowsell, H. C., Downie, H. G., Robinson, G. A., and Mustard, J. F. (1962). *Can. Med. Ass. J.* **87**, 259.

Mustard, J. F., Hegardt, B., Rowsell, H. C., and MacMillan, R. L. (1964). *J. Lab. Clin. Med.* **64**, 548.

Niewiarowski, S., Lipinski, B., Farbiszewski, R., and Poplawski, A. (1968). *Experientia* **24**, 343.

Nordøy, A., and Rødset, J. M. (1970). *Acta. Med. Scand.* **188**, 133.

O'Brien, J. R. (1963). *Nature (London)* **200**, 763.

O'Brien, J. R. (1968). *Lancet* **1**, 779.

O'Brien, J. R., Path, F. C., Heywood, J. B., and Heady, J. A. (1966). *Thromb. Diath. Haemorrh.* **16**, 752.

Olwin, J. H., and Fahey, J. L. (1950). *Ann. Surg.* **132**, 443.

Penick, G. D., Dejanov, I. I., Reddick, R. L., and Roberts, H. R. (1966). *Thromb. Diath Haemorrh., Suppl.* **21**, 543.

Poller, L., Thomason, J. M., Thomas, W., and Wray, C. (1971). *Brit. Med. J.* **1**, 705.

Poplawski, A., Skorulska, M., and Niewiarowski, S. (1968). *J. Atheroscler. Res.* **8**, 721.

Quick, A. J. (1940). *Amer. J. Clin. Pathol.* **10**, 222.

Rapaport, S. I., and Chapman, C. G. (1959). *Amer. J. Med.* **27**, 144.

Ream, V. J., Deykin, D., Gurewich, V., and Wessler, S. (1965). *J. Lab. Clin. Med.* **66**, 245.

Rodman, N. F. (1967). *Blood* **30**, 540.

Rodman, N. F., and Mason, R. G. (1967). *Fed. Proc., Fed. Amer. Soc. Exp. Biol.* **26**, 95.

Rodman, N. F., and Mason, R. G. (1970). *Thromb. Diath. Haemorrh., Suppl.* **42**, 61.

Rodman, N. F., Barrow, E. M., and Graham, J. B. (1958). *Amer. J. Clin. Pathol.* **29**, 525.

Rodman, N. F., Mason, R. G., McDevitt, N. B., and Brinkhous, K. M. (1962). *Amer. J. Pathol.* **40**, 271.

Rodman, N. F., Painter, J. C., and McDevitt, N. B. (1963a). *J. Cell Biol.* **16**, 225.

Rodman, N. F., Mason, R. G., and Brinkhous, K. M. (1963b). *Fed. Proc., Fed. Amer. Soc. Exp. Biol.* **22**, 1356.

Rodman, N. F., Mason, R. G., Painter, J. C., and Brinkhous, K. M. (1966). *Lab. Invest.* **15**, 641.

Rodman, N. F., McDevitt, N. B., and Almond, J. R. (1971a). *Fed. Proc., Fed. Amer. Soc. Exp. Biol.* **30**, 285 (abstr.).

Rodman, N. F., Mason, R. G., and Brinkhous, K. M. (1971b). *Amer. J. Pathol.* **65**, 103.

Roseman, S. (1970). *Chem. Phys. Lipids* **5**, 270.

Rozenberg, M. C., and Dintenfass, L. (1964). *Aust. J. Exp. Biol. Med. Sci.* **42**, 109.

Rutherford, R. N., Hougie, C., Banks, A. L., and Coburn, W. A. (1964). *Obstet. Gynecol.* **24**, 886.

Schneider, C. L. (1951). *Surg., Gynecol. Obstet.* **92**, 27.

Shermer, R. W., Mason, R. G., Wagner, R. H., and Brinkhous, K. M. (1961). *J. Exp. Med.* **114**, 905.

Silver, M. D., and Stehbens, W. E. (1965). *Quart. J. Exp. Physiol. Cog. Med. Sci.* **50**, 241.

Spaet, T. H., and Cintron, J. (1965). *Brit. J. Haematol.* **11**, 269.

Spaet, T. H., and Kropatkin, M. (1958). *Amer. J. Physiol.* **195**, 77.

Spain, D. M. (1968). *In* "Pathology of the Heart and Blood Vessels" (S. E. Gould, ed.), pp. 760–788. Thomas, Springfield, Illinois.

Stein, M., and Thomas, D. P. (1967). *J. Appl. Physiol.* **23**, 47.

Stemerman, M. B., Baumgartner, H. R., and Spaet, T. H. (1971). *Lab. Invest.* **24**, 179.

Sutton, D. M. C., Hauser, R., Kulapongs, P., and Bachmann, F. (1971). *Amer. J. Obstet. Gynecol.* **109**, 604.

Taichman, N. S., Uriuhara, T., and Movat, H. Z. (1965). *Lab. Invest.* **14**, 2160.

Thomas, D. P., Gurewich, V., and Stuart, R. K. (1968). *J. Lab. Clin. Med.* **71**, 955.

Thomas, D. P., Niewiarowski, S., and Ream, V. J. (1970). *J. Lab. Clin. Med.* **75**, 607.

Tranzer, J. P., and Baumgartner, H. R. (1967). *Nature (London)* **216**, 1126.

Trigg, J. W., Jr. (1964). *N. Engl. J. Med.* **270**, 1042.

Uriuhara, T., and Movat, H. Z. (1964). *Lab. Invest.* **13**, 1057.

Uriuhara, T., and Movat, H. Z. (1966). *Exp. Mol. Pathol.* **5**, 539.

Venkatachalam, M. A., and Cotran, R. S. (1970). *Lab. Invest.* **23**, 129.

Verstraete, M., Vermylen, C., Vermylen, J., and Vandenbroucke, J. (1965). *Amer. J. Med.* **38**, 899.

Vessey, M. P., and Doll, R. (1968). *Brit. Med. J.* **2**, 199.

von Kaulla, E., Droegemueller, W., Aoki, N., and von Kaulla, K. N. (1971). *Amer. J. Obstet. Gynecol.* **109**, 868.

von Kaulla, K. N. (1966). *Fed. Proc., Fed. Amer. Soc. Exp. Biol.* **25**, 57.

Warner, E. D., Hoak, J. C., and Connor, W. E. (1967). *Thromb. Diath. Haemorrh., Suppl.* **26**, 249.

Weiss, H. J., and Aledort, L. M. (1967). *Lancet* **2**, 495.

Wessler, S., Yin, E. T., Gaston, L. W., and Nicol, I. (1967). *Thromb. Diath. Haemorrh.* **18**, 12.

White, J. G. (1968). *Blood* **31**, 604.

Wilner, G. D., Nossel, H. L., and Procupez, T. L. (1971). *Amer. J. Physiol.* **220**, 1074.

Wolf, G. L., Cole, C. R., Carlisle, H. N., and Saslaw, S. (1967). *Arch. Pathol.* **84**, 486.

Ygge, J. (1970). *Scand. J. Haematol., Suppl.* **11**.

Yin, E. T., and Wessler, S. (1970). *Biochim. Biophys. Acta* **201**, 387.

Yoshikawa, T., Tanaka, K. R., and Guze, L. B. (1971). *Medicine (Baltimore)* **50**. 237.

Zucker, M. B., and Peterson, J. (1968). *Proc. Soc. Exp. Biol. Med.* **127**, 547.

AUTHOR INDEX

Numbers in italics refer to the pages on which the complete references are listed.

Duran-Reynals, F., 33, *42*, 122, 140, *145*
Duthie, E. S., 140, *145*, 273, *296*
Dutrochet, M. H., *246*

E

Eastman, N. J., 380, *389*
Eastoe, J. E., 124, *147*
Ebbecke, U., 17, *42*
Ebert, R. H., 11, *45*, 210, 217, 230, 240, *246*, 280, *297*, *299*
Eberth, J. C., 23, *42*
Edelman, I. S., 20, *42*, 100, *119*
Eeles, G. H., 374, *389*
Egeberg, O., 376, 379, *388*, *389*
Eichelberger, L., 132, *145*
Einstein, A., 99, *118*
Ekfors, T. O., 275, *296*
Ekholm, R., 9, 11, 26, *41*, *42*, *45*, 364, *389*
Elder, J. M., 256, 257, 280, *296*
Elfvin, L. G., 72, 74, *90*
Elhay, S., 166, 184, 186, 188, *203*
Eliot, T. S., 29, *43*
Ellinger, F., 310, *329*
Elliot, D. F., 271, 274, 283, *296*
Elsden, D. F., 124, *146*
Elster, S. K., 33, *42*
Engel, M. B., 123, 130, 132, 133, 134, 135, 139, 141, 143, *145*, *146*
Engelman, D. M., 65, 66, *92*
Ennis, E. G. W. *360*
Enno, T., 20, *41*
Eppinger, H., 265, *296*
Epstein, F., 206, 211, 212, 228, *246*
Erdös, E. G., 279, *296*, *301*
Erichson, R. B., 227, *248*
Ernest, T., 234, *246*
Erspamer, V., 269, 270, 283, *296*
Esnouf, M. P., 344, *360*
Eto, K., 181, 189, *204*
Evans, D. G., 217, *246*
Evans, H. M., 122, *145*

F

Fagerhol, M. K., 376, *388*
Fahey, J. L., 379, *391*
Farbiszewski, R., 365, 379, *389*, *391*
Farquhar, M. G., 21, 23, 26, *42*, 48, 66, 72, 75, 78, 79, 81, 83, *90*
Faulk, W. P., 254, *296*
Fawcett, D. W., 22, *42*, 48, 59, 63, 68, 74, 81, *90*, 164, 181, *203*

Feder, N., 81, *90*
Feldberg, W., 266, 284, *296*
Ferguson, J. H., *360*
Fernando, M. P., 15, *45*
Fernando, N. V. P., 9, 12, 22, *45*
Ferreira, S. H., 279, *296*
Fessler, J. H., 129, *145*
Fiedler, F., 275, *296*
Field, M. E., 197, *203*
Finean, J. B., 66, *90*
Fischer, M. H., 18, *42*
Fisher, F. E., *297*
Fishman, A. P., 292, *299*
Flanzy, J., 199, *204*
Flax, M., 261, *301*
Fleck, L., 241, *246*
Fleisch, A., 17, *42*
Fleischmajer, R., 127, *145*
Flemming, W., 122, *145*
Flexner, L. B., 20, *41*, 107, 108, *117*, *118*
Florey, H. W., 9, 11, 22, 23, 26, 31, 35, 36, *41*, *42*, *44*, *45*, 68, 71, 75, 76, 77, 78, *90*, *91*, 92, 106, *118*, 172, 176, 183, 192, 194, *202*, *203*, *204*, 211, 213, 214, 217, 221, 222, 223, 224, 225, 230, *246*, *247*, *248*, 251, 253, *296*, *298*, 338, 346, 354, 355, *360*
Földi, M., 162, 164, 172, 173, 181, 182, 185, 189, 192, 193, 195, 196, 197, 200, 201, *202*, *203*, *204*
Földi-Börcsök, E., 201, *202*, *203*
Folkow, B., 5, *42*, 95, *118*
Follis, R. H., Jr., 229, *246*
Fonio, A., 351, *360*
Forell, M. M., 275, *296*, *301*
Fox, R. H., 275, 290, *296*
Fraley, E. E., 35, *42*
Franciosi, R., 374, *390*
Francois, A. C., 199, *204*
Frears, J., 311, *330*
Freeman, A. R., 78, *91*
Freeman, M. E., 33, *42*
Freiman, D. G., 228, *244*, 364, *389*
French, J. E., 36, *42*, 227, 228, *246*, 338, 346, 347, 349, 350, 353, 354, 355, *360*, 364, *389*
Freund, J., 282, 283, *296*
Frey, E. K., 273, 275, *296*, *297*
Friederici, H. H. R., 139, *145*
Friedman, E. A., *246*
Friedman, L., 135, *145*
Frimmer, M., 25, *42*, 236, *246*
Fritel, D., 108, *118*

SUBJECT INDEX

A

Acetylsalicylic acid, inhibitor of platelet
function, 388
Adenosine diphosphate
in platelet aggregation, 227, 363, 367
in platelet cohesion, 352
in thrombus formation, 365
Adenyl cyclase-cyclic AMP mechanism, 15
Adhesiveness, in inflammatory response, 24
Adrenaline, in platelet cohesion, 352
Adrenalinelike substance, protective function
after injury, 7
Amines
natural role of, in inflammatory process,
281
vasoactive, 14, 265
permeability response in rabbit, 279
whealing, effect of, 284
Androgens, action on connective tissue, 139
Anticoagulants, in leukocyte adhesion, 241
Antidromic reflex, 16
Antihistamines, 267, 310
Arteriole (s)
contraction after injury, 6
pressure recordings during inflammation, 7
terminal, regulatory mechanism, 5
Artery following injury
contraction, 6
vasomotor changes, 5
Arthus reaction, 11, 236–237
thrombosis in, 386
Axon reflex, 16

B

Bacteria, platelet response to, 373
spread, lymphatic 197
Basement membrane
capillary, 81
collagenous component, 227

composition, 127
histology, 126
origin, 127
periendothelial, barrier function, 26
ultrastructure, 127
Blood
changes in, related to thrombosis, 365
clotted, constrictor substance in, 355
normal rheology 149, *see also* Blood flow
rheology of inflammation, 155
changes in, 149
high flow phase, 156
low flow phase, 156
static phase, 156
sludging, 29, 152
velocity gradients, 151
viscosity of, 150
influence of plasma proteins, 151
Blood capillary barrier, degradation, 4
Blood cells, adhesive properties, differential,
242
Blood clotting, 337
clot retraction, 354
factors, 340–345
increased vascular permeability and, 322
interaction, 343
hypercoagulability states, 378
intravascular, and adhesiveness after
injury, 26
mechanism, platelets in, 353
nomenclature, 340
proenzyme-enzyme transformations, 345
triggering events, 375
Blood coagulation, *see* Blood clotting
Blood flow
disturbance of pattern, in thrombosis, 381
high phase, in inflammation, 156
injury reactions, 9, 34
of tissue, 7